I0033884

Immune Response to Parasitic Infections

Volume 1: Protozoa

Editor
Emilio Jirillo
University of Bari
Italy

Co-Editor
Olga Brandonisio
University of Bari
Italy

Image on the cover was adapted from the website of the University of Edinburgh (Natural History Collections, at http://www.nhc.ed.ac.uk/index.php?page=24.25.366) and represents protozoan parasites of humans and domestic stock belonging to three phyla Sarcomastigophora , Ciliophora and Apicomplexa

eBooks End User License Agreement

Please read this license agreement carefully before using this eBook. Your use of this eBook/chapter constitutes your agreement to the terms and conditions set forth in this License Agreement. Bentham Science Publishers agrees to grant the user of this eBook/chapter, a non-exclusive, nontransferable license to download and use this eBook/chapter under the following terms and conditions:

1. This eBook/chapter may be downloaded and used by one user on one computer. The user may make one back-up copy of this publication to avoid losing it. The user may not give copies of this publication to others, or make it available for others to copy or download. For a multi-user license contact permission@bentham.org

2. All rights reserved: All content in this publication is copyrighted and Bentham Science Publishers own the copyright. You may not copy, reproduce, modify, remove, delete, augment, add to, publish, transmit, sell, resell, create derivative works from, or in any way exploit any of this publication's content, in any form by any means, in whole or in part, without the prior written permission from Bentham Science Publishers.

3. The user may print one or more copies/pages of this eBook/chapter for their personal use. The user may not print pages from this eBook/chapter or the entire printed eBook/chapter for general distribution, for promotion, for creating new works, or for resale. Specific permission must be obtained from the publisher for such requirements. Requests must be sent to the permissions department at E-mail: permission@bentham.org

4. The unauthorized use or distribution of copyrighted or other proprietary content is illegal and could subject the purchaser to substantial money damages. The purchaser will be liable for any damage resulting from misuse of this publication or any violation of this License Agreement, including any infringement of copyrights or proprietary rights.

Warranty Disclaimer: The publisher does not guarantee that the information in this publication is error-free, or warrants that it will meet the users' requirements or that the operation of the publication will be uninterrupted or error-free. This publication is provided "as is" without warranty of any kind, either express or implied or statutory, including, without limitation, implied warranties of merchantability and fitness for a particular purpose. The entire risk as to the results and performance of this publication is assumed by the user. In no event will the publisher be liable for any damages, including, without limitation, incidental and consequential damages and damages for lost data or profits arising out of the use or inability to use the publication. The entire liability of the publisher shall be limited to the amount actually paid by the user for the eBook or eBook license agreement.

Limitation of Liability: Under no circumstances shall Bentham Science Publishers, its staff, editors and authors, be liable for any special or consequential damages that result from the use of, or the inability to use, the materials in this site.

eBook Product Disclaimer: No responsibility is assumed by Bentham Science Publishers, its staff or members of the editorial board for any injury and/or damage to persons or property as a matter of products liability, negligence or otherwise, or from any use or operation of any methods, products instruction, advertisements or ideas contained in the publication purchased or read by the user(s). Any dispute will be governed exclusively by the laws of the U.A.E. and will be settled exclusively by the competent Court at the city of Dubai, U.A.E.

You (the user) acknowledge that you have read this Agreement, and agree to be bound by its terms and conditions.

Permission for Use of Material and Reproduction

Photocopying Information for Users Outside the USA: Bentham Science Publishers Ltd. grants authorization for individuals to photocopy copyright material for private research use, on the sole basis that requests for such use are referred directly to the requestor's local Reproduction Rights Organization (RRO). The copyright fee is US $25.00 per copy per article exclusive of any charge or fee levied. In order to contact your local RRO, please contact the International Federation of Reproduction Rights Organisations (IFRRO), Rue du Prince Royal 87, B-I050 Brussels, Belgium; Tel: +32 2 551 08 99; Fax: +32 2 551 08 95; E-mail: secretariat@ifrro.org; url: www.ifrro.org This authorization does not extend to any other kind of copying by any means, in any form, and for any purpose other than private research use.

Photocopying Information for Users in the USA: Authorization to photocopy items for internal or personal use, or the internal or personal use of specific clients, is granted by Bentham Science Publishers Ltd. for libraries and other users registered with the Copyright Clearance Center (CCC) Transactional Reporting Services, provided that the appropriate fee of US $25.00 per copy per chapter is paid directly to Copyright Clearance Center, 222 Rosewood Drive, Danvers MA 01923, USA. Refer also to www.copyright.com

CONTENTS

FOREWORD

In spite of the extraordinary breakthroughs witnessed by modern medicine during the 20th century, in particular with the discovery of extremely powerful new tools to combat microbes, infectious diseases - and among these, infections by protozoan and metazoan parasites - still constitute a major health problem for large segments of the human population. Indeed, in many countries, parasitic diseases represent a leading cause of death, the most serious impediment to well-being, and a major obstacle in the fight against poverty.

This situation occurs in spite of the fact that, as will become apparent on reading the various contributions presented in this book, our understanding of the interactions of the host with parasites has made considerable progress. Indeed, interest in the study of the immune response against parasites - and particularly against protozoan parasites - has increased steadily after the end of World War II. This can be seen in (Fig. **1**), which provides a minimal estimate of the number of publications devoted to immunological aspects of the parasitic infections discussed in the present e-book, and published over the past 50 years.

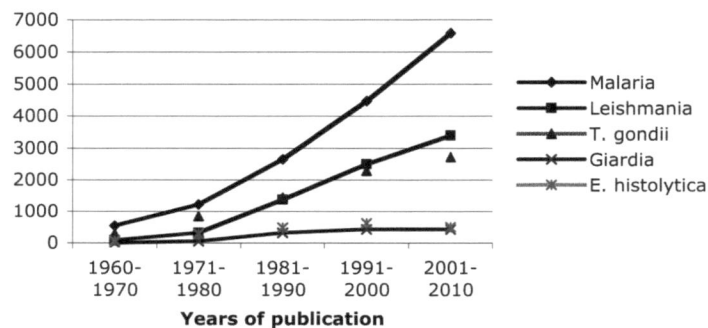

Figure 1: Minimal estimates of the number of studies relating to *immunological aspects* of parasitic infections and published in the scientific or medical literature during the period 1.1.1960-31.1.2010. The data were generated using the PubMed data base, with a series of 17 key-words with immunological connotation in association with the names of the different parasites or diseases. It will be appreciated that the figures shown will vary to some extent depending on the types, numbers and pertinence of the key-words used, and that publication numbers for the last period (2001-2010) are largely underestimated, since the search was terminated on January 31st, 2010.

Several factors have contributed to promote research on parasitic diseases, including factors far removed from basic, genuine scientific interest for these microorganisms. A strong impetus was provided by the involvement of the leading powers in new fighting areas where the prevalence of parasitic diseases represented an important challenge to the conduct of modern war (e.g. Vietnam, the Gulf countries). As quoted from the US Army doctor Stephen L. Hoffman (1996), cited in an article on US Vietnam war soldiers and malaria [1]: 'In every military campaign during this century, we had more casualties due to malaria than bullets. During World War II and the Vietnam War entire divisions ceased to be effective combat units due to malaria'.

Another reason for the current efforts to improve our understanding of host-parasite relationships is the unfortunate failure (in many places at least) of vector eradication campaigns, again illustrated by the malaria case (for a comprehensive discussion, see ref. [2]). It should be recalled that early in the second half of the 20th century, extraordinary successes were obtained in the fight against malaria due to the implementation of campaigns aimed at controlling the vector (as well as to the discovery of new and more powerful parasiticidal drugs such as chloroquine). A six-year pilot study (1946-1951) of the effects of spraying the powerful insecticide DDT (whose properties had been discovered by the Swiss chemist Paul Müller in 1939 - he was awarded the Nobel Prize in 1948) resulted in virtual elimination of malaria in the Mediterranean island of Sardinia. Similar results were obtained in Greece and, following a massive DDT-based eradication campaign, the United States were also declared malaria-free in 1952. In view of these spectacular achievements, the World Health Assembly launched its *Global Malaria Eradication Campaign* in May 1955, whose goal was to eliminate malaria world-wide through widespread use of DDT. The results were indeed astonishing. Malaria disappeared from vast territories on the Asian (Japan, Korea, Taiwan) and European continents (Spain, Italy, the Balkans) and from several South Pacific and Caribbean islands, and was drastically reduced in many other places (India, Sri Lanka, Java). While the situation was also considerably improved in northern Africa, the program could not be implemented in much of tropical Africa due to logistical constraints.

However, in the early 1970's, a growing awareness of the detrimental ecological impact of DDT and the development of resistance to this insecticide led to a discontinuation of use in agriculture and its inclusion by the Stockholm Convention on a list of *persistent organic pollutants* whose use was to be severely restricted. Malaria-control programs based on spraying DDT came to a halt. This led to malaria resurgence in certain areas were it had been nearly eliminated. For instance in Sri Lanka, whereas the number of reported cases of malaria dropped from approximately 2,8 million in 1946 to a low total of only 17 (!) in 1963, discontinuation of the DDT-based malaria control program resulted in spectacular rebound of the number of cases, which were back to initial levels (i.e. 2.5 million) as soon as 1968 [3]. Clearly, other tools had to be developed.

Finally, it is now clear that parasites challenge all possible aspects of the immune defense machinery of the host, and have developed an extraordinary array of protective mechanisms, which makes them exceedingly interesting objects of study. This in turn has many immunologists and cell biologists to choose parasites as their preferred subjects of investigations. In this connection, the establishment of research programs such as the Tropical Diseases Research (TDR) program initiated by the World Health Organization in 1975, which funds research activities in many areas of parasitic and other tropical infectious diseases, provided a very strong incentive into basic and applied research on a selected number of parasitic infections. More recently, other (non-governmental) funding agencies have similarly injected very large sums of money into parasitological research.

One of the main objectives of research programs on the immunological aspects of parasitic diseases is to discover new tools to combat these infections. The successes obtained earlier in the 20th century with campaigns of vaccination against many viral and bacterial infections had raised hopes that similar strategies could be applied to infections due to parasites, hence the current efforts to develop vaccines against parasites of medical importance. This trend is also reflected in the changing strategy advocated by WHO to combat malaria, with emphasis placed on the disease rather than on the vector (the Roll Back Malaria Initiative, see ref. [4]. Yet, the expectations that anti-parasite vaccines would be soon available have so far not been fulfilled and indeed, as shown in the following contributions, parasitic infections have proven to constitute a major challenge to the ingenuity of researchers and scientists.

It is interesting to note that the data presented in Fig.1 do not necessarily correlate with the magnitude of the public health problem created by a given parasite. For instance, comparing studies on infection by malaria parasites *vs. Leishmania*, it is clear that the latter microorganism has benefited, on the part of immunologists, of a far greater interest than would have been justified by its strict public health importance compared to other parasites (even though, of course, leishmaniasis constitutes a major health problem in many parts of the world, where it affects millions of people). Other aspects can explain such discrepancies, such as the easiness with which a given microorganism lends itself to laboratory investigations in terms of its capacity to be grown *in vitro*, to be manipulated with little risk of self-contamination, or to infect current laboratory animals. Indeed *Leishmania* fulfills several of these criteria, as many *Leishmania* species can be maintained in relatively unsophisticated culture media and can infect mice, hamsters or guinea pigs. *Leishmania* has therefore been particularly prized as a laboratory tool by immunologists, in the hands of whom it has been put to very good use indeed, since early investigations of the immune response to *L. major* in the mouse were very instrumental in delineating the respective roles of the Th1 and Th2 lymphocyte subsets in the fight against infectious agents [5]. The importance of *Leishmania* as a research tool is also reflected in the number of papers devoted to this parasite in the present e-book.

As will become apparent on reading the following chapters, the variety of tricks that parasites have developed to counteract the induction as well as the effector arm of the immune response is stupendous. It is to be hoped that the efforts of the scientists to unravel the intricacies of the host-parasite relationships will allow the development, in a not too distant future, of more successful tools to combat these infections.

Jacques Mauel
Professor Emeritus
University of Lausanne
Switzerland

REFERENCES

[1] http://veteransinfo.tripod.com/malaria.pdf. See also : Beadle C, Hoffman SL (1993) History of malaria in the United States naval forces at war : World War I through the Vietnam conflict. Clin. Inf. Dis. 16, 320.

[2] Baird, JK (2000) : Resurgent Malaria at the Millenium : Control Strategies in Crisis. Drugs 59, 719.

[3] Jukes, TH, Insecticides in health, agriculture and the environment. Naturwissenschaften 61, 6 1974, cited in ref. 2.

[4] http://www.rollbackmalaria.org/index.html

[5] Heinzel, FP, Sadick, MD, Holaday, BJ, Coffman, RL and Locksley, RM. Reciprocal expression of interferon gamma or interleukin 4 during the resolution or progression of murine leishmaniasis. Evidence for expansion of distinct helper T cell subsets J Exp Med. (1989) 169 : 59–72.

PREFACE

Diseases caused by parasitic protozoa are often emerging or uncontrolled, as in the case of human leishmaniasis, or have a heavy burden, persisting in spite of present control strategies, as for malaria. Therefore, knowledge of recent findings on host-parasite interaction is extremely important for the development of new relevant control tools, including novel vaccination strategies and possible antigenic targets of protective immune response.

In **Chapter 1** by Carolina Montes *et al.* the full spectrum of B cell response toward parasite infections will elegantly be described. As parasites interact with different B cell compartments, they usually trigger an antibody response which can be protective but often harmful for the host.

Besides their major function of producing antibodies, parasite-induced B cells may act as antigen presenting cells and secretors of cytokines, which may contribute to host protection or susceptibility. B cells also function as regulatory cells, modulating anti-parasite immune response mediated by T cells, including unwanted autoaggressive T-cell responses.

The escape mechanisms of parasites from B cell response have also been highlighted. Variation of antigenic coat, molecular mimicry, induction of apoptosis of B cells, B cell fratricide, T cell apoptosis mediated by B cells and interference with the B cell signalling constitute the strategies adopted by parasites to elude B cell responses, which ultimately drive the infection to chronicity.

In **Chapter 2** (by Clotilde Marín and Manuel Sánchez-Moreno), new insights into immune diagnosis of *Trypanosoma cruzi* infection (Chagas disease) are outlined.

Serologic testing for specific antibodies to *T. cruzi* antigens is the most commonly employed approach for diagnosing *T. cruzi* chronic infection in clinical patients as well as in blood donors, but no assay has universally been accepted as the gold standard for the serologic diagnosis This review will examine different antigenic preparations (parasite extracts, recombinant antigens and synthetic peptides), which may have different affinities for both specific and non-specific antibodies and can produce variable sensitivities. In particular, the review focuses on the usefulness of parasite excreted-secreted antigens in immunoblotting assays and ELISA as diagnostic confirmatory tests for Chagas disease. Nowadays, the trypomastigote excretory-secretory antigens (TESA) composed of surface components and excreted dismutase and purified by affinity chromatography seem to represent sensitive and specific reagents for diagnosis of Chagas disease by ELISA.

In **Chapters 3** (by Antonio Verdini *et al.*) and **4** (by Sócrates Herrera and Myriam Arévalo-Herrera) the state of the art on malaria vaccine development is pointed out.

Chapter 3 critically covers malaria vaccine development since the beginning about twenty years ago, especially focusing on two mayor strategies, i.e. recombinant proteins and synthetic peptides, and examining the basis for failure or success encountered in clinical trials. In particular, the results obtained in phase IIa and IIb efficacy evaluation trials, by using *Plasmodium falciparum* proteins or protein fragments produced by peptide synthesis or DNA recombinant technology have been reported. The purpose is to make the scientific community aware of the shortcomings of some of these constructs, with regard to their 3-dimensional structure, and the need for more stringent biological/functional requirements to be met before field evaluations are initiated. Both of these factors are largely responsible for most of the failures witnessed in the past 20 years.

Chapter 4 illustrates present vaccination strategies against *Plasmodium vivax*. In spite of the high *P.vivax* malaria burden, the increasing drug resistance and possibility of severe and lethal cases, there are relatively only few vaccination trials, in comparison with *P.falciparum* vaccines under evaluation. Among *P. vivax* antigens, only two -CSP and Pvs25- have been already tested in Phase I trials, whereas two antigens from asexual blood stages -DBP and MSP-1- are likely to reach clinical testing within the next two years. In addition, a growing number of antigens, expressed on sporozoite surface, asexual blood stages or sexual stages, are being added to the list of potential candidates. However, the availability of *P. vivax* genome and proteomic studies will certainly accelerate the development of such new vaccines.

Finally, the Authors report a recent development of successful sporozoite challenge models in malaria-naïve human volunteers with *P. vivax* strain derived from human donors, and underline the importance of these models for the understanding of mechanisms of immunity to *P. vivax* infection.

In **Chapter 5** (by Leanne Mortimer and Kris Chadee) the immune responses elicited against *Entamoeba histolytica* are discussed.

The infected host is characterized by an impaired antigenic presentation and a dramatic reduction of cytokines produced by macrophages during the parasitic invasion. Furthermore, in the infective phase, CD4+ cells are decreased and CD8+ cells are increased. Moreover, cystein protease release by *E. histolytica* degrades human IgA and cleaves IgG heavy chains. When the parasite successfully subverts both the innate and adaptive immune response, the chronic disease ensues.

An important point in the study of very complex amoeba-host interactions is to understand why most people maintain asymptomatic infections while others succumb to acute illness. A determining factor may be the level of interleukin (IL)-10, which is crucial for the maintenance of gut homeostasis at the mucosal barrier. In a mouse model, IL-10 produced by haematopoietic cells is necessary for innate resistance to amoebic invasion, and also in humans an IL-10 deficiency could weaken the mucus layer, thus promoting parasite invasion.

Further chapter sections describe in detail intestinal and liver abscess pathogenesis, with data obtained from human biopsies that mark the progress of tissue destruction. Once beyond the epithelial barrier, trophozoites move into the mucosa and engorge on host tissue, while the invading trophozoites rapidly lyse any cells they encounter, including inflammatory cells which are abundantly produced.

The heavy burden of amebiasis in terms of incidence and mortality has prompted to vaccination studies. Some attempts to prepare an anti-*E. histolytica* vaccine are illustrated also in view of the evidence that only trophozoites need to be targeted and they express highly immunogenic proteins. The surface adhesin Gal-lectin enables amoeba to colonize via attachment to colonic mucus and has many functions that are central to the pathogenicity of *E. histolytica*. During invasion, it mediates adherence to host cells, apoptosis and phagocytosis, also triggers an inflammatory response and is involved in complement resistance. A recombinant version of the Gal-lectin cysteine rich region has experimentally been used for the preparation of a vaccine devoid of side effects. At the same time, the pentapeptide Monocyte Locomotion Inhibitory Factor and the surface antigen serin rich protein, are other potential candidate for vaccination.

Giardia intestinalis is the most common protozoan cause of diarrhoea in the world. **Chapter 6** by Aleksander Keselman and Steven Singer focuses on the role of immune responses in determining the outcome of infections with *Giardia*, both in eradicating parasites from the intestinal lumen and contributing to the symptoms of infection. Colonization of the small intestine elicits an immune response, both innate and adaptive, which plays an essential role in clearing infection and suggests that vaccination may be a promising and practical route of giardiasis control.

However, *G. duodenalis* has the capacity to suppress murine bone marrow derived dendritic cell (DC) antigen presentation, by blocking induction of MHC II proteins and co-stimulatory molecules. In addition, LPS-induced IL-12 secretion by DCs is significantly diminished, while ERK1/2-dependent IL-10 release is upregulated by coincubation with *Giardia* extract.

Furthermore, several mechanisms that contribute to pathogenesis of giardiasis are described. The recently discovered role for the neurotransmitter cholecystokinin (CCK) in mediating enhanced intestinal motility following *Giardia* infection is pointed out. CCK alters muscle function by activating mast cells, and also promotes parasite replication by stimulating the intestinal release of bile which is essential for trophozoite replication. Compromised molecular ultrastructural integrity in the intestinal epithelium, including changes of tight junction proteins, and caspase 3-dependent apoptosis of epithelial cells contribute to malabsorption by causing increased epithelial permeability. Moreover, *Giardia* produces excretory-secretory products that have enterotoxic properties and induces intestinal secretion of sodium and chloride.

Toxoplasma gondii and other Apicomplexa parasites are widely distributed obligate intracellular protozoa. In **Chapters 7** and **8** the immune responses toward *T. gondii* are described.

In particular, in **Chapter 7** Felix Yarovinsky reviews the evidence for specific Toll-like receptor (TLR) function in host resistance to *T. gondii*.

IL-12 is the critical host mediator in the initiation of adaptive immune response to *T. gondii* which culminates in the release of interferon (IFN)-γ deserving a protective function in the host. However, also this parasite can evade the host immune response by impairing DC antigen presentation, reducing release of IL-12 and interfering with IFN-γ signalling pathways in the infected cells.

Concerning different host signalling pathways which contribute to innate recognition of *T. gondii*, MyD88 activation is clearly a critical step in the initiation of the IL-12-dependent response to this parasite. A potent stimulator of IL-12 production by DCs in a MyD88-dependent manner was isolated and identified as a *T. gondii* profilin, belonging to small, actin-binding proteins that regulate actin polymerization in eukaryotic cells. Profilin is required not only for parasite gliding, invasion, and egress from the host cell, but is also essential for the parasite virulence *in vivo*. Further investigations have identified TLR11 as an innate immune receptor for *T. gondii* profilin in mice, also required for DC IL-12 production. Interestingly, profilins isolated from *Cryptosporidium parvum*, *Eimeria tenella*, and *Theileria parva* induce TLR11 activation in a similar manner, thus establishing TLR11 as a common pattern-recognition receptor for apicomplexan protozoa.

Other TLRs also contribute to the host resistance to *T.gondii*. Macrophage activation strictly depends on TLR2 activation, acting on regulation of the chemokine CCL2 and *Tumor Necrosis Factor* production in response to the parasite. The definitive ligands for TLR2 are, as for *P.falciparum,* glycans and diacylglycerols isolated from purified *T. gondii* glycosylphosphatidylinositol (GPI).

Interestingly, intestinal cell damage triggered by parasitic infection allows an overgrowth of commensal bacteria in the ileum, which activate TLR2-, TLR4-, and TLR9-dependent host response and small intestine inflammation. Therefore, these TLRs are also involved in *T. gondii*-induced immunopathology.

Since apoptosis also plays a crucial role in the parasite-host interactions, the complex apoptosis processes that develop in *Toxoplasma gondii*-infected hosts are reviewed by Yoshifumi Nishikawa in **Chapter 8**.

Upon infection with *T. gondii*, apoptosis is triggered in T lymphocytes, macrophages and other leukocytes, thereby suppressing immune responses against the parasite. Among mechanisms of host immune suppression in the course of *T. gondii* infection, apoptosis of T cells should be taken into consideration even at regional level, as observed in the case of intestinal Peyer' patches lymphocytes.

On the other hand, *T. gondii* inhibits host-cell apoptosis by direct or indirect mechanisms in the infected cells to facilitate parasite survival. This dual activity of *T. gondii* to both promote and inhibit apoptosis requires tight regulation. Therefore, molecular mechanisms behind the inhibition or induction of apoptosis and their role in pathogenesis of the infection are clearly elucidated in this review. In this respect, in a mouse model abortion due to *T. gondii* infection seems to depend on the apoptotic reduction of T regulatory (Treg) cells at placenta and splenic levels.

Leishmaniasis is caused by flagellated parasites of the genus *Leishmania*, which are inoculated into the skin during the blood meal of a sandfly vector. A broad spectrum of clinical manifestations in humans, ranging from a self-limiting cutaneous infection to disseminating visceral leishmaniasis, is described.

Chapters 9, **10** and **11** deals with the host immune response against *Leishmania* antigens.

In mouse models, healing of leishmaniasis is associated with a protective Th1-type response, characterised by an early interferon-gamma production by CD4+ T cells and the expression of inducible nitric oxide synthase and other leishmanicidal molecules by activated macrophages.

It is well known that professional antigen presenting cells -such as DCs- are crucial for the induction of the protective immune response in skin-draining lymph nodes. In this context, presentation of skin-derived *Leishmania* antigens by DC subtypes is reviewed by Uwe Ritter (**Chapter 9**) in particular focusing the possible role of epidermal Langerhans cells and dermal dendritic cells in the presentation of skin-derived *Leishmania* antigens.

L. major parasites have the skin as portal of entry into the host, and, therefore, epidermal Langherans cells (LCs) should initiate adaptive immune response. However, recent findings attribute to dermal DCs a central role in the triggering of adaptive immune response. Consequently, LCs seem to play an indirect role in delivering skin-derived antigens to cutaneous lymph node-resident DCs. Moreover, based on the data from experimental leishmaniasis, it is feasible that distinct DC subtypes interact with particular T cell populations during the first days after infection: LCs with "regulatory" T cells, Langerin+ DCs with CD8+ T cells, and Langerin- DCs with CD4+ T cells, respectively.

Leishmania parasites need phagocytic cells for intracellular replication, and neutrophils and macrophages play a pivotal role as host cells for *Leishmania*. This parasite has the ability to enter host macrophages safely and replicate inside phagocytes that were recruited to destroy it.

The inability of macrophages to kill the parasite and activate cells of the adaptive immune system is a consequence of the parasite capacity to alter several key signalling pathways in the host, as reviewed by Issa Abu-Dayyeh and Martin Olivier in **Chapter 10**.

In infected macrophages, production of microbicidal molecules and activation of cytokines are inhibited, whereas secretion of immunosuppressive molecules, like PGE2, TGF-β, IL-10 and certain chemokines is increased. The main signalling molecules altered by *Leishmania* to survive inside host macrophages include PKC, JAK2, Mitogen-activated protein kinases ERK ½, JNK and p38, and several transcription factors.

One important step in this immune evasion process is the *Leishmania*-induced activation of protein tyrosine phosphatases (PTPs) such as SHP-1, which act as negative regulators of signal transduction. SHP-1 has been shown to directly inactivate JAK2 and Erk1/2, and to play a role in the negative regulation of several transcription factors involved in macrophage activation such as NF-kB, STAT-1α and AP-1. These signalling alterations contribute to an inactivation of critical macrophage functions such as the production of IFN-γ-induced nitric oxide associated with parasite killing. Moreover, recent findings also revealed a pivotal role for SHP-1 in the inhibition of TLR-induced macrophage activation through binding to a newly identified Kinase Tyrosine-based Inhibitory Motif (KTIM) and inactivating IL-1 receptor-associated kinase 1 (IRAK-1).

Finally, among the several *Leishmania* virulence factors involved in initial interaction and internalization, the glycoprotein 63 (gp63) plays a novel and important role in the cleavage and activation of several macrophage PTPs as well as in the cleavage and degradation of the key transcription factor AP-1.

There is limited information about the cytokine responses in different clinical forms of human leishmaniasis. It is generally considered that patients with cutaneous leishmaniasis present a heterogeneous cellular immune response with a predominant CD4$^+$ Th1 type response upon healing. The subsets of T cells (CD4+ or CD8+), and their function within lesions is still, however, under debate. The presence of IFN-γ is most often associated with cure of the infection and the presence of IL-4 and IL-13 are associated with non-healing lesions, analogous to results obtained in the murine model of infection with *L. major*. However, levels of IFN-γ do not always correlate with resistance and the preferential participation of Th1 or Th2 responses during human infection with *Leishmania* is not completely understood.

Therefore, the analysis by Catherine Ronet *et al.* (**Chapter 11**) of immune response in patients with localized American cutaneous leishmaniasis (LCL) due to *Leishmania guyanensis*, which is endemic in the North East of Latin America, is of particular interest.

The Authors have investigated the role of cytokines during different phases of infection with *L. guyanensis*. Cytokine production has been determined in PBMCs and at the site of infection in: i. healthy subjects who have never been exposed to *Leishmania,* ii. healthy subjects exposed recently to *Leishmania*, and iii. patients developing the disease.

PBMCs from unexposed healthy subjects, following stimulation with live *L. guyanensis,* produce IFN-γ and TGF-β but not IL-4, IL-10 and IL-13. IFN-γ is generated from naïve CD8$^+$ T cells and requires the presence of whole *L. guyanensis* parasites. Also stimulation of PBMCs with the antigen *Leishmania* homologue of Receptors of Activated C Kinase (LACK) induces IFN-γ production by CD8$^+$ T cells. However, the picture is more complex, since LACK also induces IL-10 response in purified memory CD45RA$^-$ CD4$^+$ T cells and, after neutralization of TGF-β, in CD4$^+$ and CD8$^+$ T cells.

In healthy exposed subjects, followed after their stay in the rain forest in French Guyana, IFN-γ production by PBMCs originates from both CD4+ and CD8+ cells, also in response to Soluble Leishmania Antigen (SLA), in contrast to unexposed subjects. Interestingly, LACK-induced IFN-γ production by CD4$^+$ T cells was detected in these subjects before SLA-induced IFN-γ production, suggesting that the former assay could be used as an early predictive immunological marker of exposure to *Leishmania* in healthy subjects.

In patients with LCL, peripheral blood mononuclear cells produce IFN-γ at high levels and IL-10, but not TGF-β following *L. guyanensis* stimulation. However, IFN-γ was produced in response to LACK stimulation only during the early phase of infection, probably due to recruitment of IFN-γ-producing LACK-specific T cells in the inflamed skin during the late phase of infection. Indeed, at the site of infection in LCL patients Th2 responses predominate during the early phase and precede the development of a Th1 response.

In addition, in lesions of LCL patients Treg cells accumulate during the early phase of infection and their persistence is an index of a poor response to therapy. Interestingly, IL-13 is the main cytokine expressed within the lesion at the early phase and may be responsible for the maintenance of infection.

In conclusion, the bulk of data presented through the various chapters of this E-book emphasize the predominant as well as crucial role of the full spectrum of antiprotozoan immunity elicited by the host. Moreover, advances in the understanding of the mechanisms of immunity in the course of protozoan diseases have facilitated the development of novel vaccinal strategies, also in view of the emergent resistance of parasites to currently used antiparasitic drugs.

On these grounds, it appears clear that Immunoparasitology has enormously grown as an autonomous discipline, either didactically or scientifically. Therefore, this E-book also pursues the major goal to inform scientific community, clinicians and students about the progress of this hot sector of parasitic diseases.

This is the first of two eBooks on immune response to parasitic infections. The second volume of this series will deal with immune responses to helmithic infections.

Olga Brandonisio & Emilio Jirillo
University of Bari
Italy

CONTRIBUTORS

Issa Abu-Dayyeh
Centre for the Study of Host Resistance at the Research Institute of the McGill University Health Centre, and Departments of Microbiology and Immunology and Medicine, McGill University, Montréal, Québec, Canada

Eva V. Acosta Rodriguez
Immunology, Department of Clinical Biochemistry, School of Chemical Sciences, National University of Córdoba, Córdoba, Argentina

Maria C. Amezcua Vesely
Immunology, Department of Clinical Biochemistry, School of Chemical Sciences, National University of Córdoba, Córdoba, Argentina

Myriam Arévalo-Herrera
Centro Internacional de Vacunas, AA 26020, Cali, Colombia

Daniela A. Bermejo
Immunology, Department of Clinical Biochemistry, School of Chemical Sciences, National University of Córdoba, Córdoba, Argentina

Eliane Bourreau
Immunologie des Leishmanioses, Institut Pasteur de la Guyane, 97306 Cayenne French Guyana

Olga Brandonisio
Department of Internal Medicine, Immunology and Infectious Diseases, University of Bari, Medical School, 70124 Bari, Italy

Kris Chadee
Department of Microbiology and Infectious Diseases, Faculty of Medicine, University of Calgary, Calgary, Alberta Canada

Giampietro Corradin
Department of Biochemistry, University of Lausanne, 1066 Epalinges, Switzerland

Nicolas Fasel
Department of Biochemistry, University of Lausanne, Chemin des Boveresses 155, 1066 Epalinges, Switzerland

Adriana Gruppi
Immunology, Department of Clinical Biochemistry, School of Chemical Sciences, National University of Córdoba, Córdoba, Argentina

Sócrates Herrera
Immunology Institute, Universidad del Valle, AA 25574, Cali, Colombia

Annette Ives
Department of Biochemistry, University of Lausanne, Chemin des Boveresses 155, 1066 Epalinges, Switzerland

Emilio Jirillo
Department of Internal Medicine, Immunology and Infectious Diseases, University of Bari, Medical School, 70124 Bari, Italy

Aleksander Keselman
Department of Biology, Georgetown University, Washington, DC

Pascal Launois
1) WHO-IRTC, Chemin des Boveresses 155, 1066 Epalinges, Switzerland; 2) Department of Biochemistry, University of Lausanne, Chemin des Boveresses 155, 1066 Epalinges, Switzerland; 3) Special Programme for Research and Training in Tropical Diseases (TDR), Avenue Apia, 20, 1211 Geneva 27

Clotilde Marín
Department of Parasitology, Faculty of Sciences, University of Granada, Severo Ochoa s/n, E-18071 Granada, Spain

Slavica Masina
Department of Biochemistry, University of Lausanne, Chemin des Boveresses 155, 1066 Epalinges, Switzerland

Jacques Mauel
Professor Emeritus University of Lausanne, Faculty of Biology and Medicine, Department of Biochemistry, Ch. des Boveresses 155, CH-1066 Epalinges, Switzerland

Carolina L. Montes
Immunology, Department of Clinical Biochemistry, School of Chemical Sciences, National University of Córdoba, Córdoba, Argentina

Leanne Mortimer
Department of Microbiology and Infectious Diseases, Faculty of Medicine, University of Calgary, Calgary, Alberta Canada

Yoshifumi Nishikawa
National Research Center for Protozoan Diseases, Obihiro University of Agriculture and Veterinary Medicine, Inada-cho, Obihiro, Hokkaido 080-8555, Japan

Martin Olivier
Centre for the Study of Host Resistance at the Research Institute of the McGill University Health Centre, and Departments of Microbiology and Immunology and Medicine, McGill University, Montréal, Québec, Canada

Sope Olugbile
Seattle Biomedical Research Institute, Seattle, WA, USA

Richard Pink
Department of Biochemistry, University of Lausanne, 1066 Epalinges, Switzerland

Uwe Ritter
Department of Immunology, University of Regensburg, Regensburg, Germany

Catherine Ronet
WHO-IRTC, Chemin des Boveresses 155, 1066 Epalinges, Switzerland

Manuel Sánchez-Moreno
Department of Parasitology, Faculty of Sciences, University of Granada, Severo Ochoa s/n, E-18071 Granada, Spain

Steven Singer
Department of Biology, Georgetown University, Washington, DC, USA

Antonio Verdini
Department of Biochemistry, University of Lausanne, 1066 Epalinges, Switzerland

Felix Yarovinsky
Department of Immunology, University of Texas Southwestern Medical Center, 5323 Harry Hines Blvd, Dallas, TX 75390-9093, USA

CHAPTER 1

B Cell Response to Parasite Infections: A Survival Battle Between Hosts and Parasites

Carolina L Montes, Daniela A Bermejo, Maria C Amezcua Vesely, Eva V Acosta Rodriguez, and Adriana Gruppi*

Immunology, Department of Clinical Biochemistry, School of Chemical Sciences, National University of Córdoba, Córdoba, Argentina

Abstract: Parasites interact with different B cell compartments triggering, in most cases, a vigorous antibody response. Unfortunately, this response is not necessarily protective; indeed, it can be harmful for the host. In this chapter we describe how protozoan parasites and helminths induce mature B cell responses and how B cells influence the characteristics of T cell response involved in parasite control. To protect themselves, the parasites develop unique ways to evade B cell responses, including changes in their antigenic coat and induction of immunosuppression and apoptosis of B cells. We discuss how parasites elude B cell immunity establishing a favourable balance that drives the infection to chronicity.

INTRODUCTION

The rate of elimination and/or neutralization of microorganisms has critical importance for the survival of the host during the evolution of infectious challenges. Antibody (Ab) responses are a key aspect of circulating-microorganism immunity helping to clear acute infections, to protect against reinfection, and to control reactivation of persistent pathogens. Definitely, Abs are key host-protective molecules responsible of pathogen clearance, but they can also be harmful if they recognize self-antigens (Ags).

Ab immunity is mediated by specific types of Abs secreted by terminally differentiated Ab-secreting B cells known as plasma cells. Plasma cells derive from activated mature B cells that are sub-classified as conventional (B2), B1 and marginal zone B cells. The first wave of Ab-secreting cells that arise after Ag encounter mainly secretes IgM and produces a low affinity Ab response. This response does not require T cell help. In secondary lymph organs, activated B cells receive co-stimulation by specialized CD4+ T helper cells and form germinal centres in which class switching recombination (CSR), affinity maturation and somatic hypermutation occur. T cell-dependent Ab responses then generate a humoral memory provided by long-lived plasma cells and/or memory B cells. In contrast to T-dependent Ab response, T-independent responses do not generate detectable germinal centres and, apparently, neither do they generate memory [1] (Fig. **1**).

Even though the most popular function assigned to B cells is Ab production, they also participate in the immune response through Ab-independent mechanisms. The Ab-independent B cell activities include the secretion of proinflammatory cytokines and chemokines, and antigen presentation. B cells are able to function as accessory and regulatory cells [2, 3] since they regulate dendritic cells and T-cell subsets. The diverse mature B cell subsets present different phenotypes and topographic locations suggesting that they have distinct functional roles [4, 5]. Indeed, they have the abilities to produce different immunoglobulins and cytokines under the same stimulus [6], and then each B cell subset can influence the immune response in a different way, promoting protection or driving pathogenesis.

Innate-like B cell Response in Parasite Infections

Among the mature B cells, MZ and B1 B cells appear to be evolutionarily selected and maintained to facilitate prompt Ab responses. Since they respond quickly by producing the first wave of Abs required to control replicating microorganisms, MZ and B1 B cells provide a bridge between the innate and the adaptive arms of the anti-pathogen immune response.

***Corresponding Author:** Adriana Gruppi, Inmunología, Departamento de Bioquímica Clínica, Facultad de Ciencias Químicas, Universidad Nacional de Córdoba. Haya de la Torre y Medina Allende, Ciudad Universitaria, Córdoba (5000), Argentina; Tel: +54 351-4344973, Fax: +54 351-4333048, E-mail: agruppi@ fcq.unc.edu.ar

Emilio Jirillo (Ed)
All rights reserved - © 2010 Bentham Science Publishers Ltd.

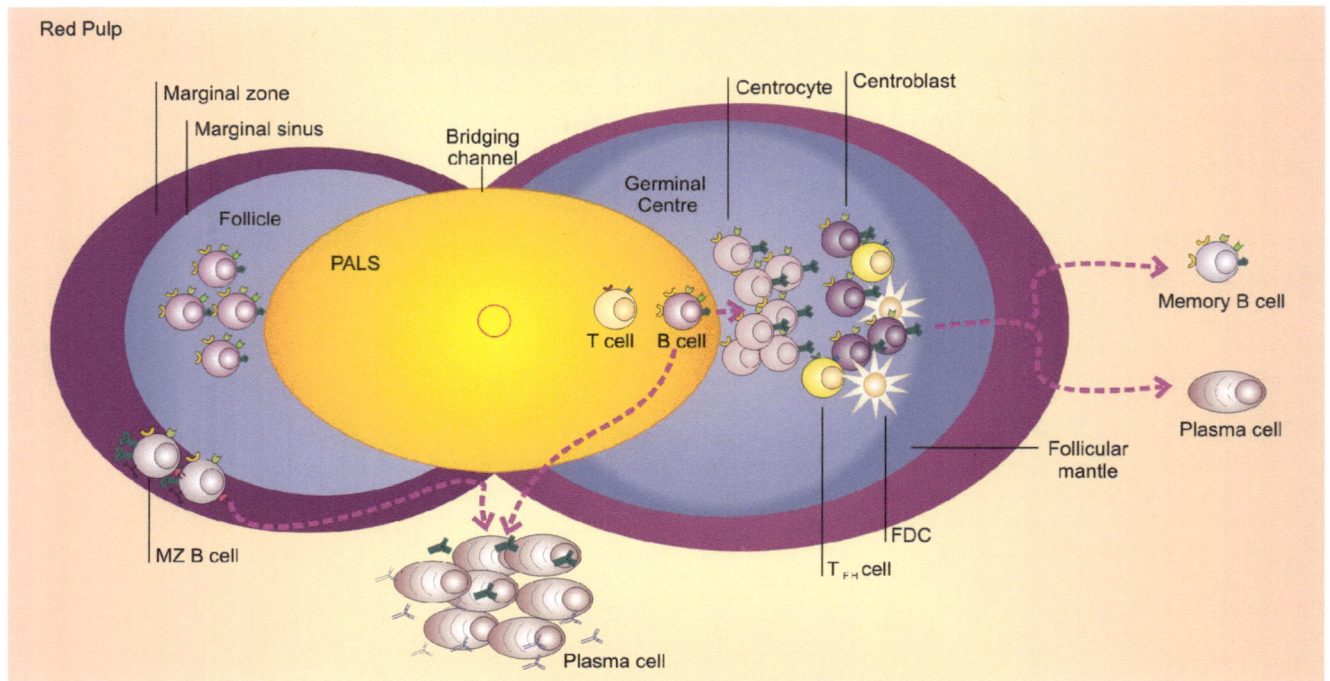

Figure 1: Schedule of follicular and extrafollicular Ab response development in spleen.

MZ: marginal zone

PALS: periarteriolar lymphoid sheath

FDC: follicular dendritic cell

B1 B cells, which are characterized by the expression of $CD5^+CD23^{neg}Mac-1^+IgM^+$ and mainly located in the peritoneal cavity, proliferate continuously *in vivo* in apparent absence of Ag generating persistent levels of low-affinity multispecific Abs. Their low threshold of activation might be exploited to induce an accelerated Ab response to pathogens that cause rapid disease. B1 B cells and the Abs produced by them participate in various activities: they are involved in immune regulation [7], clearance of senescent and apoptotic cells [8] and resistance to infection [4] particularly to blood and airborne virus and bacteria.

Intriguingly, B1 B cells have been clearly involved in the parasite burden control of nematodes such as *Brugia malayi* [9] and trematodes such as *Schistosoma mansoni* [10] infections; however, B1 B cells apparently do not participate in the control of protozoan parasite replication [11, 12]. For example, BALB/c Xid mice carrying an X-linked mutation (that prevents B1 B cell development) infected with *Trypanosoma cruzi*, display poor B cell responses to the infection, accompanied by low levels of specific and non-specific immunoglobulins (Igs) in the serum. Surprisingly, these studies showed that Xid mice infected with *T. cruzi* were able to control parasitemia, but they did not show the wasting syndrome observed in wild type mice. In addition, they developed almost no pathology early in the chronic phase. These results suggested that B1 B cells play a key role in Chagas' disease pathology rather than protective immunity.

B1 B cells, as a source of IL-10, can contribute to the susceptibility of BALB/c mice to *Leishmania major* infection by skewing the T helper cell network towards a Th2 phenotype. In this way, it has been demonstrated that susceptible BALB/c mice infected with *L. major* show a significant increase, more than three-fold, in the proportion of peritoneal B1 B cells compared with non-infected BALB/c mice [12]; whereas resistant C57Bl/6 mice (with predominant Th1 response) do not have any change in the proportion of peritoneal CD5+ B cells, compared with uninfected mice. It has been observed that *L. major* infection of B cell-defective BALB/c Xid mice induces less severe disease compared to wild type control mice. In contrast, experimentally B1 B cell-depleted BALB/c mice showed similar or even worse disease progression compared with control BALB/c mice [12] suggesting that the B1 B cells do not contribute to the susceptibility of BALB/c mice to *L. major* infection. The behavior of *L. major* infected Xid mice can be explained more by the high endogenous interferon-gamma (IFN-gamma) production in Xid immune deficiency than by the lack of B-1 cells [13].

Early resistance to *B. malayi* infection is mediated by humoral immune response with a significant attrition of the incoming infectious larval load. Sterile clearance of the remaining parasite burden appears to require cell mediated immunity. The early response can be exerted by B1 B cells since they are necessary to mediate host resistance to Brugian infection. Mice bearing the Xid mutation are as permissive to *B. malayi* and *B. pahangi* infection as those lacking all B cells, suggesting that the B1 B cell subset is responsible for host protection. This hypothesis was confirmed by reconstitution of immunodeficient recombination activating gene (Rag)-1 -/- mice with B1 B cells which conferred resistance, even in the absence of conventional B2 lymphocytes and most T cells [9].

B1 B cell-deficient animals also display a higher susceptibility to *S. mansoni* infection as revealed by an increase in the tissue egg loads and a significantly elevated mortality, as well as an increase in the granuloma densities. Larger amounts of IFN-gamma and IL-4 are observed in infected BALB/c Xid mice while IL-10 production is reduced. Infected BALB/c Xid mice show higher amounts of specific IgE and IgG1 Abs and lower amounts of IgM and IgA. These observations support the idea that B1 B cells provide IgA that may help to control *S. mansoni* infection and that a Th1 response is self-defeating for the host [10].

MZ B cells represent a distinct lineage of naive B lymphocytes involved in early humoral response apart from peritoneal B1 B cells, and consequently, are considered a significant source of natural IgM Abs. Moreover, they have been described as cells endowed with natural memory which provide a bridge between innate and adaptative B cell response. Splenic MZ B cells can be distinguished from the other splenic B cells by $CD24^{high}$, IgM^{high}, IgD^{high}, $CD23^-$ expression, as well as by their higher expression of CD21. It is known that these B cells mediate humoral immune responses against blood-borne type 2 T-independent antigens [4] but their role in parasite infection has been scarcely studied.

Induction of a T-independent anti-trypanosome IgM response has been shown to be a crucial factor in *T. brucei* parasite elimination. Even when the increased splenic cellularity [14] occurs after *T. brucei* infection, a significant reduction of splenic IgM+ MZ B cell numbers takes place right after the first week of infection. The infection-associated disappearance of the MZ B cells from the spleen could be explained by two independent mechanisms, namely cell differentiation and/or cell death. Supporting the first possibility is the observation that the rapid disappearance of MZ B cells coincided with the temporary accumulation of IgM+plasma cells. However, a direct link between these two events remains speculative as no specific markers exist that allows cell fate analysis that would determine the MZ B cell origin of the occurring plasma cells. The analysis of MZ B cells that remain in the spleen in the days following the clearance of the first peak of parasitemia, revealed that these cells upregulated Annexin V expression. In addition, these cells exhibit caspase 3 gene expression as well as the conversion of pro-caspase 3 into the cleaved 12 kD and 17 kD caspase 3 activation products suggesting the induction of trypanosomiasis-associated apoptosis in the splenic MZ B cell population [15]. Probably, apoptosis-induction of MZ B cells can be used by the parasite as strategy to avoid early IgM protective response.

As in African trypanosomes, after *Plasmodium chabaudi chabaudi* infection B cells are absent from the MZ for at least 30 days after the peak of infection, although flow cytometry shows their continued presence in the spleen throughout infection [16]. Unexpectedly, unlike other B cell subsets, MZ B cells show faster expansion on re-infection than in the first encounter with the parasite [17]; however, their protective role has not been studied.

Parasites Trigger Massive B Cell Response in Secondary Lymph Organs

In leishmaniasis, like in other parasite diseases described below, a strong polyclonal B-cell activation develops. This is reflected in hypergammaglobulinemia, as well as in a marked increase in the B cells number, not only in peripheral blood but also in lesion-draining lymph nodes of both *L. major*-susceptible and -resistant mouse strains. This polyclonal B cell activation is mediated by CD4+T cells since purified L3T4+ T cells obtained from lymph nodes draining the lesions of *L. major* infected BALB/c mice polyclonally stimulate B cells of infected mice to undergo proliferation and differentiation into immunoglobulin-secreting cells [18]. A link between B-cell expansion, circulating Abs and virulence enhancement has been reported in *Leishmania* infections. Mice depleted of B cells by continuous administration of anti-IgM, mice that were B-cell mutants (µMT mice) and mice lacking circulating Abs (JhD mice) infected with different *Leishmania* species showed enhanced resistance compared with control BALB/c mice. Moreover, susceptibility to leishmaniasis is recovered when the B-cell population is reconstituted [19;20].

T. cruzi infected mice also present increased cellularity of spleen and lymph node cells in the acute phase of infection. A rapid blast transformation and proliferative activity of B cells and CD4+ and CD8+T cells is observed. At 2 weeks of *T.*

cruzi infection most cells in these organs are enlarged and more than half are dividing. By 2 and 6 months after infection (chronic phase of resistant strains), large numbers of activated B lymphocytes and, to a lesser extent, of CD8+ T cells are still detected. Similar results were obtained in C57BL/6 (resistant) and C3H/HeJ (susceptible) mouse strains [21]. In *T. congolense* infection a relationship between polyclonal activation and infection susceptibility was tested in eight inbred strain of mice. In all of the strains studied the mice present a marked increase in splenic B cells resulting in a non-specific polyclonal activation of lymphocytes that affects primarily B cells. In strains of mice which survived longest, i.e. C57B1/6J and AKR/A, the increase in splenic B cells is less marked. Whether this is associated with a decreased susceptibility of these strains to polyclonal activation induced by trypanosome infection, or is the result of lower levels of parasitemia, remains to be determined. Surgically splenectomized mice are more susceptible to *T. congolense* infection than intact mice of the same strain. However, the effect of splenectomy was much less pronounced in C57B1/6J mice than in the relatively more susceptible BALB/c/A mice [22]. Ultimately, these protozoan infections result in a strong production of non-parasite specific Abs characterized by the predominance of IgG2a- and IgG2b isotypes.

Intraperitoneal inoculation of *Neospora caninum* tachyzoites into BALB/c mice induces an acute response characterized by a rapid increase in the numbers of CD69-expressing peritoneal and splenic B cells. This early B-cell stimulatory effect preceded an increase in the numbers of total and immunoglobulin-secreting splenic B cells and a rise in serum levels of *N. caninum*-specific immunoglobulins, predominantly of the IgG2a and IgM isotypes. The B-cell stimulatory effect observed in mice challenged with *N. caninum* tachyzoites was reduced in mice challenged with gamma-irradiated parasites indicating that polyclonal B cell activation is triggered by live parasites. In contrast with the peripheral B-cell expansion, a depletion of B-lineage cells was observed in the bone-marrow of the *N. caninum*-infected mice [23]. Likewise, *T. cruzi* induces a marked loss of immature B cells in the bone-marrow, which also compromises recently emigrated B cells in the periphery. The depletion of bone-marrow immature B cells is associated with an increased rate of apoptosis mediated by a parasite-indirect mechanism in a Fas/FasL-independent fashion [24].

A detailed analysis of splenic B cell response was performed in malaria. B cells and Abs play a key role in controlling the erythrocytic stage of malaria. *P. chabaudi chabaudi* causes major, but temporary changes in the distribution of leukocytes in the spleen. Malaria infection triggers vigorous extrafollicular growth of plasmablasts and germinal center formation. Early in the response, the lymphocytes in the T zone and follicles become widely spaced and the limits of these compartments distort. This effect is maximal around the peak of parasitemia. Initially, the plasma cells have a conventional red pulp distribution, but by day 10 they are unconventionally sited in the periarteriolar region of the white pulp. In this region they form clusters occupying part of the area normally filled by T cells. Relatively normal splenic architecture is regained by day 60 of infection [16]. Similar behavior is observed in *T. cruzi* infected mice (Bermejo *et al.* manuscript in preparation).

A destruction of the structure of the splenic lymphoid follicles is reported in *S. japonicum* infection. This disruptive effect is correlated with a severely impaired T cell-dependent Ab response upon challenge with ovalbumin [25]. Schistosomal infection also triggers a polyclonal B-cell activation and modulation of Ig isotype production, compatible with the alternate predominance of Th2 and Th1 lymphocyte subsets in the acute and the chronic phases of the disease, respectively [26]. Apparently, the polyclonal B cell activation triggered by parasites leads to a strong germinal center response with unshaped follicules that do not seem to interfere with the development of the humoral response but affect Ab response to a secondary challenge with heterologous antigens [27-29].

Different roles are proposed for polyclonal B cell activation, which can be crucial for early host defense against rapidly dividing microorganisms by contributing Abs specific for a spectrum of conserved structures present in the pathogens. In addition, polyclonal B cell activation can be responsible for maintenance of memory B cell responses) because of the continuous, unrestricted stimulation of memory B cells whose Ab production may be sustained in the absence of the antigen binding-specific B Cell Receptor (BCR) [30]. Conversely, polyclonal activation can be triggered by microorganisms to avoid the host-specific immune response by activating B cell clones which produce non-microorganism-specific Abs. Additionally, some reports suggest a deleterious role for polyclonal activation, arguing that it could potentially turn on anti-self-responses and lead to autoimmune manifestations during chronic infections. Based on these considerations, the study of specific components of each microorganism, ultimately responsible for the polyclonal B cell response, has acquired new relevance as these components can be potential targets to control the infection's undesired effects or they can be used to enhance a natural Ab response. The polyclonal activators derived from microorganisms are usually components of the cell membranes, the cytosol, or excretion/secretion products. For example, two soluble *T. cruzi*-derived proteins, a mitochondrial malate dehydrogenase [31] and a glutamato dehydrogenase (GDH) [32] are able to induce polyclonal B cell response. Furthermore, other *T. cruzi* proteins described as *T. cruzi* polyclonal activators are an excretory/secretory antigen of 24 kDa [33] and two cell surface proteins: a proline racemase [34] and a trans-sialidase [35]. Other parasitic proteins also acting as polyclonal B cell activators are the soluble proteins from *S. japonicum* eggs [36], the *L. major* ribosomal protein S3a homologue [37] and a cystein-rich interdomain region 1-alpha of the *P. falciparum* erythrocyte membrane protein [38].

B Cells Regulate Anti-Parasite Immune Response Mediated by T Cells

As regulatory cells, B cells can favour the T cell response involved in the progression of parasite infection or restraining unwanted autoaggressive T-cell responses. In secondary lymph organs, once activated, CD4 T cells migrate toward the B cell zone where they form conjugates with B cells at the junction of the T and B cell regions [39]. B cells support continued CD4 T cell expansion, which is required for a sustained response leading to effector and memory function [40;41]. B cells preferentially favor the development of IL-4-producing Th2 cells; however, some studies suggest that B cells may down-regulate the level of IL-12 released by DC, thereby inhibiting the development of IFN-gamma producing Th1 cells [42]. The B cell participation in T cells-priming and migration to the infection site was demonstrated in JhD mice (which do not display B cells and Abs). After *L. amazonensis* infection, these mice show a delayed onset of disease and develop small tissue lesions. At the infection site, a significant decrease in CD4+ and CD8+ T cells, but not in MAC1+ macrophages, is observed. In addition, no or minimal signs of necrotic foci is observed. The participation of B cells in this process was confirmed after adoptive transfer of B cells or Abs which restores CD4+ T cell activation and migration in infected JhD mice. These mice also present a marked reduction in CD4+ T cell proliferation and cytokine (IFN-γ and IL-10) in comparison with WT [20].

B cells also participate in the generation of effector/memory T cells. In *T. cruzi* infection skeletal muscle inflammatory infiltrate shows a predominance of CD8+CD45Rb^{low} in B-cell-sufficient C57Bl/6 mice, whereas the preponderant cell type in mu MT knockout mice (mice lacking mature B cells) skeletal muscle inflammatory infiltrate was predominantly CD4+ T cells. B cells are crucial in the maintenance of central and effector memory CD8+T cell, as well as the determination of the T cell cytokine functional pattern. *T. cruzi* infection in C57Bl/6m mu MT knockout mice is intensified in relation to control mice and this exacerbation is related to low levels of inflammatory cytokines produced and the lower numbers of central and effector memory CD4+ and CD8+ T cells generated during the acute phase of the infection. In summary, the tissue inflammatory response was much less intense in the acute phase of the infection of B cell deficient mice, consistent with a deficit in the generation of effector T cells [43]. Accordingly, both OBF-1 knockout mice (mice with reduced number of peripheral B cells) and mu MT mice develop severely reduced hepatic granulomas at five weeks post-infection with *S. japonicum* compared to their wild-type counterparts. In contrast, they display no significant difference in granuloma pathology at eight weeks post infection. B cells and Abs accumulate in the hepatic granulomas early in schistosomiasis, indicating a contribution of the B cell response to the granulomatous inflammation in early infection [44].

The progression from a Th1-regulated to a Th2-regulated immune response fails to occur in B-cell-depleted mice (by treatment with anti-u Abs) infected with *P. chabaudi chabaudi* indicating that B cells are required for the downregulation of Th1-mediated and/or the generation of Th2-mediated protective immunity to *P. chabaudi chabaudi*. Infected B cell depleted mice mount a significant Th1 response which is manifested as an enduring inability of splenic CD4+ T cells to produce significant levels of IL-4 and IL-10. IL-2 and IFN-y levels remain significantly elevated throughout the 50-day observation period, and there was sustained production of nitric oxide [45]. On the contrary, in *Trichuris muris* the host protective mucosal Th2 response is inhibited in B cell-deficient mice, whereas a Th1 response is sustained. Administration of anti-IL-12 Ab restored the resistance, suggesting that B cells block IL-12 thereby promoting the Th2 response [46]. Similar results were obtained following parenteral immunization of B cell-deficient mice with *S. mansoni* eggs in that immune deviation from a Th2 to a Th1 response was observed [47].

It is still unknown how B cells influence Th response. B cells can exert their regulatory functions in an Ab-independent way as cytokine producers or through Ab production. B cell cytokine production apparently is influenced by the type of parasite, via ligands of Toll like receptor or other pathogens pattern receptors. In the case of Abs, Abs coating of *Leishmania* stimulate dendritic cells to produce high levels of IL-10 and increase their ability to prime naive CD4+ T cells. Then, B cells influence negatively the protective response in Leishmaniasis since a correlation between B cell activation and lesion progress in immunocompetent infected mice has been documented [20].

Suppression and Evasion of Immune B Cell Response

In immunoparasitology it is generally accepted that the survival and degree of pathogenicity of parasites is coupled to their ability to escape and resist immune responses. As the host displays sophisticated mechanisms that give it protection from parasites, the parasite develops countermeasures. In consequence, different strategies have been developed for parasites to avoid immune surveillance and to persist within the host. Parasites can use different devices to evade host immune attack since they are able to manipulate dendritic cell function [48] as well as effector and memory T cell activities [49-51]. The escape from B cell response has been less studied; however, it has been reported that parasites can evade Abs and B cell immunity by penetrating and multiplying within cells, eliminating their protein coat, varying their surface antigens, affecting B cell signal pathway and/or deleting progenitors and mature B cells (Fig. 2). Immunomodulation of host response can be exerted directly by parasites or by molecules produced by them.

African Trypanosomiasis is a textbook example of an extracellular parasitic infection where antigenic variation of the variant-specific surface glycoprotein (VSG) coat occurs. During the process of antigenic variation, one homogeneous surface coat is replaced over a period of time by a new homogeneous coat. Replacement of this coat occurs at rapid regular time intervals allowing the parasite to escape from an effective host Abs response. For the parasite, this lengthened time is required to increase the chance of successful parasite transmission through the tsetse vector. The kinetics of Ab responses to VSG surface coats displayed by trypanosomes at the first peak of parasitemia and the kinetics of Ab responses to different VSG coats displayed by variant antigenic types in subsequent waves of parasitemia are similar. However, VSG double expressers arise naturally during the process of antigenic variation. In this sense, Dubois *et al.* [52] demonstrated that B cells exposed to a mosaic VSG coat during infection mount a significantly reduced T-independent antibody response to VSG epitopes. This result suggests that the process of antigenic variation not only provides the trypanosome with a new immunological identity upon completion of coat switching but also provides the parasite with an immunological "stealth coat" during the intermediate stages of coat switching, when two VSG species coexist in the glycoprotein surface coat [52].

The development of an effective immune response in Malaria is hampered by the fact that stage-specific proteins tend to be highly polymorphic or antigenically variable. Sequence polymorphism is common in several *Plasmodium* proteins, especially in those with extensive repetitive regions, such as the circumsporozoite protein (CSP), an antigen with multiple tandem repeats and that is located on the surface of malaria sporozoites [53]. In addition, when an Ab response does develop against sporozoites, plasmodia overcome the response by sloughing off their surface CSP coat, rendering the Abs ineffective [54].

Interestingly, it has been reported that a phosphorylcholine (PC)-containing glycoprotein (ES-62) released by the rodent filarial parasite *Acanthocheilonema viteae* interferes with B cell activation, promoting down-regulation of PKC isoforms in B cells, mainly by stimulating proteolytic degradation. ES-62 also disrupts the normal activation and nuclear translocation patterns of the alpha and iota/lambda isoforms of PKC following ligation of BCR [55]. In vivo and in vitro studies show that this parasite antigen is able to reduce B cell ability to proliferate upon BCR stimulation [56]. As PC-containing secreted products (PC-ES) are also released by human filarial parasites, it has been suggested that PC-ES, by interfering with B cell function, could play a role in prolonging filarial infection in parasitized individuals.

Taking into account that B cell apoptosis is an immune-regulatory mechanism triggered by the host to control the excessive expansion of these cells, it is likely that parasite-induced massive B lymphocyte activation would be an evasive mechanism developed by pathogens to trigger host homeostatic control and interfere with protective Ab response. Moreover, it has been demonstrated that cell apoptosis may have an additional negative effect because the clearance of apoptotic bodies by *T. cruzi*-infected macrophages promotes parasite replication favoring the chronic establishment of the parasite in the host [57]. Infection with *T. cruzi* induces FasL expression in B cells and FasL mediated B cell fratricide, affecting the specificity of the Abs produced [58]. IL-4 rescues B cells from apoptosis and favors differentiation of memory B cells by a mechanism that reduces the expression of FasL [59] and requires expression of galectin-3 [60] providing effectors B cells for a re-encounter with *T. cruzi*. At the same time, infection with *S. mansoni* increases FasL expression by B1a cells and contributes to CD4+ T-cell apoptosis [61]. Moreover, in culture, SEA (Schistosoma soluble egg antigen) induced splenic and granuloma CD4+T-cell apoptosis and stimulated expression of FasL on splenic but not granuloma CD4+T cells, CD8+T cells, and CD19+B cells. SEA-stimulated splenocytes and granuloma cells preferentially lysed a Fas-transfected target cell line. Depletion of B cells from SEA-stimulated splenic cultures decreased CD4+T cell apoptosis. Coculture of purified splenic B cells with CD4+T cells and adoptive transfer of purified B cells indicated that antigen-stimulated B cells can kill CD4+Th cells. However, CD4+T cells were the dominant mediators of apoptosis in the granuloma [62].

Finally, parasites specific B cell response sometimes involves antigenic mimicry, in which Abs directed to parasite are cross-reactive with host mammalian Ags. This is the case of *T. cruzi* infection in which cruzipain, the main cystein protease of the parasite, induces in mice Abs cross reactive with cardiac myosin of the host [63] altering immune recognition and inducing autoimmune disease.

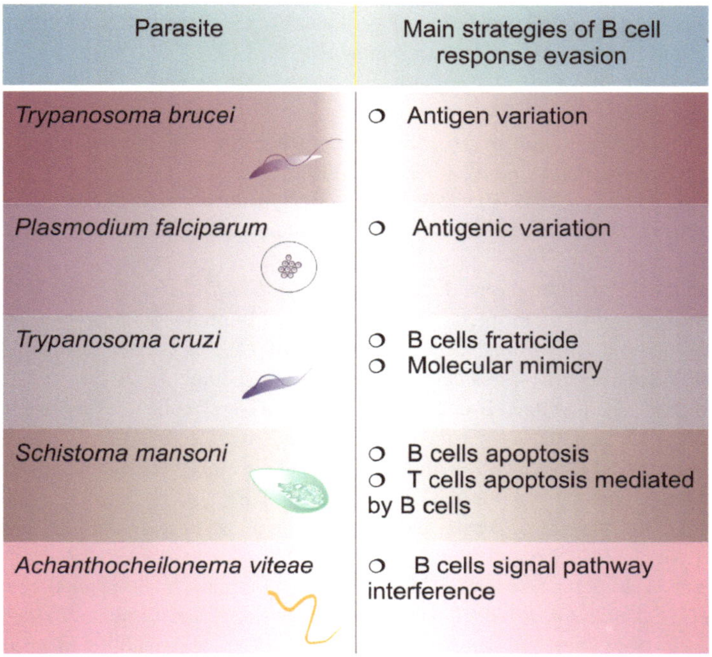

Parasite	Main strategies of B cell response evasion
Trypanosoma brucei	○ Antigen variation
Plasmodium falciparum	○ Antigenic variation
Trypanosoma cruzi	○ B cells fratricide ○ Molecular mimicry
Schistoma mansoni	○ B cells apoptosis ○ T cells apoptosis mediated by B cells
Achanthocheilonema viteae	○ B cells signal pathway interference

Figure 2: Main strategies employed by parasites to avoid Abs and B cell response.

CONCLUDING REMARKS

Parasites induce a strong B cell response and, consequently, a high Abs production; however, this response is not enough to control parasite invasion capacity and replication, and they establish chronically in the host. The complex life cycle of parasites which involves more that one host, in addition to parasites' ability to avoid immune response has made more difficult the identification of target antigens used in vaccine design. Parasite control requires the orchestration of humoral and cellular mechanisms; therefore, one of the most important challenges in parasitology is the identification of molecules, adjuvants and immunization pathways able to generate an efficient anti-parasite response.

REFERENCES

[1]   MacLennan IC. Germinal centers. Annu Rev Immunol 1994; 12: 117-39.
[2]   Zuniga E, Rabinovich GA, Iglesias MM, Gruppi A. Regulated expression of galectin-1 during B-cell activation and implications for T-cell apoptosis. J Leukoc Biol 2001; 70: 73-79.
[3]   Mauri C, Gray D, Mushtaq N, Londei M. Prevention of arthritis by interleukin 10-producing B cells. J Exp Med 2003; 197: 489-501.
[4]   Martin F, Oliver AM, Kearney JF. Marginal zone and B1 B cells unite in the early response against T-independent blood-borne particulate antigens. Immunity 2001; 14: 617-29.
[5]   Berland R, Wortis HH. Origins and functions of B-1 cells with notes on the role of CD5. Annu Rev Immunol 2002; 20: 253-300.
[6]   Genestier L, Taillardet M, Mondiere P, Gheit H, Bella C, Defrance T. TLR agonists selectively promote terminal plasma cell differentiation of B cell subsets specialized in thymus-independent responses. J Immunol 2007; 178: 7779-86.
[7]   Szczepanik M, kahira-Azuma M, Bryniarski K, et al. B-1 B cells mediate required early T cell recruitment to elicit protein-induced delayed-type hypersensitivity. J Immunol 2003; 171: 6225-35.
[8]   Shaw PX, Horkko S, Chang MK, et al. Natural antibodies with the T15 idiotype may act in atherosclerosis, apoptotic clearance, and protective immunity. J Clin Invest 2000; 105: 1731-40.
[9]   Paciorkowski N, Porte P, Shultz LD, Rajan TV. B1 B lymphocytes play a critical role in host protection against lymphatic filarial parasites. J Exp Med 2000; 191: 731-36.
[10]   Gaubert S, Viana da CA, Maurage CA, et al. X-linked immunodeficiency affects the outcome of Schistosoma mansoni infection in the murine model. Parasite Immunol 1999; 21: 89-101.
[11]   Minoprio P, Coutinho A, Spinella S, Hontebeyrie-Joskowicz M. Xid immunodeficiency imparts increased parasite clearance and resistance to pathology in experimental Chagas' disease. Int Immunol 1991; 3: 427-33.

[12]   Babai B, Louzir H, Cazenave PA, Dellagi K. Depletion of peritoneal CD5+ B cells has no effect on the course of Leishmania major infection in susceptible and resistant mice. Clin Exp Immunol 1999; 117: 123-29.

[13]   Hoerauf A, Solbach W, Lohoff M, Rollinghoff M. The Xid defect determines an improved clinical course of murine leishmaniasis in susceptible mice. Int Immunol 1994; 6: 1117-24.

[14]   Igbokwe IO, Nwosu CO. Lack of correlation of anaemia with splenomegaly and hepatomegaly in Trypanosoma brucei and Trypanosoma congolense infections of rats. J Comp Pathol 1997; 117: 261-65.

[15]   Radwanska M, Guirnalda P, De TC, Ryffel B, Black S, Magez S. Trypanosomiasis-induced B cell apoptosis results in loss of protective anti-parasite antibody responses and abolishment of vaccine-induced memory responses. PLoS Pathog 2008; 4: e1000078.

[16]   Achtman AH, Khan M, MacLennan IC, Langhorne J. *Plasmodium chabaudi chabaudi* infection in mice induces strong B cell responses and striking but temporary changes in splenic cell distribution. J Immunol 2003; 171: 317-24.

[17]   Stephens R, Ndungu FM, Langhorne J. Germinal centre and marginal zone B cells expand quickly in a second Plasmodium chabaudi malaria infection producing mature plasma cells. Parasite Immunol 2009; 31: 20-31.

[18]   Lohoff M, Matzner C, Rollinghoff M. Polyclonal B-cell stimulation by L3T4+ T cells in experimental leishmaniasis. Infect Immun 1988; 56: 2120-24.

[19]   Smelt SC, Cotterell SE, Engwerda CR, Kaye PM. B cell-deficient mice are highly resistant to Leishmania donovani infection, but develop neutrophil-mediated tissue pathology. J Immunol 2000; 164: 3681-88.

[20]   Wanasen N, Xin L, Soong L. Pathogenic role of B cells and antibodies in murine *Leishmania amazonensis* infection. Int J Parasitol 2008; 38: 417-29.

[21]   Minoprio PM, Eisen H, Forni L, Imperio Lima MR, Joskowicz M, Coutinho A. Polyclonal lymphocyte responses to murine *Trypanosoma cruzi* infection. I. Quantitation of both T- and B-cell responses. Scand J Immunol 1986; 24: 661-68.

[22]   Morrison WI, Roelants GE, Mayor-Withey KS, Murray M. Susceptibility of inbred strains of mice to *Trypanosoma congolense*: correlation with changes in spleen lymphocyte populations. Clin Exp Immunol 1978; 32: 25-40.

[23]   Teixeira L, Marques A, Meireles CS, *et al.* Characterization of the B-cell immune response elicited in BALB/c mice challenged with *Neospora caninum* tachyzoites. Immunology 2005; 116: 38-52.

[24]   Zuniga E, Acosta-Rodriguez E, Merino MC, Montes C, Gruppi A. Depletion of immature B cells during *Trypanosoma cruzi* infection: involvement of myeloid cells and the cyclooxygenase pathway. Eur J Immunol 2005; 35: 1849-58.

[25]   Ji F, Liu Z, Cao J, *et al.* B cell response is required for granuloma formation in the early infection of *Schistosoma japonicum*. PLoS One 2008; 3: e1724.

[26]   el-Cheikh MC, Dutra HS, Minoprio P, Borojevic R. Increase of B-lymphocyte number and activity during experimental murine schistosomiasis mansoni. Braz J Med Biol Res 1994; 27: 1605-17.

[27]   Yamashita T, Watanabe T, Saito S, Araki Y, Sendo F. *Schistosoma japonicum* soluble egg antigens activate naive B cells to produce antibodies: definition of parasite mechanisms of immune deviation. Immunology 1993; 79: 189-95.

[28]   Guobadia EE, Fagbemi BO, Oyejide A. The immune response of *Trypanosoma gambiense*-infected mice to Schistosoma whole worm antigens. Afr J Med Med Sci 1996; 25: 347-52.

[29]   Goumard P, Vu DN, Maurois P, Camus D. Influence of malaria on a pre-existing antibody response to heterologous antigens. Ann Immunol (Paris) 1982; 133D: 313-26.

[30]   Bernasconi NL, Traggiai E, Lanzavecchia A. Maintenance of serological memory by polyclonal activation of human memory B cells. Science 2002; 298: 2199-2202.

[31]   Montes CL, Zuniga EI, Vazquez J, Arce C, Gruppi A. *Trypanosoma cruzi* mitochondrial malate dehydrogenase triggers polyclonal B-cell activation. Clin Exp Immunol 2002; 127: 27-36.

[32]   Montes CL, Acosta-Rodriguez EV, Mucci J, Zuniga EI, Campetella O, Gruppi A. A Trypanosoma *cruzi* antigen signals CD11b+ cells to secrete cytokines that promote polyclonal B cell proliferation and differentiation into antibody-secreting cells. Eur J Immunol 2006; 36: 1474-85.

[33]   Da Silva AC, Espinoza AG, Taibi A, Ouaissi A, Minoprio P. A 24,000 MW *Trypanosoma cruzi* antigen is a B-cell activator. Immunology 1998; 94: 189-96.

[34]   Reina-San-Martin B, Degrave W, Rougeot C, *et al.* A B-cell mitogen from a pathogenic trypanosome is a eukaryotic proline racemase. Nat Med 2000; 6: 890-97.

[35]   Gao W, Wortis HH, Pereira MA. The *Trypanosoma cruzi* trans-sialidase is a T cell-independent B cell mitogen and an inducer of non-specific Ig secretion. Int Immunol 2002; 14: 299-308.

[36]   Yamashita T, Watanabe T, Saito S, Araki Y, Sendo F. *Schistosoma japonicum* soluble egg antigens activate naive B cells to produce antibodies: definition of parasite mechanisms of immune deviation. Immunology 1993; 79: 189-95.

[37]   Cordeiro-Da-Silva A, Borges MC, Guilvard E, Ouaissi A. Dual role of the *Leishmania major* ribosomal protein S3a homologue in regulation of T- and B-cell activation. Infect Immun 2001; 69: 6588-96.

[38]   Donati D, Mok B, Chene A, *et al.* Increased B cell survival and preferential activation of the memory compartment by a malaria polyclonal B cell activator. J Immunol 2006; 177: 3035-44.

[39]   Garside P, Ingulli E, Merica RR, Johnson JG, Noelle RJ, Jenkins MK. Visualization of specific B and T lymphocyte interactions in the lymph node. Science 1998; 281: 96-99.

[40]   Linton PJ, Harbertson J, Bradley LM. A critical role for B cells in the development of memory CD4 cells. J Immunol 2000; 165: 5558-65.

[41]   Bradley LM, Harbertson J, Biederman E, Zhang Y, Bradley SM, Linton PJ. Availability of antigen-presenting cells can determine the extent of CD4 effector expansion and priming for secretion of Th2 cytokines *in vivo*. Eur J Immunol 2002; 32: 2338-46.

[42]   Moulin V, Andris F, Thielemans K, Maliszewski C, Urbain J, Moser M. B lymphocytes regulate dendritic cell (DC) function in vivo: increased interleukin 12 production by DCs from B cell-deficient mice results in T helper cell type 1 deviation. J Exp Med 2000; 192: 475-82.

[43]   Cardillo F, Postol E, Nihei J, Aroeira LS, Nomizo A, Mengel J. B cells modulate T cells so as to favour T helper type 1 and CD8+ T-cell responses in the acute phase of *Trypanosoma cruzi* infection. Immunology 2007; 122: 584-95.

[44]   Ji F, Liu Z, Cao J, *et al.* B cell response is required for granuloma formation in the early infection of *Schistosoma japonicum*. PLoS One 2008; 3: e1724.

[45]   Taylor-Robinson AW, Phillips RS. B cells are required for the switch from Th1- to Th2-regulated immune responses to *Plasmodium chabaudi chabaudi* infection. Infect Immun 1994; 62: 2490-98.

[46]   Blackwell NM, Else KJ. B cells and antibodies are required for resistance to the parasitic gastrointestinal nematode *Trichuris muris*. Infect Immun 2001; 69: 3860-68.

[47]   Hernandez HJ, Wang Y, Stadecker MJ. In infection with *Schistosoma mansoni*, B cells are required for T helper type 2 cell responses but not for granuloma formation. J Immunol 1997; 158: 4832-37.

[48]   Millington OR, Di LC, Phillips RS, Garside P, Brewer JM. Suppression of adaptive immunity to heterologous antigens during Plasmodium infection through hemozoin-induced failure of dendritic cell function. J Biol 2006; 5: 5.

[49]   Achtman AH, Bull PC, Stephens R, Langhorne J. Longevity of the immune response and memory to blood-stage malaria infection. Curr Top Microbiol Immunol 2005; 297: 71-102.

[50]   Semnani RT, Nutman TB. Toward an understanding of the interaction between filarial parasites and host antigen-presenting cells. Immunol Rev 2004; 201: 127-38.

[51]   Donelson JE, Hill KL, El-Sayed NM. Multiple mechanisms of immune evasion by African trypanosomes. Mol Biochem Parasitol 1998; 91: 51-66.

[52]   Dubois ME, Demick KP, Mansfield JM. Trypanosomes expressing a mosaic variant surface glycoprotein coat escape early detection by the immune system. Infect Immun 2005; 73: 2690-97.

[53]   Ramasamy R. Molecular basis for evasion of host immunity and pathogenesis in malaria. Biochim Biophys Acta 1998; 1406: 10-27.

[54]   Frevert U. Heparan sulphate and RNA-binding motifs in the malaria circumsporozoite protein. Biochem Soc Trans 1999; 27: 482-87.

[55]   Deehan MR, Harnett MM, Harnett W. A filarial nematode secreted product differentially modulates expression and activation of protein kinase C isoforms in B lymphocytes. J Immunol 1997; 159: 6105-11.

[56]   Wilson EH, Deehan MR, Katz E, *et al.* Hyporesponsiveness of murine B lymphocytes exposed to the filarial nematode secreted product ES-62 *in vivo*. Immunology 2003; 109: 238-45.

[57]   Freire-de-Lima CG, Nascimento DO, Soares MB, *et al.* Uptake of apoptotic cells drives the growth of a pathogenic trypanosome in macrophages. Nature 2000; 403: 199-203.

[58]   Zuniga E, Motran CC, Montes CL, Yagita H, Gruppi A. *Trypanosoma cruzi* infection selectively renders parasite-specific IgG+ B lymphocytes susceptible to Fas/Fas ligand-mediated fratricide. J Immunol 2002; 168: 3965-73.

[59]   Acosta Rodriguez EV, Zuniga E, Montes CL, Gruppi A. Interleukin-4 biases differentiation of B cells from *Trypanosoma cruzi*-infected mice and restrains their fratricide: role of Fas ligand down-regulation and MHC class II-transactivator up-regulation. J Leukoc Biol 2003; 73: 127-36.

[60]   Acosta-Rodriguez EV, Montes CL, Motran CC, *et al.* Galectin-3 mediates IL-4-induced survival and differentiation of B cells: functional cross-talk and implications during *Trypanosoma cruzi* infection. J Immunol 2004; 172: 493-502.

[61]   Lundy SK, Boros DL. Fas ligand-expressing B-1a lymphocytes mediate CD4(+)-T-cell apoptosis during schistosomal infection: induction by interleukin 4 (IL-4) and IL-10. Infect Immun 2002; 70: 812-19.

[62]   Lundy SK, Lerman SP, Boros DL. Soluble egg antigen-stimulated T helper lymphocyte apoptosis and evidence for cell death mediated by FasL(+) T and B cells during murine *Schistosoma mansoni* infection. Infect Immun 2001; 69: 271-80

[63]   Giordanengo L, Maldonado C, Rivarola HW, *et al.* Induction of antibodies reactive to cardiac myosin and development of heart alterations in cruzipain-immunized mice and their offspring. Eur J Immunol 2000; 30: 3181-89.

CHAPTER 2

Excreted/Secreted Antigens in the Diagnosis of Chagas' Disease

Clotilde Marín & Manuel Sánchez-Moreno*

Department of Parasitology, Faculty of Sciences, University of Granada, Severo Ochoa s/n, E-18071 Granada (Spain)

Abstract: *Trypanosoma cruzi* is a blooded-flagellated protozoan transmitted to humans either by blood-sucking triatomine vectors, by blood transfusion or by congenital transmission causing the Chagas' disease or American Trypanosomiasis. Serologic testing for specific antibodies to *T. cruzi* antigens is the most common employed approach for diagnosing chronic infection with this protozoan parasite in clinical patients as well as in blood donors. No assay has been universally accepted as the gold standard for the serologic diagnosis of *T. cruzi* infection, and likewise no assay is viewed as a definitive confirmatory test. Therefore, the antigen fractions (antigenic extract form, recombinant antigens and/or synthetic peptides) may have different affinities for both specific and non-specific antibodies and can produce variable sensitivities. To date, excreted-secreted antigens by the parasites have been proposed as antigen fractions for the detection of this parasite: Trypomastigote Excretory-Secretory Antigens (TESA), composed mainly of surface components such as SAPA, Gala1-3Gal, Tc-85 and T-DAF epitopes and excreted dismutase (SODe) appears to provide good sensitivity and specificity as reagents for the diagnosis of Chagas' disease. This chapter revises the research on excreted/secreted antigens and their utility to establish an ideal diagnostic confirmatory Chagas test.

INTRODUCTION

Chagas' disease or American Trypanosomiasis, one of the world's serious and neglected tropical diseases, is endemic to Central and South America as well as Mexico. The prevalence is around 13 million, with 3.0–3.3 million symptomatic cases and an annual incidence of 50,000 new cases [1]. The aetiological agent is the flagellated protozoa *Trypanosoma cruzi*, a hemo-flagellate protozoan transmitted to humans either by blood-sucking triatomine vectors, blood transfusion or congenitally [2, 3]. *T. cruzi* has four morphologically and physiologically distinct stages. The bloodstream trypomastigotes and intracellular amastigote stages of parasites appear in the mammalian host, whereas epimastigotes and metacyclic trypomastigotes develop in the insect vector [4].

According to the Division for the Control of Tropical Diseases of the WHO, Chagas' disease is still considered an important world public health problem [5, 6]. The traditional epidemiological pattern of Chagas' disease has changed due to process of urbanization in Latin America and migratory population movements: rural-to-urban and from endemic countries to developed countries. Thus, the disease has changed from a rural condition to an urban infection that can be transmitted by blood transfusion or organ transplantation or vertical transmission [7]. This kind of transmission has allowed neglected tropical disease to emerge and re-emerge in non-endemic areas, such as Europe, Asia, and the United States. During the last few decades emigration to the United States from countries where Chagas' disease is endemic has increased markedly. Approximately 13 million such immigrants now live in the United States, and an estimated 80,000 to 120,000 of these persons are infected with *T. cruzi* [8].

Chagas' disease has two successive phases, acute and chronic. The acute phase lasts 6 to 8 weeks. Once the acute phase subsides, most of the infected patients recover an apparent healthy status, where no organ damage can be demonstrated by the current standard methods of clinical diagnosis. The infection can be verified only by serological or parasitological tests. This form of the chronic phase of Chagas' disease is called indeterminate form. Most patients remain in this form of the disease. However, after several years after the onset of the chronic phase, 20% to 35% of the infected individuals, depending on the geographical area will develop irreversible lesions of the autonomous nervous system in the heart, oesophagus, colon and peripheral nervous system. The chronic phase lasts the rest of the life of the infected individual.

Chagas' disease represents the first cause of cardiac lesions in young, economically productive adults in the endemic countries of Latin America. The specific differential characteristics of chronic chagasic cardiopathy, lack of knowledge of the disease among many healthcare workers, and the fact that arrhythmia or sudden death is frequently the first manifestation of disease make accurate diagnosis essential [7].

Corresponding Author: Manuel Sánchez-Moreno, Department of Parasitology, Faculty of Sciences, University of Granada, Severo Ochoa s/n, E-18071 Granada, Spain; Email: msanchem@ugr.es

Emilio Jirillo (Ed)
All rights reserved - © 2010 Bentham Science Publishers Ltd.

CURRENT DIAGNOSIS OF CHAGAS' DISEASE

Several strategies exist to diagnose Chagas' disease. The combination of clinical, epidemiological, and serologic findings offers a highly accurate definition of the chagasic patient. Direct detection of the parasite in the blood by microscopy, hemoculture, xenodiagnosis, or PCR is highly specific and confirms the existence of an infection [9]. However, these procedures are technically and operationally demanding. In addition, as a consequence of the pathology of the disease, direct detection is not very sensitive during the indeterminate and chronic phases of Chagas' disease [9]. The direct parasitological examination provides evidence of the trypomastigote forms of *T. cruzi* only when the parasitemia is raised, at the time of the acute phase, reactivation and congenital phases. Normally, the smear or thick drop by direct examination is used. The examination using concentration techniques (microhematocritic and enrichment by buffy coat) provides more sensitivity. The major drawback of the parasitological examination by hemoculture or xenodiagnosis is the need for specialized laboratories and a considerable length of time to have the results. Xenodiagnosis needs a high number of healthly triatomines which have to feed on the patient's blood directly or indirectly and the insect faeces must be examined. The sensitivity of xenodiagnostic tests ranges from 9% to 87.5% [10] and that of haemoculture from 0 to 94% in the chronic phase of the disease [11]. The inoculation of animals and the hemocultures are less used after the tuning of the polymerase chain reaction (PCR). The PCR is a highly specific technique but a large variation in sensitivity has been reported in patients with chronic disease – from 45% to 96.5% - [12-14] and in individuals with inconclusive serology – from 0.0% to 46.2% [15, 16]. Furthermore, PCR is an expensive method, cannot be used on a large scale and needs appropriate facilities as well as highly trained technicians.

Given the absence of fast and reliable diagnostic methods, the main diagnosis of Chagas' disease is the detection of anti-*T. cruzi* immunoglobulin by serologic analysis. The most common methods used for this technique are the indirect haemagglutination assay (IHA), the indirect immunofluorescence assay (IFA), and the enzyme-linked immunosorbent assay (ELISA). Serodiagnosis may give different results according to the kind of antigen, the disease phase (acute, intermediate, chronic), and the Ig class (IgM and IgG) [17-20].

Depending on the tests applied for blood screening, the percentage of inconclusive samples is high [17, 18, 20-22], and thus it is advisable to combine two or three tests, which may give contradictory results and consequently a number of inconclusive samples.

None of these techniques give 100% sensitivity and specificity. Actually, is recommended to carry out at least two tests (based on different methodologies). If the results are discordant, another confirmation test is required.

CHOOSING A SEROLOGIC ASSAY FOR CHAGAS' DISEASE

Although the diagnosis of Chagas' disease in patients with high anti-*T. cruzi* antibody levels and/or positive parasitemia is very reliable, there are, to our knowledge, no known gold-standard methods for diagnosis of the disease in patients with low levels of such antibodies or in individuals with inconclusive serological tests. The ideal serologic test must be able to detect antibodies specific for antigens which are expressed by the different developmental stages of the parasite and which are well-suited for a fast and easy diagnosis of the disease.

However, in blood donors as well as in clinical patients, the laboratory diagnosis of chronic infection is based on serologic assays [23]. Among the existing serologic procedures, the ELISAs are the tests of choice due to their capacity to be automated and to permit the testing of a great number of serum samples in a short time. Additionally, the results are precise, since readings are objective and test validation criteria as well as the interpretation of results are rigorous. In 2006, the US Food and Drug Administration approved a serologic ELISA for screening donated blood for Chagas' disease (Ortho *T. cruzi* ELISA Test System, Ortho-Clinical Diagnostics, Raritan, NJ) and subsequently the American Red Cross, as well as other entities involved in US blood banking, began screening donated units for markers of Chagas' disease [24].

The majority of the commercially available ELISAs employ as antigens crude sonicated epimastigote (non- infective form) [25-28], proteins extracted from epimastigotes [29-32], fixed whole epimastigotes [33-36], fixed and sonicated amastigotes [37], sonicated and purified trypomastigote glycoconjugate antigens [26, 38], recombinant or synthetic peptides [26, 39-45, 46] or whole-trypomastigote (infective form) of *T. cruzi* grown in liquid culture [47-49]. ELISA using epimastigote antigens are sensitive but less specific in the chronic phase [50-52]. These high-sensitivity and high-specificity ELISA methods need to be validated in populations with a low prevalence of *T. cruzi* antibodies.

Nevertheless, these tests are sensitive but often fail to distinguish between *T. cruzi*-specific and *Leishmania* sp.-specific antibodies, thus leading frequently to false-positive results [45]. Furthermore, parasite culture conditions and antigen purification protocols are difficult to standardize. In addition, contradictory results have been found by different methods and laboratories, probably due to the use of different strains of *T. cruzi*, different antigenic fractions, and non-standardized procedures, causing variations in sensitivity and specificity [53].

THE LOOKING FORWARD NEW ANTIGENS

As mentioned above, whole epimastigotes or epimastigote fractions (antigenic extracts, recombinant antigens and/or synthetic peptides) are commonly used in the serological diagnosis due to ease of culture and good antigen yield. These forms may have different affinities for both specific and non-specific antibodies and can produce variable sensitivities [54]. Also, these antigens may give rise to false-positive reactions mainly due to cross-reactivity with antibodies developed against other parasitic diseases [55]. These problems may be overcome by using defined antigens containing specific *T. cruzi* epitopes that can be recognized by the majority of chagasic patients. The World Health Organization has long emphasized the need for defined antigens to improve serodiagnosis of Chagas' disease. In an attempt to solve this problem, several research groups have used recombinant and/or synthetic and biochemically purified antigens [47, 56-60]. To be useful, these antigens must meet the following criteria: (i) they should be present in *T. cruzi* isolates from different areas of endemicity and absent in other infectious disease agents; (ii) they should be highly immunogenic in populations with different immunogenetic backgrounds, regardless of the clinical phase of Chagas' disease; and (iii) they should be stable and easily amenable to quality control tests, to guarantee reproducibility [61, 62].

A variety of recombinant antigens have been proposed in order to optimise the diagnosis of the infection, particularly in terms of specificity. However, most of them proved not to be as sensitive as native antigens [41, 53]. Attempts to replace parasite extracts by proteins purified from the parasites that present higher sensitivity and specificity scores have been made, and a variety of native molecules have been evaluated [21, 26, 31, 63-66]. However, direct purification of proteins from total extracts of the parasite is generally difficult because of their low relative quantities and need for multiple purification steps, which generally lead to low yields of purified proteins [67]. In this context, simplified methods have been developed that can easily be scaled up to obtain antigens for diagnosis.

To date, several molecules of the parasite itself have been proposed as antigen fractions for the detection of this parasitoses: a lectin-purified GP90 [68], a cysteine proteinase (GP57/51) released in the metacyclogenesis [69], a grp78 heat-shock protein produced by the parasite during the infection [70] and a high-specific ubiquitin [71], together with some recombinant molecules (rAgs), such as an acute-phase transialidase [72].

Recently, a 67-kDa galactose binding protein has been described, defined as a 67-kDa lectin-like glycoprotein or LLGP-67. LLGP-67 is present in epimastigote and tripomastigote stages of the parasite, and has been shown to be involved in the host-cell invasion and host-cell receptor recognition in the endothelial cells of the mammary artery, atrium and right ventricle [73]. The identification and purification of this protein has been previously achieved on the basis of its specific interactions with galactose residues displayed on the surface of desialylated human erythrocytes. However, this method has no practical value to obtain the amounts of protein required to perform assays such as an evaluation of its antigenic profile for human diagnosis of *T. cruzi* infection. A major disadvantage is the relatively low stability of erythrocyte columns. In 2003, Mancipar *et al.* showed that this protein can be purified from *T. cruzi* in a direct way using non-derivatized agarose as a chromatographic ligand [74]. This shows the relevance of LLGP-67 as an antigen for human diagnosis of chagasic infection. Sensitivity and specificity for this antigen were calculated as being 98% and 98.11%, respectively.

THE OUTSIDE PEPTIDES OF *T. CRUZI*: EXCRETED/SECRETED ANTIGENS

The existence of excreted or secreted antigens probably involved in the mechanisms of parasite dissemination, resistance to the host immunological defences, and serologically detectable even when the parasitemia level was the lowest, urged the scientific community to find these proteins for diagnosis of Chagas' disease in both acute/chronic phases and congenital forms, and follow-up of treated chagasic patients (Table **1**).

Table 1: Excerted/Secreted antigens of *T. Cruzi*.

Detection	Year	Author	Name	Molecular mass (kDa)	Isoelectric point	Reference
Culture medium	1965	Tarrant et al.	Exoantigen	-	4.6	73
	1974	Dzbbnski et al.				79
Sera from infected animals	1979	De Siquierea et al.				80
	1982	Araujo et al.	-	-	-	81
	1985	Moretti et al.				82
	1981	Araujo et al.				83
Sera from human patients	1983	Kahn et al.	-	-	-	85
	1987	Freilij et al.				86
Urine from infected acutely mice and dogs	1981	Bongertz et al.	-	-	-	87
Urine from patients with acute, congenital and chronic Chagas' disease	1987	Freilij et al.				86
	1989	Katzin et al.				88
	1989	Katzin et al.	-	-	-	89
Plasma of acutely infected Balb/C mice	1987	Moretti et al.	Exoantigen	200	-	90
Tissues and organs in the chronic phase of experimental infection	1988	Ben Younes-Chennoufi et al.	-	-	-	92
Patients in the disease's chronic phase	1989	Gruppi et al.	Exoantigen	-	5 6	91
Supernatant fluid of epimastigote culture and in the sera of patients in the disease's acute phase	1989	Martin et al.	EF	-	-	97
Trypomastigote culture medium and in blood of acutely infected mice	1989	Affranchino et al.	SAPA	160-200	-	54
Trypomastigote culture medium	1990	Ouassi et al.	ES	160 130 80-110 (Tc-85)	5.4-6.7	98
Acute phase	1991	Jazin et al.	Exoantigen	150-200 45-55	-	99
Chronic phase				160-170		
Actively release surface antigens	1991	Gonçalves et al.	-	160-170	-	100
Supernatant fluid of epimastigote culture, polyclonal sera of infected mice and chagasic' patients	2005	Villagrán et al.	SODe-CRU	25	3.8	119

The first report on exoantigens in *T. cruzi* dates to 1965 by Tarrant et al. [75]. This study showed the existence of serologically active antigens in the culture medium of *T. cruzi*, as well as in other parasites: *Trichinella spiralis* [76], *Fasciola hepatica* [77], *Angiostrongylus cantonensis* [78], *Schistosoma mansoni* [79] and *T. brucei* [80]. This goal revealed a substance complex (possibly a glycoprotein) with a pI of 4.6 and truly an exoantigen, and not simply a somatic antigen released as a result of lysis or breakdown of dead *T. cruzi*.

Since the 1970s, circulating antigens have been demonstrated in sera from animals infected by *T. cruzi* [81-84] and from human patients with Chagas'disease [85-88]. Also, presence of parasite antigens were reported in the urine from acutely infected mice and dogs [89] and from patients with acute, congenital, and chronic Chagas' disease, even when the parasitemia becomes negative during the course of specific treatment [88, 90, 91].

The physicochemical properties of exoantigens from the plasma of acutely infected BALB/c mice showed that it was composed of peptide and carbohydrate moieties, with the epitopes located in the sugar moieties and a molecular mass of approximately 200 kDa [92]. Also, in sera from patients with chronic Chagas' disease antibodies against exoantigens were detected and differentiated into two distinct groups of antigens at pI around 5 and 6. The exoantigens of lower pI share epitopes with components of the cell surface of epimastigotes of *T. cruzi*, whereas exoantigens of higher pI share epitopes with normal human heart tissue [93].

The detection by Ben Younes-Chennoufi *et al.* [94] of parasite antigens in tissues and organs in the chronic phase of experimental infection suggested that the adsorption of *T. cruzi* antigens to uninfected cells may lead to damage of these cells by the immune response directed to the parasite [95, 96]. Thus is, the circulating antigens either free or in the form of immunocomplexes could play a major role in the pathology of the disease, contributing to processes of self-aggression or immunosuppression [97, 98].

In a study dated in 1989, Martin et *al.* [99] detected an antigen factor (EF) in the supernatant fluid of epimastigote cultures of *T. cruzi* and in the sera of patients in the acute phase of the disease. The EF proved be highly immunogenic and present on the fibroblast surface membranes of infected rats. However, the authors were not able to establish whether the EF was the result of an excretion-secretion or simply a result of the parasite death. However, they suggested that EF was associated with the process of parasite proliferation and could be used by *T. cruzi* in the process of cell penetration.

Again, it was evidenced that the trypomastigote stage shed an antigen into the culture medium and was detected in blood of acutely infected mice: SAPA (Shed Acute Phase) [56]. SAPA is a pool of five protein bands with apparent molecular masses ranging from 160 to 200 kDa, and the nucleotide sequence of the 3' end revealed the presence of 14 tandemly arranged 12-amino acid-long repeats. Therefore, SAPA does not react with control sera nor with sera positive for Leishmaniasis (Kala-azar) and it was possible to detect antibodies against SAPA as early as 15 days after the appearance of clinical manifestations in humans and 15 days post-infection in rabbits and mice.

Excretory-secretory immunogens of *T. cruzi* trypomastigotes were characterized and identified as potential protective antigens by Ouassi et *al.* [100]. These immunogens, called ES, showed a molecular mass of 160 kDa, 130 kDa and 80-110 kDa and pI between 5.4 and 6.7. The ES of 85 kDa or Tc-85 (pI 5.7 and 6.5-6.6) was also identified on the cell surface and in serum from patients with acute and chronic Chagas' disease.

In 1991, it was found exoantigens from trypomastigotes and epimastigotes of *T. cruzi* RA and CAI strains and it was found that there was a progressive change in the immunogens throughout the disease. In the acute phase a family of 150 to 200 kDa bands was detected together with a very strong pair of 45 to 55 kDa bands. Meanwhile, in the chronic phase a 160 or 170 kDa band was detected. The researchers speculated that the 160 to 170 kDa exoantigen might be the same antigen that they found in the membranes and suggested that this protein might be involved in attachment to host-cell receptors [101].

In the same year, the Gonçalves group [102] demonstrated that trypomastigotes of *T. cruzi* (four strains: Y, YuYu, CAI and RA) actively released surface antigens by a spontaneous process of membrane vesicles. Despite the differences in the amounts of polypeptides released, the four strains released a set of surface polypeptides ranging in molecular mass from 70 to 150 kDa. However, other antigens may be released by a different mechanism and/or the same antigen could be released by different mechanisms. This is suggested by the presence of glycophosphatidylinositol (GPI) -anchored proteins in epimastigotes and metacyclic trypomastigotes of *T. cruzi,* and enzymes (phospholypase C-like and others hydrolases) that solubilize the membrane and could be involved in mechanisms of solubilisation of surface antigens [103]. The 160 to 170 kDa exoantigen discovery coincides with the previous research and confirmed their role in the establishment of a chronic infection and the resistance to reinfection.

Perhaps research on major excreted/secreted enzymes, such as superoxide dismutases (SODs, EC 1.15.1.1), has followed a more directed strategy. SODs are a group of antioxidant metalloenzymes with an important role in the defence from superoxide radicals to protect normal cells as well as a number of pathogens from reactive oxygen species (ROS) [104-106]. Thus is, these enzymes are considered virulence factors that protect the parasites from the attack of the host cells [107], and can even confer immunological capacities [108]. SOD activity has been detected in the main species belonging to the family Trypanosomatidae, in *Trypanosoma cruzi* [109], in *T. brucei brucei* [110], in several species of the genus *Leishmania* [111], in some lower trypanosomatids, and in plant trypanosomes [112-114]. Due to the important role of this enzyme family, extracellular SODs (EcCu/ZnSODs) have been evidenced in animal Kingdom (*Brugia pahangi* [115], *Onchocerca volvulus* [116], *Caenorhabditis elegans* [117], *Callinectes sapidus* [118], etc). Also, in mammals, several researchers have studied an extracellular SOD (EC-SOD), which is the major extracellular antioxidant enzyme and plays a critical role in the pathogenesis of a variety of pulmonary, neurological, and cardiovascular diseases [119, 120].

In the epimastigote cellular extract four iron superoxide dismutase (SODI, SODII, SODIII, and SODIV) [121, 122] were isolated and purified. The molecular masses of the different SODs were 20 kDa (SOD I), 60 kDa (SOD II), 50 kDa (SOD III), and 25 kDa (SOD IV), whereas the isoelectric points were 6.9, 6.8, 5.2, and 3.8, respectively. Subcellular location and digitonin experiments have shown that these SODs are mainly cytosolic, with small amounts in the low-mass organelles (SOD II and SOD I) and the mitochondrion (SOD III). However, around 20% of the SOD activity was not solubilized even at high digitonin concentrations, indicating that part of the SODs could be associated with membranes or even excreted by the parasite.

Following this clue for the first time in 2005, it was detected an excreted SOD activity (SODe-CRU) in Grace's medium without serum containing *T. cruzi* epimastigotes [121]. This excreted activity coincided with the cellular enzyme SODIV.

The SODe excreted into the medium by the parasite was immunogenic and able to produce polyclonal antibodies. The role of SODe is related to the establishment of the parasite within the host, and its high immunogenicity and specificity make it a useful molecular marker in diagnosing infection with this parasite. Thus is, it was possible to obtain polyclonal antibodies anti-SODe-CRU in BALB/c mice which showed reactivity up a dilution of 1: 2,500 by western blot. As a result, SODe-CRU was detected by sera from chagasic patients. These results support the existence of a SOD excreted by *T. cruzi*, which has a role in the establishment of the parasite in the host. This SOD is highly immunogenic and specific, and therefore should be a useful tool in the diagnosis of Chagas' disease.

THE EXCRETED/SECRETED ANTIGENS APPLICATIONS

Progressively, the interest in exoantigens is derived from the study of their applications. On one hand, they act as protectives molecules, such as the purified exoantigen Ea 4.5 (pI 4.5), which was able to induce in mice a partial protection against *T. cruzi* infection [123]. On the other hand, the issue of paramount importance is the diagnosis.

As described above, trypomastigote excreted-secreted antigens (TESA) are composed mainly of surface components such as SAPA, Gala1-3Gal, Tc-85, and T-DAF (Trypomastigote Decay-Accelerating Factor) epitopes [20, 56, 101, 102]. With TESA proteins, both enzyme-linked immunosorbent assay (TESA-ELISA) and immunoblot assays (TESA-blot) have been reported for the diagnosis of Chagas' disease. TESA-blot has typically been used in parasite diagnostics to rule out false-positive ELISA results. For example, the TESA-blot performed using of *T. cruzi* Y strain was proposed as a sensitive and specific diagnostic assay in cases of suspected acute or congenital *T. cruzi* infection and as a general confirmatory test for conventional Chagas' disease serology [20]. In the same way, the assay of chronic chagasic patient sera by TESA-blot, showed that a 150–160 kDa band was recognized by 100% of sera and did not react with sera from patients with leishmaniasis [21]. However, immunoblots are expensive, difficult to standardize, and time-consuming. In contrast, the ELISA format is inexpensive, simple to automate, and rapid [49]. To date, the TESA proteins evaluated for use in the diagnosis of Chagas' disease have been complex mixtures that cross-react with sera from subjects with other parasitic diseases, particularly leishmaniasis. Thus, TESA-ELISA resulted in high sensitivity with chronic and acute chagasic patient sera but the specificity of the assay was impaired [124, 125].

Unfortunately, the antigens from *T. cruzi* epimastigotes may give rise to false-positive reactions mainly due to cross-reactivity with antibodies developed against other parasitic diseases [55]. However, these problems may be overcome by using defined antigens containing specific *T. cruzi* epitopes that can be recognized by most of chagasic patients. To resolve this matter, Berrizbeitia *et al.* [126] have purified by immunoaffinity chromatography a extract of excretory-secretory antigens (TESA$_{IA}$) which has been tested by western blot and ELISA. By TESA$_{IA}$-blot a series of polypeptide bands with molecular masses ranging from 60 to 220 kDa were recognized by pooled sera positive for Chagas' disease. TESA$_{IA}$-ELISA had a slightly lower sensitivity (98.6%) but an improved specificity (100%) compared to the sensitivity and specificity of the total TESA protein-based ELISAs.

The SODe-CRU was validated by western blot against 1,029 sera of individuals from 11 municipalities in the state of Queretaro (Mexico) [121]. The results were compared with those for the same sera with three conventional serologic methods: an ELISA, indirect hemagglutination (IHA), and indirect immunofluorescence assay (IFA). Samples that were positive by these three techniques were also positive by western blot method. The comparison of the values obtained with two of the conventional serologic tests (ELISA and IFA), showed a seroprevalence values of 5.64%. However, when we compared the results of the ELISA with those of the western blot, the seroprevalence increased to 8.16% and the concordance between the two techniques reached nearly 100%.

CONCLUSIONS

Among TESAs proteins, transialidases have been also recognized, which, like the SOD enzyme, may be virulence factors and are strong immunogens that elicit polyclonal antibody responses and are involve in both inflammation and autoimmunity [127, 128]. The estimated molecular mass for the TESA proteins is from 60 to 220 kDa for TESA$_{IA}$ [126], from 85 to 170 kDa for transialidases [129] and 67 kDa for a lectin-like protein that binds to human erythrocyte membranes in a galactose-dependent way [130], contrary to the relatively low molecular mass of the SODe-CRU (25 kDa) [121]. Therefore, a serological diagnosis performed with the highly specific SODe-CRU is the the better choice for diagnostic of Chagas' disease.

ACKNOWLEDGEMENTS

We are thankful to MEC, Junta de Andalucía and University of Granada for their financial support of general project and grants to improving knowledge in the Family Trypanosomatidae. We are very grateful to David Nesbitt for his kind and patient revising of the English manuscript.

REFERENCES

[1]   Kirchhoff LV. In: Guerrant RL Walter DL, Weller PF, Eds. tropical infectious disease: principles, pathogens, and practice. Churchill Living-stone, New Cork, NY. 2006; pp. 1082-94.

[2]   Mocayo A. Chagas' disease. Epidemiology and prospects for interruption of transmission in the Americas. World Health Stat Q 1992; 45: 276-9.

[3]   Schmunis GA. Prevention of transfusional *Trypanosoma cruzi* infection in Latin America. Mem Inst Oswaldo Cruz 1999; 94(Suppl. I): 93-101.

[4]   Tyler KM, Engman DM. The life cycle of *Trypanosoma cruzi* revisited. Int J Parasitol 2001; 3: 472-81.

[5]   Mocayo A. Chagas' disease. Epidemiology and prospects for interruption of transmission in the Americas. World Health Stat Q. 1992; 45:276–279.

[6]   Schimunis G A. Prevention of transfusional *Trypanosoma cruzi* infection in Latin America. Mem Inst Oswaldo Cruz. 1999; 94(Suppl. I):93-101.

[7]   Gascón J, Albajar P, Cañas E, *et al*. Diagnosis, management and treatment of chronic Chagas' heart disease in areas where *Trypanosoma cruzi* infection is not endemic. Rev Esp Cardiol 2007; 60: 285-93.

[8]   Kirchhoff LV, Paredes P, Lomeli-Guerrero A, *et al*. Transfusion-associated Chagas' disease (American trypanosomiasis) in Mexico: implications for transfusion medicine in the United States. Transfusion 2006; 46: 298-304.

[9]   Ferreira AW, Avila SLM. (Eds.). Diagnóstico laboratorial das principais doenças infecciosas e auto-imunes, 2rd ed. Guanabara Koogan S. A., Rio de Janeiro, Brazil. 2001.

[10]   Barbosa W, Czerewuta AC, Oliveira RL. Tentativa de isolamento primário de pacientes crônicos de doença de Chagas por hemocultura agentes bloqueadores. Rev Patol Trop 1983; 12:155-63.

[11]   Luz LMP, Coutinho MG, Cançado JR, Krettli AU. Hemocultura: técnica sensível na detecção do *Trypanosoma cruzi* em pacientes chagásicos na fase crônica da doença de Chagas. Rev Soc Bras Med Trop 1994; 27: 143-8.

[12]   Wincker P, Brito C, Pereira JB, Cardoso MA, Oelemann W, Morel CM. Use of a simplified polymerase chain reaction procedure to detect *Trypanosoma cruzi* in blood samples from chronic chagasic patients in a rural endemic area. Am J Trop Med Hyg 1994; 51: 771-7.

[13]   Britto C, Silveira C, Cardoso MA, *et al*. Parasite persistence in treated chagasic patients revealed by xenodiagnosis and polymerase chain reaction. Mem Inst Oswaldo Cruz 2001; 96: 823-6.

[14]   Portela-Lindoso AA, Shikanai-Yasuda MA. Chronic Chagas' disease: from xenodiagnosis and hemoculture to polymerase chain reaction. Rev Saude Publica. 2003; 37: 107-15.

[15]   Gomes ML, Galvão LM, Macedo AM, Pena SD, Chiari E. Chagas disease diagnosis: comparative analysis of parasitologic, molecular, and serologic methods. Am J Trop Med Hyg 1999; 60: 205-10.

[16]   Ribeiro-dos-Santos G, Nishiya AS, Sabino EC, Chamone DF, Sáez-Alquézar A. An improved, PCR-based strategy for the detection of *Trypanosoma cruzi* in human blood samples. Ann Trop Med Parasitol 1999; 93: 689-94.

[17]   Salles NA, Sabino EC, Cliquet MG, *et al*. Risk of exposure to Chagas disease among seroreactive Brazilian blood donors. Transfusion 1996; 36: 969-73.

[18]   Wendel S. Transfusion-transmitted Chagas disease. Curr Opin Hematol 1998; 5: 406-11.

[19]   Umezawa ES, Luquetti A, Levitus G, *et al*. Serodiagnosis of chronic and acute Chagas' disease with *Trypanosoma cruzi* recombinant proteins: results of a collaborative study in six Latin American countries. J Clin Microbiol 2004; 42: 449-52.

[20]   Umezawa ES, Nascimento MS, Kesper N, *et al*. Immunoblot assay using excreted-secreted antigens of *Trypanosoma cruzi* in serodiagnosis of congenital, acute, and chronic Chagas' disease. J Clin Microbiol 1996; 34: 2143-7.

[21]   Oelemann WMR, Teixeira MGM, Verissimo-da-Costa GC, *et al*. Evaluation of three commercial enzyme-linked immunosorbent assays for diagnosis of Chagas disease. J Clin Microbiol 1998; 36: 2423-7.

[22]   Marcon GE, Andrade PD, de Albuquerque DM, *et al*. Use of a nested polymerase chain reaction (N-PCR) to detect *Trypanosoma cruzi* in blood samples from chronic chagasic patients and patients with doubtful serologies. Diagn Microbiol Infect Dis 2002; 43: 39-43.

[23]   Schmunis GA, Cruz JR. Safety of the blood supply in Latin America. Clin Microbiol Rev 2005; 18: 12-29.

[24]   Blood donor screening for Chagas disease—United States, 2006-2007. MMWR Morb Mortal Wkly Rep 2007; 56: 141-3.

[25] Breniere SF, Carrasco R, Miguez H, Lemesre JL, Carlier Y. Comparisons of immunological tests for serodiagnosis of Chagas disease in Bolivian patients. Trop Geogr Med 1985; 37: 231-8.

[26] Almeida IC, Covas DT, Soussumi LM, Travassos LR. A highly sensitive and specific chemiluminescent enzyme-linked immunosorbent assay for diagnosis of active *Trypanosoma cruzi* infection. Transfusion 1997; 37: 850-7.

[27] Monteon VM, Guzman-Rojas L, Negrete-Garcia C, Rosales-Encinas JL, Lopez PA. Serodiagnosis of American trypanosomosis by using nonpathogenic trypanosomatid antigen. J Clin Microbiol 1997; 35: 3316-9.

[28] Pinho RT, Pedrosa RC, Costa-Martins P, Castello-Branco LR. Saliva ELISA: a method for the diagnosis of chronic Chagas disease in endemic areas. Acta Trop 1999; 72: 31-8.

[29] Schechter M. Evaluation of a monoclonal antibody affinity purified antigen for zymodeme specific serological diagnosis of *Trypanosoma cruzi* infection. Mem Inst Oswaldo Cruz 1987; 82: 81-85.

[30] Cuna WR, Rodriguez C, Torrico F, Afchain D, Loyens M, Desjeux P. Evaluation of a competitive antibody enzyme immunoassay for specific diagnosis of Chagas disease. J Parasitol 1989; 75: 357-9.

[31] Solana ME, Katzin AM, Umezawa ES, Miatello CS. High specificity of *Trypanosoma cruzi* epimastigote ribonucleoprotein as antigen in serodiagnosis of Chagas disease. J Clin Microbiol 1995; 33: 1456-60.

[32] Partel CD, Rossi CL. A rapid, quantitative enzyme-linked immunosorbent assay (ELISA) for the immunodiagnosis of Chagas disease. Immunol Invest 1998; 27: 89-96.

[33] De Hubsch RM, Chiechie N, Comach G, Aldao RR, Gusmao RD. Immunoenzyme assay using micro Dot on nitrocellulose (Dot-ELISA) in the diagnosis of Chagas disease. I. Comparative study of 2 antigenic preparations of *Trypanosoma cruzi*. Mem Inst Oswaldo Cruz 1988; 83: 277-85.

[34] De Hubsch RM, Chiechie N, Comach G, Aldao RR, Gusmao RD. The Dot immunoenzymatic assay on nitrocellulose (Dot-ELISA) in the diagnosis of Chagas disease. II. Seroepidemiologic study in 4 rural communities of Venezuela. Mem Inst Oswaldo Cruz 1989; 84: 401-8.

[35] Carbonetto CH, Malchiodi EL, Chiaramonte MG, Zwirner NW, Margni RA. Use of formalinized epimastigotes for the detection of anti-*Trypanosoma cruzi* antibodies using immunoenzyme technics. Rev Argent Microbiol 1989; 21: 79-83.

[36] Antas PR, Azevedo EN, Luz MR, *et al*. A reliable and specific enzyme-linked immunosorbent assay for the capture of IgM from human chagasic sera using fixed epimastigotes of *Trypanosoma cruzi*. Parasitol Res 2000; 86: 813-20.

[37] Araujo FG, Guptill D. Use of antigen preparations of the amastigote stage of *Trypanosoma cruzi* in the serology of Chagas disease. Am J Trop Med Hyg 1984; 33: 362-71.

[38] Aznar, C., Liegeard, P., Mariette C, Lafou S, Levin MJ, Honteberyrie MC. A simple *Trypanosoma cruzi* enzyme-linked immunoassay for control of human infection in nonendemic areas. FEMS Immunol Med Microbiol 1997; 18: 31-7.

[39] Cetron MS, Hoff R, Kahn S, Eisen H, Van Voorhis WC. Evaluation of recombinant trypomastigote surface antigens of *Trypanosoma cruzi* in screening sera from a population in rural northeastern Brazil endemic for Chagas disease. Acta Trop 1992; 50: 259-66.

[40] Godsel LM, Tibbetts RS, Olson CL, Chaudoir BM, Engman DM. Utility of recombinant flagellar calcium-binding protein for serodiagnosis of *Trypanosoma cruzi* infection. J Clin Microbiol 1995; 33: 2082-5.

[41] da Silveira JF, Umezawa ES, Luquetti AO. Chagas disease: recombinant *Trypanosoma cruzi* antigens for serological diagnosis. Trends Parasitol 2001; 17: 286-91.

[42] Matsumoto TK, Cotrim PC, da Silveira JF, Stolf AM, Umezawa ES. *Trypanosoma cruzi*: isolation of an immunodominant peptide of TESA (Trypomastigote Excreted-Secreted Antigens) by gene cloning. Diagn Microbiol Infect Dis 2002; 42: 187-92.

[43] Chang CD, Cheng KY, Jiang LX, *et al*. Evaluation of a prototype *Trypanosoma cruzi* antibody assay with recombinant antigens on a fully automated chemiluminescence analyzer for blood donor screening. Transfusion 2006; 46: 1737-44.

[44] Carmo MS, Santos MR, Cummings LM, *et al*. Isolation and characterization of genomic and cDNA clones coding for a serine-, alanine-, and proline-rich protein of *Trypanosoma cruzi*. Int J Parasitol 2001; 31: 259-64.

[45] Cheng KY, Chang CD, Salbilla VA, *et al*. Immunoblot assay using recombinant antigens as a supplemental test to confirm the presence of antibodies to *Trypanosoma cruzi*. Clin Vaccine Immunol 2007; 14: 355-61.

[46] Ferreira AW, Belem ZR, Lemos EA, Reed SG, Campos-Neto C. Enzyme-Linked inmunosorbent assay for serological diagnosis of Chagas' disease employing a *Trypanosoma cruzi* recombinant antigen that consists of tour different peptides. J Clin Microbiol 2001; 39: 4390-5

[47] Umezawa ES, Bastos SF, Camargo ME, *et al*. Evaluation of recombinant antigens for serodiagnosis of Chagas' disease in South and Central America. J Clin Microbiol 1999; 37: 1554-60.

[48] Leiby DA, Wendel S, Takaoka ST, Fachinj RM, Oliveira LC, Tibbals MA. Serologic testing for *Trypanosoma cruzi*: Comparison of radioimmuno precipitation assay with commercially available indirect immunofluorescence assay, indirect hemaglutination assay, and enzyme-Linked immunosorbent assay kits. J Clin Microbiol 2000; 38: 639-42.

[49] Nakazawa M, Rosa DS, Pereira VR, *et al*. Excretory-secretory antigens of *Trypanosoma cruzi* are potentially useful for serodiagnosis of chronic Chagas disease. Clin Diag Lab Immunol 2001; 8: 1024-7.

[50]   Pirard M, Iihoshi N, Boelaert M, Basanta P, Lopez F, Van der Stuyft P. The validity of serologic tests for *Trypanosoma cruzi* and the effectiveness of transfusional screening strategies in a hyperendemic region. Transfusion 2005; 45: 554-61.

[51]   Salomone OA, Basquiera AL, Sembaj A, *et al*. *Trypanosoma cruzi* in persons without serologic evidence of disease, Argentina. Emerg Infect Dis 2003; 9: 1558-62.

[52]   Silveira-Lacerda EP, Silva AG, Junior SF, *et al*. Chagas' disease: application of TESA blot in inconclusive sera from a Brazilian blood bank. *Vox Sang* 2004; 87: 204-7.

[53]   Gomes YM. PCR and sero-diagnosis in chronic Chagas' disease: biotechnological advances. Appl Biochem Biotechnol 1997; 66: 107-19.

[54]   Caballero ZC, Sousa OE, Marques WP, Saez-Alquezar A, Umezawa ES. Evaluation of serological tests to identify *Trypanosoma cruzi* infection in humans and determine cross-reactivity with *Trypanosoma rangeli* and *Leishmania* spp. Clin Vaccine Immunol 2007; 14: 1045-9.

[55]   Camargo ME. 1992. In: Wendel S, Brener Z, Camargo ME, Rassi A. (Eds.). Chagas' disease (American trypanosomiasis): its impact on transfusion and clinical medicine. ISBT Brazil'92, Sáo Paulo, Brazil1992; pp. 165-8.

[56]   Affranchino JL, Ibanez CF, Luquetti AO, *et al*. Identification of a *Trypanosoma cruzi* antigen that is shed during the acute phase of Chagas' disease. Mol Biochem Parasitol 1989; 34: 221-8.

[57]   Goldenberg S, Krieger MA, Lafaille JJ, Almeida E, Oelemann W. Use of *Trypanosoma crnzi* antigens in the immunological diagnosis of Chagas' disease. Mem Inst Butantan 1991; S3: 71-6.

[58]   Krieger MA, Almeida E, Oelemann W, *et al*. Use of recombinant antigens for the accurate immunodiagnosis of Chagas' disease. Am J Trop Med Hyg 1992; 46: 427-34.

[59]   Lafaille JJ, Linss L, Krieger MA, Souto-Padron T, de Souza W, Goldenberg S. Structure and expression of two *Trypanosoma* crnzi genes encoding antigenic proteins bearing repetitive epitopes. Mol Biochem Parasitol 1989; 35: 127-36.

[60]   Luquetti AO. Use of *Trypanosoma crnzi* defined proteins for diagnosis-multicentre trial. Serological and technical aspects. Mem 1nst Oswaldo Cruz 1990; 85: 497-505.

[61]   Stolf MAS. In: Wendel S, Brener Z, Camargo ME, Kassi A (Eds.). Chagas' disease (American trypanosomiasis): its impact on transfusion and clinical medicine. lSBT Brazil'92, Sáo Paulo, Brazil 1992; pp. 195-205.

[62]   Zingales B, Gruber A, Ramalho CB, Umezawa ES, Colli W. Use of recombinant proteins of *Trypanosoma cruzi* in the serological diagnosis of Chagas. disease. Mem Inst Oswaldo Cruz 1990; 85: 519-22.

[63]   Kircchoff LV, Gam AA, Gusmao RA, Goldsmith RS, Rezende JM, Rassi A. Increased specificity of serodiagnosis of Chagas' disease by detection of antibody to the 72- and 90-kilodalton glycoproteins of *Trypanosoma cruzi*. J Infect Dis 1987; 155: 561-4.

[64]   Scharfstein J, Schechter M, Sena M, Peralta JM, Mendonca-Previato L, Miles MA. *Trypanosoma cruzi*: characterization and isolation of a 57/51,000 m.w. surface glycoprotein (GP57/51) expressed by epimastigotes and bloodstream trypomastigotes. J Immunol 1988; 137: 1336-41.

[65]   Martinez J, Campetella O, Frasch ACC, Cazzulo JJ. The major cysteine proteinase (Cruzipain) from *Trypanosoma cruzi* is antigenic in human infections. Infect Immun 1991; 59: 4275-7.

[66]   Aguillon JC, Harris R, Molina MC, *et al*. Recognition of an immunogenetically selected *Trypanosoma cruzi* antigen by seropositive chagasic human sera. Acta Trop 1997; 63: 159-66.

[67]   Carbonetto CH, Malchiodi EL, Chiaramonte M, Durante de Isola E, Fossati CA, Margni RA. Isolation of a *Trypanosoma cruzi* antigen by affinity chromatography with a monoclonal antibody. Preliminary evaluation of its possible application in serological tests. Clin Exp Immunol 1990; 82: 93-6.

[68]   Schechter M, Voller A, Marinkelle CJ, Flint JE, Guhl F, Miles M. A purified *Trypanosoma cruzi* specific glycoprotein for discriminative serological diagnosis of South American trypanosomiasis (Chagas disease). Lancet 1983; 22: 939-41.

[69]   Ronaldo MC, D'Escoffier LN, Salles JM, Goldenberg S. Characterization and expression of proteases during *T. cruzi* metacyclogenesis. Exp Parasitol 1991; 73: 44-51.

[70]   Krautz GM, Peterson JD, Godsel LM, Krettli AU, Engman DM. Human antibody responses of *Trypanosoma cruzi* 70-kD heat-shock proteins. Am J Trop Med Hyg 1998; 58: 137-43.

[71]   Telles S, Abate T, Slezynger T, Henriquez DA. *Trypanosoma cruzi* Ubiquitin as an antigen in the differential diagnosis of Chagas disease and Leishmaniasis. FEMS Immunol Med Microbiol 2003; 37: 23-8.

[72]   Frash ACC. Transialidase SAPA amino acid repeats and the relationship between *Trypanosoma cruzi* and the mammalian host. Parasitology 1994; 108: 37-44.

[73]   Silber AM, Marcipar IS, Roodveldt C, *et al*. *Trypanosoma cruzi*: identification of a galactose-binding protein that binds to cells surface of human erythrocyte and is involved in cell invasion by the parasite. Exp Parasitol 2002; 100: 217-25.

[74]   Marcipar IS, Welchen E, Roodveldt C, Marcipar AJ, Silber AM. Purification of the 67-kDa lectin-like glycoprotein of *Trypanosoma cruzi*, LLGP-67, and its evaluation as a relevant antigen for the diagnosis of human infection. FEMS Microbiol Lett 2003; 220: 149-54.

[75]   Tarrant CJ, Fifeeh JR, Anderson RI. Serological characteristics and general chemical nature of the in vitro exoantigens of *T. cruzi*. J Parasitol 1965; 51: 277-85.

[76]   Sadun E, Norman L. Metabolic and somatic antigens in the determination of the response of rabbits to graded infections with *Trichinella spiralis*. J Parasitol 1957; 43: 236-45.

[77]   Minning W, Newsome J, Robinson DL. Trematoden-Stoffwechsel-produkte als antigene, Ztshr Tropenmed Parasit 1958; 9: 335-42.

[78]   Anderson RI, Sadun EH, Rosen L, Weinstein PP, Sawyer T. The detection of antibodies in eosinophilic meningitis. J Parasitol 1962; 48: 162-7.

[79]   Kagan IG, Oliver-Gonzalez J. Hemagglutination studies with schistosome antigens. J Parasitol 1958; 44: 457-60.

[80]   Weitz B. A soluble protective antigen of *Trypanosoma brucei*. Nature 1960; 195: 788.

[81]   Dzbbnski TH. Exoantigens of *Trypanosoma cruzi* in vivo. Ztshr Tropenmed Parasit 1974; 25:485-91.

[82]   De Siquiera AF, Ferriolifilho F, Ribeiro R. Early immunological aspects in rats infected by *Trypanosoma cruzi*. II. Soluble antigen circulation and the modifications of serum complement from animals in sucessive days of the infection (author's transl). Rev Bras Pesqui Med Biol 1979; 12: 75-9.

[83]   Araujo FG. Detection of circulating antigens of *Trypanosoma cruzi* by enzyme immunoassay. Ann Trop Med Parasitol 1982; 76: 25-36.

[84]   Moretti ER, Basso B, Vottero-Cima E. Exoantigens of *Trypanosoma cruzi*. I. Conditions for their detection and immunogenic properties in experimental infections. J Protozool 1985; 32: 150-3.

[85]   Araujo FG, Chiari E, Dias JCP. Demonstration of *Trypanosoma cruzi* antigen in serum from patients with Chagas' disease. Lancet 1981; 1: 246-9.

[86]   Arcipar A, Barnes S, Lentwoit E, Brown G. Immunoenzyme determination of antibody-bound soluble antigens of *Trypanosoma cruzi*. Appl Biochem Biotechnol 1982; 7: 459-62.

[87]   Kahn T, Corral R, Freilij H, Grinstein S. Detection of circulating immune complexes, antigens and antibodies by enzyme-linked immunosorbent assay in human *Trypanosoma cruzi* infection. IRCS Med Sci 1983; 12: 949-50.

[88]   Freilij HL, Corral RS, Katzin AM, Grinstein S. Antigenuria in infants with acute and congenital Chagas' disease. J Clin Microbiol 1987; 25: 133-7.

[89]   Bongertz V, Hungerer K, Galvao Castro M. *Trypanosoma cruzi* circulating antigens. Mem Inst Oswaldo Cruz 1981; 76: 71-82.

[90]   Katzin AM, Marcipar A, Freilij HL, Corral R, Yanovsky JF. Rapid determination of *Trypanosoma cruzi* urinary antigens in human chronic Chagas disease by agglutination test. Exp Parasitol 1989; 68: 208-15.

[91]   Katzin AM, Alves MJ, Abuin G, Colli W. Antigenuria in chronic chagasic patients detected by a monoclonal antibody raised against *Trypanosoma cruz*i. Trans R Soc Trop Med Hyg 1989; 83: 341-3.

[92]   Moretti ER, Gruppi A, Basso B, Vottero-Cima E. Exoantigens of *Trypanosoma cruzi*. II. Physicochemical properties. Rev Argent Microbiol 1987; 90: 139-44.

[93]   Gruppi A, Gea S, Moretti ER, Vottero-Cima E. Human antibodies against *Trypanosoma cruzi* exoantigens recognizing parasite surface antigens and heart tissue components. Int Arch Allergy Appl Immunol. 1989; 90: 119-23.

[94]   Ben Younes-Chennoufi A, Hontebeyriejoskowicz M, Tricottet V, Eisen H, Reynes M, Said G. Persistence of *Trypanosoma cruzi* antigens in the inflammatory lesions of chronically infected mice. Trans R Soc Trop Med Hyg 1988; 82: 77-83.

[95]   Ribeiro Dos Santos R, Hudson L. *Trypanosoma cruzi*: Binding of parasite antigens to mammalian cell membranes. Parasite Immunol 1980; 2: 1-10.

[96]   Williams GT, Fielder L, Smith H, Hudson L. Adsorption of *Trypanosoma cruzi* proteins to mammalian cells *in vitro*. Acta Trop 1985; 42:33-38.

[97]   Brener Z. Pathogenesis and immunopathology of chronic Chagas' disease. Mem Inst Oswaldo Cruz 1987; 82: 205-13.

[98]   Petry K, Eisen H. Chagas' disease: A model for the study of autoimmune diseases. Parasitol Today. 1989; 5: 111- 6.

[99]   Martín UO, Afchain D, Loyens M, Maidana C, Caprón A. *Trypanosoma cruzi*: circulating polysaccharide factors excreted *in vitro* and *in vivo*. Medicina 1989; 49: 33-6.

[100]   Ouaissi MA, Taibi A, Cornette J, *et al*. Characterization of major surface and excretory-secretory immunogens of *Trypanosoma cruzi* trypomastigotes and identification of potential protective antigen. Parasitology 1990; 100: 115-24.

[101]   Jazin EE, Luquetti AO, Rassi A, Frasch ACC. Shift of excretory-secretory immunogens of *Trypanosoma cruzi* during human Chagas' disease. Infect Immun 1991; 59: 2189-91.

[102]   Gonçalves MF, Umezawa ES, Katzin AM, *et al*. *Trypanosoma cruzi*: Shedding of surface antigens as membrane vesicles. Exp Parasitol 1991; 72: 43-53.

[103]   Schenkman S, Yoshida N, Almeida MLC. Glycophosphatidylinositol-anchored proteins in metacyclic trypomastigotes of *Trypanosoma cruzi*. Mol Biochem Parasitol 1988; 29: 141-52.

[104]   Fridovich I. Superoxide dismutases: an adaptation to a paramagnetic gas. J Biol Chem 1989; 264: 7761-4.

[105]   McCord JM, Fridovich I. Superoxide dismutase: the first twenty years (1968-1988) Free Radic Biol Med 1998; 5:363-9.

[106]   Bannister JV, Bannister WH, Rottilio G. Aspects of the structure, function and application of superoxide dismutase. CRC Crit Rev Biochem 1987; 22: 111-80.

[107] Paramchuck WJ, Ismail SO, Bhatia A, Gedamu L. Cloning, characterization and overexpre-ssion of two iron superoxide dismutase cDNAs from *Leishmania chagasi*: role in pathogenesis. Mol Biochem Parasitol 1997; 90: 203-21.

[108] Pérez-Fuentes R, Guégan JF, Barnabé C, *et al*. Severtity of chronic Chagas disease is associated with citokine/antioxidant imbalance in chronically infected individuals. Int J Parasitol 2003; 33: 293-9.

[109] Ismail SO, Paramchuk W, Yasir A, *et al*. Molecular cloning and characterization of two iron superoxide dismutase cDNAs from *Trypanosoma cruzi*. Mol Biochem Parasitol 1997; 86: 87-97.

[110] Kabiri M, Steverding D. Identification of a developmentally regulated iron superoxide dismutase of *Trypanosome brucei*. J Biochem 2001; 360: 173-7.

[111] Ismail SO, Skeiky YA, Bhatia A, Omara-Opyene LA, Gedamu L. Molecular cloning, characterization, and expression in *E. coli* of iron superoxide dismutase cDNA from *Leishmania donovani chagasi*. Infect Immun 1994; 62: 657-64.

[112] Quesada JM, Entrala E, Fernández-Ramos C, Marín C, Sánchez-Moreno M *Phytomonas spp.*: superoxide dismutase in plant trypanosomes. Mol Biochem Parasitol 2001; 115: 123-7.

[113] Marín C, Rodríguez-González I, Hitos AB, Rosales MJ, Dollet M, Sánchez-Moreno M. Purification and characterization of two iron superoxide dismutases of *Phytomonas* sp. isolated from E*uphorbia characias* (Plant Trypanosomatids). Parasitology 2004; 129: 79-86.

[114] Marín C, Hitos AB, Rodríguez-González I, Dollet M, Sánchez-Moreno M. *Phytomonas* Iron Superoxide dismutase: A possible molecular marker. FEMS Microbiol Lett 2004; 234: 69-74.

[115] Tang L, Ou X, Henkle-Duhrsen K, Selkirk ME. Extracellular and cytoplasmic CuZn superoxide dismutases from Brugia lymphatic filarial nematode parasites. Infect Immun 1994; 62: 961-7.

[116] James ER, McLean DC, Perler F. Molecular cloning of an *Onchocerca volvulus* extracellular Cu–Zn superoxide dismutase. Infect Immun 1994; 62: 713-6.

[117] Fujii M, Ishii N, Joguchi A, Yasuda K, Ayusawa D. A novel superoxide dismutase gene encoding membrane-bound and extracellular isoforms by alternative splicing in *Caenorhabditis elegans*. DNA Res 1998; 5: 25-30.

[118] Brouwer M, Hoexum Brouwer T, Grater W, Brown-Peterson N. Replacement of a cytosolic copper/zinc superoxide dismutase by a novel cytosolic manganese superoxide dismutase in crustaceans that use copper (haemocyanin) for oxygen transport. Biochem J 2003; 374: 219-28.

[119] Fukai T, Folz R J, Landmesser U, Harrison DG. Extracellular superoxide dismutase and cardiovascular disease. Cardiovasc Res 2002; 55: 239-49.

[120] Suliman HB, Ryan LK, Bioshop L, Folz RJ. Prevention of influenza-induced lung injury in mice overexpressing extracellular superoxide dismutase. Am J Physiol Lung Cell Mol Physiol 2001; 280: 169-78.

[121] Villagrán ME, Marín C, Rodríguez-González I, De Diego JA, Sánchez- Moreno M. An iron Superoxide Dismutase (Fesode) excreted by *Trypanosoma cruzi* useful in the diagnosis of Chagas disease: Seroprevalence of this infection in rural zones of the State of Queretaro (Mexico). Am J Trop Med Hyg 2005; 73: 510-6.

[122] Mateo H, Marín C, Pérez-Cordón G, Sánchez-Moreno M. Purification and biochemical characterization of four iron superoxide dismutases in *Trypanosoma cruzi*. Mem Inst Oswaldo Cruz 2008; 103: 271-6.

[123] Gruppi A, Pistoresi-Palencia MC, Ordoñez P, Cerbán F, Vottero-Cima E. Enhancement of natural antibodies in mice immunized exoantigens of pI 4.5 from *Trypanosoma cruzi*. Immunol Lett 1994; 42: 151-9.

[124] Nakazawa M, Rosa DS, Pereira VR, *et al*. Excretory-secretory antigens of *Trypanosoma cruzi* are potentially useful for serodiagnosis of chronic Chagas' disease. Clin Diagn Lab Immunol 2001; 8: 1024-7.

[125] Umezawa ES, Nascimento MS, Stolf AM. Enzyme-linked immunosorbent assay with *Trypanosoma cruzi* excreted-secreted antigens (TESA-ELISA) for serodiagnosis of acute and chronic Chagas' disease. Diagn Microbiol Infect Dis 2001; 39: 169-76.

[126] Berrizbeitia M, Ndao M, Bubis J, *et al*. Purified excreted-secreted antigens from *Trypanosoma cruzi* trypomastigotes as tools for diagnosis of Chagas' disease. J Clin Microbiol 2006; 44: 291-6.

[127] Pestel J, Defoort JP, Gras-Masse H, *et al*. Polyclonal cell activity of a repeat peptide derived from the sequence of an 85-kilodalton surface protein of *Trypanosoma cruzi* trypomastigotes. Infect Immun 1992; 60: 715-9.

[128] Weston D, Patel B, Van Voorhis WC. Virulence in *Trypanosoma cruzi* infection correlates with the expression of a distinct family of sialidase superfamily genes. Mol Biochem Parasitol 1999; 98: 105-16.

[129] Pinho RT, Vannier-Santos MA, Alves CR, Marino AP, Castello Branco LR, Lannes-Vieira J. Effect of *Trypanosoma cruzi* released antigens binding to non-infected cells on anti-parasite antibody recognition and expression of extracellular matrix components. Acta Trop 2002; 83: 103-15.

[130] Silber AM, Marcipar IS, Roodveldt C, Cabeza Meckert P, Laguens R, Marcipar AJ. *Trypanosoma cruzi*: identification of a galactose-binding protein that binds to cell surface of human erythrocytes and is involved in cell invasion by the parasite. Exp Parasitol 2002; 100: 217-25.

CHAPTER 3

Malaria Vaccine Development: 20 Years of Hopes, Hypes and Limited Achievements

Antonio Verdini, Sope Olugbile, Giampietro Corradin* and Richard Pink

Department of Biochemistry, University of Lausanne, 1066 Epalinges, Switzerland

Abstract: This review critically examines the development of malaria vaccine candidates and the results obtained in phase IIa and IIb efficacy evaluations since the first human trial till date. It is restricted only to proteins or protein fragments produced by peptide synthesis or DNA recombinant technology, for the simple reason that these are the only products that could be structurally evaluated. It is meant to make the scientific community aware of the shortcomings of some of these constructs with regard to their 3-dimensional structure and the need for more stringent biological/functional requirements to be met before field evaluations are initiated. Both of these factors are largely responsible for most of the failures witnessed in the past 20 years.

INTRODUCTION

Malaria remains the most important parasitic infection in the world. Up to 40% of the world population is estimated to be at risk of contracting malaria; this figure may however increase in the future with increasing temperature brought about by global warming. The majority of the over 1 million annual deaths that result from *Plasmodium falciparum* infection (the most lethal of the *Plasmodium* species) occur among young children living in sub-Saharan Africa [1, 2].

But what is frequently overlooked is the pain and suffering young children living in malaria-endemic areas go through, often every month, sometimes more frequently, till they reach early adulthood when they achieve partial immunity against the debilitating symptoms of malaria. The impact is so immense and is best described by one of the authors of this review (S. Olugbile) who grew up in a malaria-endemic region of south-west Nigeria and also treated several cases of malaria as a doctor before being inspired to get involved in malaria vaccine development. He used to miss two to three school days almost every month due to malaria. The joint pains and the high fever were most distressing and equally harsh were the bitter medications, which on their own induce vomiting thus delaying the onset of drug action. So each episode had to be 'extinguished' by parenteral antimalarials, while another one was only a few weeks away. Majority of children that present at the health facilities are also as a result of malaria and its complications. Not uncommon were complications that arose from treatments given at home before presentation at the hospital. These complications might be side-effects of orthodox medications or bizarre herbal concoctions 'prescribed' by neighbors and older family members. So, the impact of malaria in its entirety is the sum of the mortality mostly in young children and the frequent periodic morbidities that extend up into early adulthood.

In the past few years, there has been an unprecedented increase in interest in malaria with concomitant funding aimed at the development of novel interventions. Scientists are trying to better understand the biology of *Plasmodium* and its interaction with the host immune system. New drugs are being developed, so also are different combinations of new and old drugs being formulated in order to overcome drug resistance. Awareness is also being generated for the use of insecticide treated nets. The encouraging results being observed are making some optimists to start hinting about complete eradication even if this seems farfetched as there is no objective rationale to suggest this is achievable in the nearest future. It is however apparent that a malaria vaccine will form the backbone of the effort to drastically reduce the morbidity and mortality associated with malaria.

It is on this human suffering background that efforts to develop an efficacious vaccine should be undertaken. This should also inspire a closer collaboration between all the players in vaccine development. But research and development of a vaccine has been hampered for many years, not only by the lack of adequate resources, but also of an earnest and effective global collaboration among the various academic groups, industrial partners and funding agencies. The latter aspect is still

*Corresponding Author: Giampietro Corradin, Department of Biochemistry, University of Lausanne, 1066 Epalinges, Switzerland; Tel: +41 21 692 5731; Email: giampietro.corradin@unil.ch

Emilio Jirillo (Ed)
All rights reserved - © 2010 Bentham Science Publishers Ltd.

missing with tendencies towards development of the same candidates even after repeated trial failures, and the most advanced but not necessarily the most promising candidates or formulations. Some funding agencies also selectively sponsor only projects using supposedly 'latest' technologies with sparse evidence on efficacies in human. The nonexistence of a licensed malaria vaccine till date may be attributed in part to this fragmented approach. Of note however is a laudable effort promoted by the European Community through EMVDA (European Malaria Vaccine Development Association) consisting of several European laboratories involved in malaria vaccine development. They are currently comparing a number of vaccine candidates side by side with the aim of selecting the best 3 for further clinical development.

In this review we critically examine the results obtained in phase IIa and IIb trials over the past 20 years with the aim of elucidating the likely reasons for most of the failures and few partial successes in order to further refine vaccine development strategies and ensure development of an effective vaccine in the nearest future. We will focus on recombinant and synthetic proteins (or protein fragments) whose vaccine efficacy may largely be determined by the 3-dimensional identity (mimicry) with the native antigen. This fundamental criterion currently receives minimal attention from the scientific community and funding agencies. The other area of our focus will be on the formulation of a rigorous, pragmatic and systematic process of selecting the most promising candidates and the threshold of biological/functional activities obtained from phases Ia and IIa studies that will merit the progression into field trials. Finally, we will conclude the review by highlighting new opportunities that are currently or will shortly be available with potentials of accelerating the development of a safe and efficacious malaria vaccine.

SYNTHETIC MALARIA SUBUNIT VACCINE CANDIDATES

The logical approach to subunit malaria vaccine candidates has been the selection of key peptide antigens involved in the complex molecular interactions at the interface between parasite and host. In the majority of cases, candidate antigens have been expressed as recombinant proteins and formulated with adjuvants for evaluation in animals and human.

Over the past two decades a number of antigens produced by chemical synthesis have also been used in pre-clinical studies and in Phase I and II clinical trials. To date, synthetic or recombinant candidate vaccines have provided only marginal protection against malaria infection. The only notable exception is the recombinant RTS,S, a particulate formulation of large segments of the CS protein fused with the hepatitis B surface antigen. RTS,S in combination with AS02A, which contains the immunostimulants MPL and QS21 in an oil-in-water emulsion, has shown partial efficacy [3, 4, see next Section].

There are several reasons why synthetic vaccine candidates have yet to fulfill the expected promises. Apart from the limited number of antigens that have been assessed compared with the more than 5300 proteins predicted to be present in the *Plasmodium falciparum* genome [5], the main limitations on malaria vaccine development include: 1) the high polymorphism in the regions of immunological interest; 2) the low immunogenicity without the use of powerful adjuvants; 3) the short duration of the immune responses and 4) the lack of bio-assays able to predict protection and hence guide pre-clinical investigations.

Very little attention has been paid to the conformational properties of the peptide portions incorporated into vaccine constructs and formulations. Indeed, the failure of most vaccine candidates in human clinical trials may be traced to poor structural mimicry of the corresponding segments present in the native proteins.

In particular, designing peptide-based constructs to be target of a protective antibody response is like sailing a boat between Scylla and Charybdis. On one side, the three-dimensional conformation of the peptide should closely mimic that of the same fragment in the native protein in order to obtain conformation-dependent neutralizing antibodies; on the other side, the peptide should be simple, quickly assembled and purified through a reproducible chemical process. It should also be stable in storage and prepared at a reasonable cost in sufficient quantities to perform pre-clinical and clinical testing.

Pre-Erythrocytic Stage Synthetic Malaria Vaccines

Most malaria vaccine research has been focused on *Plasmodium falciparum*, as this species is responsible for the vast majority of deaths and severe morbidities. Pre-erythrocytic *Plasmodium falciparum* vaccine candidates are mostly based on the most abundant protein on the surface of the sporozoite, the circumsporozoite (CS) protein [6, 7], which was the first sequenced malaria protein. The CS protein's relatively simple repeat domain, located in the middle of the chain and composed of 41 tandem repeats of tetrapeptide sequences (37 NANP repeats and 4 NVDP repeats at positions 2, 4, 6 and 22) immediately inspired structure proposals and synthesis of peptide mimetics for the preparation of vaccine constructs. Within a few months peptide chemists were able to prepare $(NANP)_{40}$, a long sequential polypeptide closely mimicking the central protein domain, as well as shorter analogues containing NANP or NANP and NVDP repeats [8].

Theoreticians calculated the three-dimensional structure of tandemly repeated NANP or NPNA motifs. Two low-energy helical structures were predicted: a right-handed helix of three repeats (12 residues) per turn with a pitch of 9.91 A° [9], and an unprecedented 12_{38} right-handed helix with 12 residues per turn, an intrachain hydrogen-bond loop containing 38 atoms, a diameter of ca. 17 A° and a pitch of 4.95 A°, corresponding to a rise of 1.65 A° per tetrapeptide unit [10]. The latter structure (Fig. **1 A** and **1 B**) is highly stabilized by extensive hydrogen bonding and has an energy of about 20 kcal/mol of tetramer lower than that reported in [9]. The side-chain amide groups of the asparagine residues are parallel to the helical axis, allowing for the formation of inter-repeat H bonds. Each tetrapeptide unit acts as an acceptor for five hydrogen bonds to residues in adjacent turns and forms four weak internal hydrogen bonds.

The discoverers of the 12_{38} helix were the first to propose a vaccine candidate with a precise tridimensional structure. They suggested that a polypeptide vaccine candidate should have more than 36 residues (9 repeats) to mimic the native conformation, since more than three turns were required to impart stability to the 12_{38} helix. The polypeptide should also include: a) replacements of alanyl-asparagine with valyl-aspartic acid motifs, which were thought to be essential for ordering the entire hydrogen bond array in a specific manner and b) some of the lead-in sequence adjacent to the repeat segment to aid in the selection of the correct helical structure among the class of almost isoenergetic calculated 12_{38} helical structures. The tridimensional structure of the central repeat domain of the CS protein has thus far eluded experimental determination.

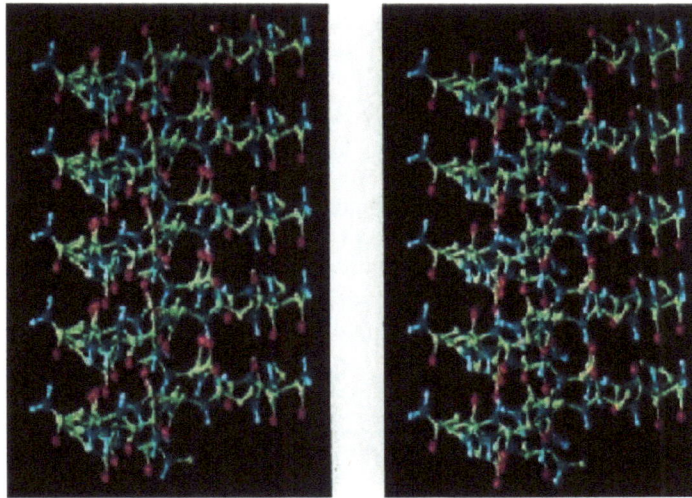

Figure 1A: Stereo side view of the most favorable calculated structure for an oligomer of the Pf CS protein repeating tetrapeptide having 15 Asn-Pro-Asn-Ala units. The helical axis is aligned vertically with the N terminus at the bottom. Adapted from [10].

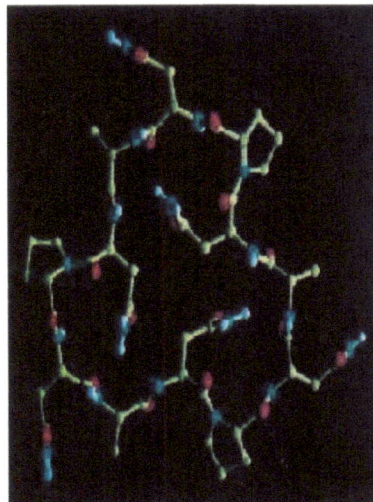

Figure 1B: End view down the helical axis of the most favorable calculated structure for an oligomer of the PfCS protein repeating tetrapeptide having nine Asn-Pro-Asn-Ala units. Adapted from [10].

Malaria researchers have largely overlooked this significant proposal. Rather, all their efforts focused on the promise of simpler subunit vaccines. The first synthetic sporozoite vaccine candidate was indeed prepared by conjugation of the short linear peptide Ac-Cys-(NANP)$_3$ with maleimidopropionyl-tetanus toxoid (TT) [11]. The rationale for trying such a vaccine was based on the recognition that the immunodominant epitope of the *Plasmodium falciparum* CS protein was the repetitive NANP sequence and that monoclonal antibodies directed against it could neutralize sporozoite infectivity *in vitro*. If the levels of the antibodies induced by the vaccine were sufficiently high, they would block invasion of hepatocytes and prevent infection [12].

Volunteers who were injected with (NANP)$_3$-tetanus toxoid produced pathogen-reactive antibodies. However, some individuals produced antibodies that did not react with the pathogen. Only one of the three vaccinated individuals did not develop a blood infection when challenged by the bite of infected mosquitoes. The other two had detectable parasitemia 11 days after challenge, while the four controls developed parasitemia 8.5 days (mean) following challenge. An important disadvantage of the conjugate was the lack of malaria T-cell epitopes present in the TT-conjugate vaccine. Thus, the immune response to the vaccinees will most likely not be boosted in endemic areas following exposure to sporozoites. Furthermore, the immune response was lower than expected probably because all volunteers had previously been vaccinated with tetanus toxoid (epitopic suppression, 13).

The limited efficacy of the (NANP)$_3$-tetanus toxoid construct could also be explained, at least in part, by the extreme conformational flexibility of the short NANP chains in water and hence the lack of a preferred structure. Conjugation of the synthetic peptide to the carrier resulted in (NANP)$_3$ chains linked at various positions on the carrier molecule. Thus, the highly flexible peptide chains may have experienced different conformational perturbations by closely spaced protein segments. The sensitivity of the (NANP)$_3$ extensions to serum proteases could also have played a role.

Shortly after the conclusion of a second disappointing human trial in volunteers injected with a recombinant DNA *Plasmodium falciparum* sporozoite vaccine [14], mono- and bi-dimensional NMR studies of the peptide models (NANP)$_2$-NA and (NANP)$_6$ showed that both molecules were unstructured in water. In less solvating media (alcohol-water mixtures), (NANP)$_2$-NA folded and adopted a structure consisting of a mixed sequence of type I β-turns and half turns (γ-turns) at the N_{i-1}-P_i-N_{i+1} chain segments, in rapid dynamic equilibrium with unfolded forms [15].

These earlier observations were confirmed, in part, by high-resolution proton NMR studies of two models with different repeat cadences, Ac-(NANP)$_3$-NH$_2$ and Ac-(NPNA)$_3$-NH$_2$. The NMR results suggested the presence of helical and/or β-turn-like structures based only on the NPNA cadence, in rapid equilibrium with random coil chains [16].

The presence of transient secondary structures in short NPNA peptides in water suggested that perhaps antipeptide antibodies with higher affinity could be generated by restricting the conformation of the peptides to a shape resembling that of the natural immunogen. An examination of space-filling molecules of NPNA in a reverse-turn conformation revealed that the side chains of asparagines might readily form amide-amide hydrogen bonds. Hence, the first shaped conformationally restricted malarial peptide was obtained by mimicking the hydrogen bond -HN-CO...NH-CO- of a couple of asparagine side chains by joining them with an ethylene moiety, -CH$_2$-CH$_2$- [17].

The cyclic analogues of linear Cys-(NPNA)$_3$-NH$_2$ and Cys-(NANP)$_3$-NH$_2$, with all the hydrogen bonds linking the asparagine side chains (flanking proline and alanine, respectively) replaced with -CH$_2$-CH$_2$- (Fig. **2**)

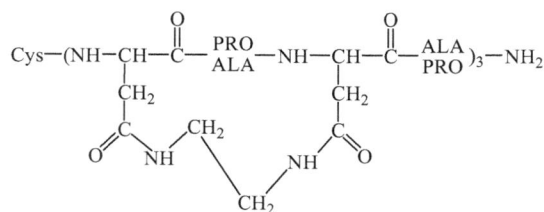

Figure 2: Ethylene bridged, conformationally restricted Cys-(NPNA)$_3$-NH$_2$ and Cys-(NANP)$_3$-NH$_2$. Adapted from [17].

were conjugated to maleimidobenzoylated keyhole lympet haemocyanin (KLH) and injected into rabbits. The polyclonal antiserum raised against cyclic Cys-(NPNA)$_3$-NH$_2$ reacted strongly with the recombinant CS protein and glutaraldehyde-fixed sporozoites. To confirm that the anti-cyclopeptide serum cross-reacted with the native form of the CS protein, it was titrated against living sporozoites with an immunofluorescent assay (IFA). A strong reaction was observed, suggesting that chemically modified, conformationally restricted NANP peptides can mimic the structure of the native repeat domain and serve as effective immunogens. NMR experiments, although not reported, demonstrated a rigid structure in water for both cyclic peptides.

This result stimulated scientists to focus on small cyclic NPNA peptides as the antigenic targets of possible protective immune responses and to develop subunit vaccines and vaccine delivery systems that induced such protection. About two decades were spent on understanding how to prepare by chemical synthesis conformationally constrained malarial peptides with precise shapes. The research on small cyclic peptides culminated in 2007 with the synthesis of an internally cyclized peptide of five NPNA repeats (see below) and its virosomal formulation as a malaria vaccine candidate [18].

An interesting cyclopeptide was prepared from (NANP)₃ by joining the amino terminal group of asparagine and the carboxyl group of the terminal proline to a residue of γ-protected diamino butyric acid (Dab; Fig. 3). After elimination of the protecting group and coupling to cysteine, the derivative was conjugated to maleimidobenzoylated tetanus toxoid protein [19].

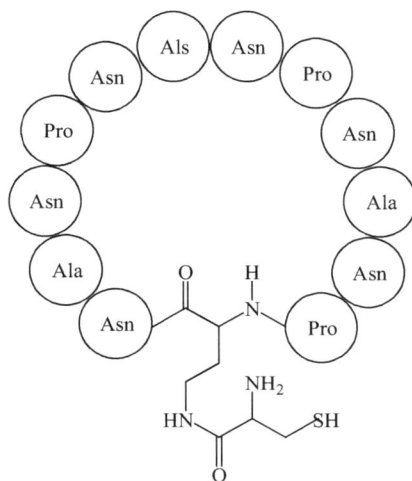

Figure 3: Cyclic (NANP)₃-Dab-Cys. Adapted from [19].

Thirty five percent (35%) of the monoclonal antibodies to the linear (NANP)₃ peptide were unreactive with the parasite. In contrast, all monoclonal antibodies to the cyclized peptide were found to react with the parasite suggesting that a likely contributor to the formation of epitopes that give rise to pathogen-unreactive antibodies is the free terminal proline which is not a terminal residue in the native protein.

In parallel, much of the continuing basic work on short linear peptides has been devoted to their conformational characterization *in vacuo* and in complex macromolecular constructs. An interesting outcome of the research on short linear peptides were the results of multidimensional solution NMR spectroscopy of (NANP)₃ displayed on the surface of filamentous bacteriophage by insertion in the N-terminal region of the major coat protein (p VIII). The peptide structure, never seen before, consisted largely of two extended and non-hydrogen bonded NPNA loops [20].

The α carbon dihedral angle was found to be approximately 10° for the N^6-A^9 loop and 0° for the N^{10}-A^{13} loop. Residues N^6 and N^8 were in the β region while residues A^9, N^{10}, N^{12} and A^{13} were in the α region of the φ/ψ Ramachandran map. Furthermore, high-resolution solid-state NMR spectra demonstrated that the NANP repeat was structured in the context of the N-terminal region of the coat protein with nearly all residues immobile on the time scale of the ^{15}N chemical shift interaction (10^4 Hz).

Distance geometry (DG) and molecular dynamics (MD) simulations of (NPNA)₃ and (NP^MeNA)₃ have reinforced the view that the NPNA motif adopts the format of a type I-β turn. In fact, in both peptides the central unit prefers to fold in a type I-β turn, while the outer motifs display more conformational flexibility [21, 22]. These results have suggested how a peptide containing multiple tandemly linked copies of a stable NPNA type I β-turn might adopt a folded stem-like structure conceivably of biological relevance in the native CS protein. Nevertheless, linear and highly flexible (NANP)$_3$ sequences continued to be incorporated into polypeptide constructs.

The encouraging results obtained with ethylene- and Dab-bridged cyclopeptides prompted the investigations of template-bound cyclic peptidomimetics containing the sequence ANPNAA (Fig. **4A**; 23) and a larger loop with two intact NPNA motifs (Fig. **4B**; 24).

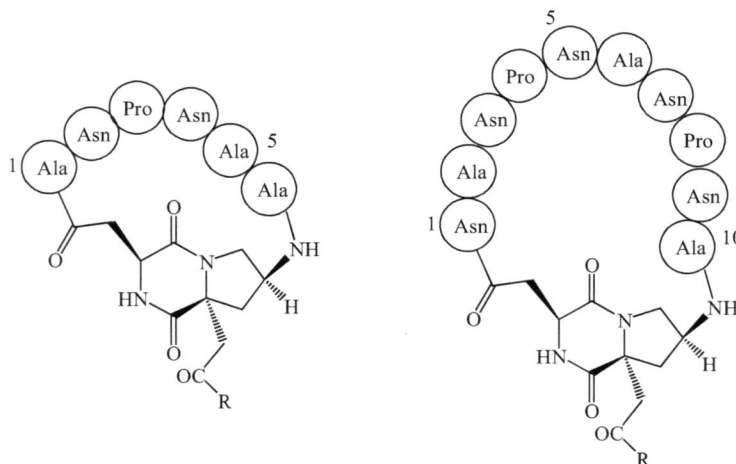

Fig. 4A   Fig. 4B

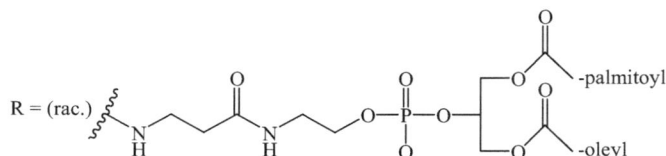

Figure 4: ANPNAA template-bound cyclic Peptide 1 linked to phosphatidylethanolamine (PE). çB. NANPNANPNA template-bound cyclic Peptide 2 linked to phosphatidylethanolamine (PE). Figures 4A and B were adapted from [18].

The backbone of Peptide 1 was shown to adopt a stable β-I turn conformation at the NPNA sequence. In contrast with the ethylene-bridged peptides, the molecule retained a significant degree of flexibility due to the flipping of pyrrolidine rings and amide planes. To see whether the cyclic mimetic was able to elicit antibodies capable of binding with *Plasmodium falciparum* sporozoites, it was incorporated into a construct together with a universal T helper cell epitope derived from tetanus toxin (Construct A). A similar construct was prepared by coupling the linear ANPNAA sequence to the termini of the tetrabranched lysyl scaffold linked to the same tetanus toxoid T helper cell epitope (Construct B). Both constructs were adjuvanted with QS-21 and injected in BALB/c mice. The sera from 12/15 mice immunized with Construct A showed specific IgG responses against the immunogen and some of the sera cross-reacted with *Plasmodium falciparum* sporozoites. The sera from none of of the mice immunized with construct B cross-reacted with sporozoites. The specificity of the cross-reaction was analysed by competition experiments. Both construct A and Peptide 1 completely abolished the antibody reactivity of positive sera with sporozoites. In control experiments, cyclic peptides with different sequences linked to the same template were unable to inhibit antibody binding to sporozoites in IFA.

The results indicated a specific recognition of sporozoites by anti-Peptide 1 antibodies in the sera. In addition, antibody responses to Peptide 1 mounted on the tetrabranched lysyl scaffold (adjuvanted with alum) or loaded on IRIVs (immunopotentiating reconstituted influenza virosomes) were compared in BALB/c mice. The IRIVs are similar to liposomes, but contain membrane-bound hemagglutinin and neuraminidase, which impart fusogenic activity and facilitate antigen delivery to immunocompetent cells [25] and provide T cell help to specific B cells. Sera from all immunized animals contained mimetic-specific antibodies. The IRIVs formulation elicited significant anti-sporozoite responses in all animals immunized. In contrast, half of the animals immunized with the alum formulation generated no detectable anti-sporozoite antibody response and in the others the IFA titers were very low.

The solution conformation of Peptide 2 was investigated by NMR spectroscopy in aqueous solution and by MD simulations [22]. The preferred conformation of this peptidomimetic was found to be quite different from that of Peptide 1. Its chain, with a β-turn at residues N^3-P^4-N^5-A^6, adopted a *helical turn conformation* in which the β-turn was extended by one asparagine residue to create a five-residue conformational unit NPNAN, with the alanine in a helical state. The molecule was found to be highly flexible. Peptide 2 was superior to peptide 1 in eliciting a high proportion of parasite cross-reactive antibodies when loaded in IRIVs. Only a subset of monoclonal antibodies elicited against the peptidomimetic cross-reacted with the CS protein on the sporozoite. The preferred conformation of Peptide 2 in aqueous solution suggested that the repeated conformational motif in the folded CS protein could not just be NPNA in a β turn structure, but rather NPNAN forming a helical turn. Tandemly repeated helical turns were in fact observed in a computer model built for the linear sequence Ac-NPNANPNANPNANPNANPNA-NH$_2$ in which each residue of the P-N-A segments was placed in the helical region of the φ/ψ space (-60°/-40°) and all asparagine residues preceding prolines were blocked in the β region (-120°/+120°) [26]. The resulting folded conformation was quite different from the 12_{38} helical structure reported above.

The computer model suggested that within the linear peptide containing five NANP motifs Ac-N^1PNAN^{5}AproNANP^{10}NANPN^{15}ENPNA^{20}-NH$_2$, three repeating helical turns at the three central NANP repeats could be stabilized by an amide cross-link between the γ amino group of Apro^6 [(2S, 4S)-4-amino proline] and the spatially adjacent side chain of the glutamic acid^{16} caboxyl.

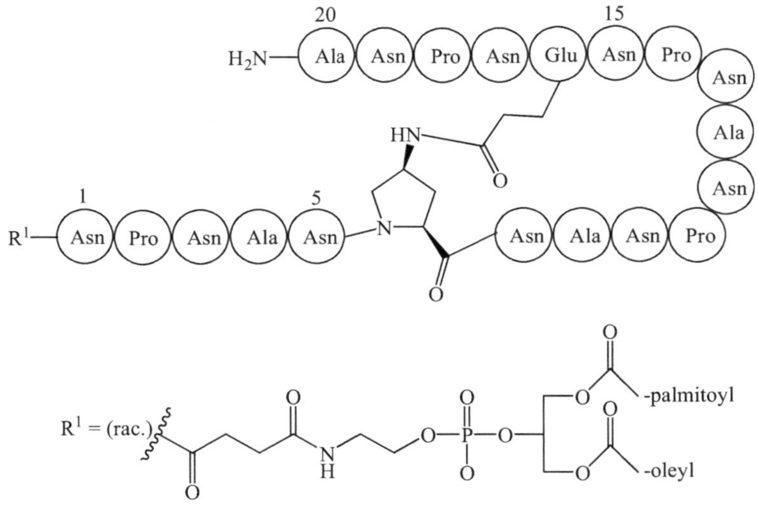

Figure 5: Structure of peptidomimetic UK-39 adapted from [18].

The acetyl derivative of the linear 20-mer peptide precursor was first assembled stepwise on resin and then cyclized in solution by coupling the γ amino group of Apro^6 to the free glutamic acid^{16} carboxyl (Fig. 5). The conformation of the cyclic peptidomimetic (designated UK-40) was investigated in water by NMR spectroscopy [18, 26]. The results indicated the existence of a major and two minor forms interconverting slowly on the NMR timescale due to the cis-trans isomers at the N-P peptide bonds. Similar cis-trans isomers were found in linear peptides containing NPNA repeats and in the cyclic compound containing a (2S, 3R)-3-amino proline residue (designated BP-66). The major form has been assigned to the all-trans conformation. The N^5PNA^8 and N^9PNA^{12} units within the UK-40 cycle were found to have a conformation similar both to the helical turn found in the computer model of Ac-(NPNA)$_5$-NH$_2$ and to the β-turn found in the crystal structure of the pentapeptide Ac-ANPNA-NH$_2$. In the crystal, the NPNA unit adopts a type-I β-turn stabilized by hydrogen bonding between the CO of N^2 and the NH of A^5 as well as between the O(δ) of N^5 and the NH of N^4 [27]. The helical turn is adopted much less frequently, or not at all, in the N^{13}-E^{16} unit of UK-40. Extended (β) chain forms at E^{16}-N^{17} have been revealed by the NMR experiments, suggesting the presence of multiple rapidly interconverting helical and β conformations within the cycle. Thus, the backbone of the macrocyclic peptide was significantly flexible as found for Peptides 1 and 2.

For immunological studies, des-acetylated BP-66 and UK-40 were coupled to 1-palmitoyl-3-oleylphosphatydilethanolamine (PE) and the resulting products (denominated BP-65 and UK-39 respectively) inserted on the surface of IRIVs. The preparation of peptide-loaded virosomes is reported in [18]. Both virosomally formulated cyclic peptides were found to be strongly immunogenic in mice and rabbits. Cross-reactivity analysis with a set of 12 monoclonal antibodies raised against *Plasmodium falciparum* sporozoites demonstrated that all monoclonal antibodies cross-reacted strongly with UK-39 indicating that this compound better reflects the native structure of the CS protein repeat region. Purified IgG from rabbits immunized with UK-39 inhibited sporozoite invasion of hepatocytes *in vitro* and parasite gliding mobility.

Two monoclonal antibodies EP 3 and EP 9 prepared from spleen cells of mice immunized with BP-65 were found to bind both the mimetic UK-39 and *Plasmodium falciparum* sporozoites. The scarce cross-reactivity of both monoclonals with an analogue lacking the C-terminal and N-terminal exocyclic segments (Fig. **6**; designated BP-125; 18, 26) demonstrated that UK-39 represents the minimal essential epitopic structure.

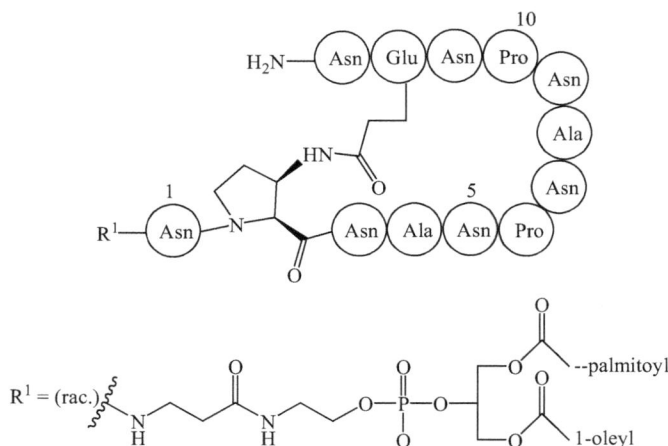

Figure 6: Structure of peptidomimetic BP-125. Adapted from [18].

Only EP 9 recognized $(NANP)_{50}$ in ELISA. Since $(NANP)_{50}$ is known to be disordered in dilute aqueous solutions, the EP 9 monoclonal antibody was likely able to recognize only linear epitopes in the central domain of the parasite CS protein. Conversely, the binding of EP 3 to UK-39 and to the parasite surface, and the scarce cross-reactivity with UK-125, taken together, suggest that EP3 recognizes conformational determinants different from single- or contiguous double β-turns. The cross-reactivity studies, which add further support to the conclusion suggested by the NMR experiments on UK-40, indicated that the main conformational epitope of UK-39 could span the entire N^5-N^{17} sequence comprehending two helical turns followed by an extended strand of five amino acid residues [18].

In summary, all cyclic and linear peptidomimetics were found to be flexible and able to elicit antibodies reactive with the CS protein. It is however unclear whether the increased frequency of anti-cyclic peptide antibodies that react with the pathogen results from a better mimicry of the native structure or from the elimination of free termini.

Finally, UK-39 was selected as a vaccine candidate because of its structural and antigenic similarity to the NPNA-repeat region of native CS protein. A randomized placebo-controlled phase I malaria vaccine trial with virosome-formulated UK-39 (PEV 302) in healthy adult volunteers demonstrated that three immunizations were safe and well tolerated. At appropriate antigen doses a seroconversion rate of 100% was achieved. Two injections were sufficient for eliciting an appropriate immune response, at least in individuals with pre-existing anti-malarial immunity [28]. A detailed analysis of the antibody response against UK-39 has also been reported [29].

Three vaccinations with a 10 µg dose of UK-39 induced high titers of sporozoite-binding antibodies in all 46 healthy malaria-naive adults immunized with the virosomal formulation of UK-39. The IgG response was affinity matured and long-lived. Purified total IgG from UK-39 immunized volunteers inhibited sporozoite migration and invasion of hepatocytes in vitro. Inhibition closely correlated with titers measured in immunogenicity assays.

This result was considered as a confirmation that the conformationally restrained peptide UK-39 was "very close to the natural conformation of the NANP repeats as already indicated by NMR analysis of UK-39 and the crystal structure of NPNA" (see below the conformational properties of long tandemly repeated NANP sequences; 29).

These results encouraged the development of a virosomal vaccine formulation (PEV3A) designed to target two different life-cycle stages of *Plasmodium falciparum*. In the bivalent PEV3A vaccine, separate IRIVs, which are mixed together in the final formulation, are used for the delivery of both UK-39 and a 49-aminoacid synthetic peptide mimicking the semi conserved loop I of domain III of AMA-1, the apical membrane antigen-1 of the K1 isolate of *Plasmodium falciparum* [30].

Immunization with PEV3A was ineffective according to the primary outcome measure of protection (namely, sterile immunity); lower rates of parasite growth were however observed in volunteers vaccinated with PEV3A. The combination of PEV3A with the multi-epitope-thrombospondin–related adhesion protein vaccine (ME-TRAP) was equally ineffective [30, 31]. Thus, a vaccine construct based on a conformationally constrained stretch of five NPNA repeats did not offer striking improvements in protective efficacy over the linear, conformationally scrambled (NANP)$_3$ peptide bound to TT adjuvanted with alum.

The lesson that could be learnt from the failure of PEV3A candidate vaccine is that short and conformationally constrained mimetics of NANP repeats can reproduce, at best, only a few epitopes with a preferred local conformation out of the many present in the structure of the CS protein repeat domain. More appropriate mimics of the immunodominant domain might be high molecular weight and folded NPNA-based polypeptides as proposed earlier by the discoverers of the 12_{38} helix. Only long polypeptide chains could present to the immune system, in a repetitive structure, a vast array of linear and conformational epitopes very similar to those of the native protein.

LONG SYNTHETIC PEPTIDE MODEL OF *P. FALCIPARUM* CS PROTEIN

Circular dichroism (CD) and Fourier transform infrared spectroscopy (FTIR) have indeed shown that long, tandemly repeated NANP peptides have a marked propensity to fold and form helical structures in solutions [32]. As in linear and cyclic NANP peptides, (NANP)$_{40}$ chains, which are essentially disordered in water, can rapidly sample many locally folded states. However, their unfolded structure is not necessarily characterized by random backbone and side-chain dihedral angles. Long NANP chains may harbor conformational preferences due to specific interactions such as short polyproline II stretches of 2-5 residues and structures in which individual residues are in α or β regions of the Ramachandran map, rapidly interconverting [33-35]. Residual structures persisting under denaturing conditions (water for NANP peptides) can influence the folding and the stability of the chains when the denaturing conditions are removed. Indeed, the addition of trifluoroethanol (TFE) to aqueous solutions of (NANP)$_{40}$ was observed to induce a gradual ordering of the polypeptide chains. TFE is known to be less effective than water in solvating the peptide backbone, and as a result, destabilizes the coil state of both short and long peptides.

In TFE-water 99%-1% v/v (NANP)$_{40}$ is indeed completely folded. The isodichroic point at 195 nm seen in the CD spectra indicates a two-state coil-helix transition induced by the addition of the organic solvent. The helical structure is reached and stabilized in the above solvent mixture only for polypeptide chains containing not less than 20 NANP repeats, while for the theoretical 12_{38} helix, 15 NANP repeats (five full turns of the helix) were found to be required to impart stability to the helix. Helices of (NANP)$_{40}$ are constituted solely by β-extended segments and β-turns, as shown by the FTIR bands appearing in the C=O stretching region. Since the synthetic long NANP sequential polypeptides are composed of all-β secondary structural elements, their structures are (or closely reproduce) that of β-solenoid proteins *(β-solenoids)* whose folds are generated by the alternation of linear parallel β-strand segments with tilted turns called β-arcs [36, 37].

The (NANP)$_n$ low-energy-β-solenoidal structure differs from that of the 12_{38} helix reported before (Verdini A, Corradin G, Kajava AV, unpublished results). The conformation of the repeating unit NPNA (pplb) contains the standard conformation of the N-P-N β-arc (ppl) that allows the peptide chain to turn by as much as 120°. Here, the Latin letters b, p and l indicate backbone conformations in corresponding regions of the Ramachandran map (b = β_E; p = β_P and l = α_L). The N-P-N residues are exposed to the solvent while the alanines are located inside the solenoid. Main chain-main chain and side chain-side chain hydrogen bonds stabilize the solenoidal structure. Among about 175 identified three-residue-β-arcs in proteins, the majority (55%) are ppl arcs. Conversely, the conformation of the NPNA repeating unit (bpll) in the 12_{38} helix reported above has not been observed in the solenoidal structures of proteins.

As recently shown by dynamic light scattering and velocity sedimentation experiments [38], recombinant CS proteins produced by expression both in *Escherichia coli* and in *Pichia pastoris* appear as highly extended proteins. High resolution atomic force microscopy revealed flexible, rod-like structures with a ribbon-like appearance [38]. Furthermore, molecular modeling of $(NPNA)_{43}$ (residues 103-274 of the native sequence) showed that the chain forms a superhelix (about 21-25 nm in length and 1.5 nm in width) composed of regular β-turns with a pitch of about 28 residues or 7 NPNA units [38].

CD, FTIR and molecular modeling results have indicated that, probably, long polypeptides containing not less than 20 NANP units closely mimic the structure of the CS protein repeat domain. Instead, both short linear and engineered cyclic peptides included in candidate vaccine constructs reproduce only NPNA linear epitopes and local folding at short chain segments. The nine repeat $(NVDPNANP)_3$-$(NANP)_3$-NA polypeptide shows a CD spectrum closely similar in shape and intensity to that of $(NANP)_{40}$ in TFE rich water-TFE mixtures while the close analogue $(NANP)_{10}$ is only partially folded [32]. Thus, as earlier suggested for the theoretical 12_{38} helix, the variant NVDP repeats greatly stabilize the helical structure in solution. The ionized carboxylate groups establish hydrogen bonds with the amide NH_2 of the asparagine side chains in the adjacent turns of the helix.

High molecular weight NANP polypeptides bind Ca^{++} when folded ($Ka=1.8.10^6$ per repeat), while conformationally scrambled $(NANP)_2NA$, $(NANP)_3NA$ and $(NANP)_{40}$ are unable to bind the alkali ion [32]. An ordered structure, again exclusively composed of β-turns and extended β segments, was induced by Ca^{++} binding. The very intense FTIR band at 1668 cm $^{-1}$ reflected a dramatic increase of the number of β turns in the chain, suggesting that calcium ions may have further stabilized the β-solenoidal structure by complexing at external asparagine side chains. Variant repeats of folded $(NVDPNANP)_3$-$(NANP)_3$-NA bind Ca^{++} preferentially [32]. Remarkably, in native *Plasmodium falciparum* CS protein variant repeats are sequentially very close to region I, a conserved sequence of amino acids important for parasite infectivity [39].

An anti-$(NANP)_{40}$ monoclonal antibody, inhibiting penetration of *Plasmodium falciparum* sporozoites into liver cells *in vitro*, and giving consistently negative results in an immunofluorescent assay on *Plasmodium falciparum* sporozoites, produced a positive fluorescent pattern surrounding the sporozoites when the parasites were placed in media containing Ca^{++} [40].

An astonishing solubility in water has been found for $(NANP)_{20}$. A solution containing 50 mg of peptide in 50 micro litres of water (H_2O: peptide molar ratio 5:1) was observed to transform with time into a visually transparent dense hydrogel. The FTIR spectrum of the gelified polypeptide closely resembled that registered in the presence of calcium ions [32]. Also the short peptide $(NANP)_3$-NA, devoid of structure in all TFE-water mixtures, formed a transparent gel on standing in TFE-water = 98-2% v/v. The FTIR spectrum of the gel was found to be indistinguishable from that of the hydrogel obtained from highly concentrated and "aged" aqueous solutions [32]. Thus, both short and long NANP tandemly repeated peptides were found to have an intrinsic propensity to fold and self-associate. The self-association of single β-solenoids has been observed to form several triple-stranded β-solenoids in which the three chains wind around a common axis [36].

The results reported above clearly indicate that folded tandemly repeated NANP chains can adopt supersecondary structures depending on the environment. The repeat domain of the CS protein can probably also assume similar supersecondary structures on the sporozoite surface. It has been observed that the shed material in the CSP reaction (the shedding of the parasite surface coat when it is cross-linked by antibodies) is not amorphous: it resembles a sheath and it resists the shearing forces which develop during centrifugation [12]. Perhaps the shed material consists of layers of CS molecules on the parasite surface self-assembled through the associated NPNA β-solenoids of the central repeat domains.

Immunization with sonicated sporozoites leading to the production of antibodies but not to protection can be explained by the "extraction" of the CS protein molecules from the sporozoite surface and their solubilization in water as individual chains [12]. In water, the huge CS protein repeat domain which is essentially unstructured as seen in long NANP peptides, should be able to elicit a non-protective antibody response similar to that induced by short and conformationally scrambled NANP peptides. The peculiar properties of the high molecular weight NANP peptides suggest a variety of functional roles for the central repeat domain of the CS protein directly correlated to the supersecondary structure that this particular sequence may adopt. Thus, folded synthetic NANP polypeptides could contain structural antigens that might induce the sterilizing immune responses of vaccination observed with whole parasites.

We favor the idea that the efficacy of antibody responses to NANP-based vaccines may be greatly improved by preserving as much as possible the specific structural determinants that are formed by association/aggregation of β-solenoidal NANP chains. As discussed above, the mimetic $(NVDPNANP)_3$-$(NANP)_3$-NA is *per se* conformationally stable in dilute aqueous solutions. Thus, a possibility to induce association/aggregation of the folded polypeptide without perturbing its structure could be the formulation on IRIVs of PE-$(NVDPNANP)_3$-$(NANP)_3$-NH_2. It should be also interesting to formulate PE-$(NANP)_{20}$ on IRIV and compare its immunological properties with those of short linear and cyclic NANP peptides. A second possibility is offered by peptide nanoparticles with regular polyhedral symmetry that can be used as repetitive antigen display systems both for $(NVDPNANP)_3$-$(NANP)_3$-NA and for $(NANP)_{20}$ [41, 42].

CS C-TERMINAL DOMAIN

Another approach aimed at mimicking the protective immune response induced by injection of irradiated sporozoites was based on the use of long polypeptides containing various T-helper and T-cytotoxic epitopes. Long fragments of the CS protein provided epitopes capable of binding to the various MHC class I and II molecules, thus overcoming the MHC restriction observed in response to smaller epitopes. The 102-mer precursor corresponding to residues 282-383 of the *Plasmodium falciparum* CS protein (NF54 strain), which contains 4 Cys residues, was assembled stepwise on a solid support with two unprotected and two tert-buthylthio- protected cysteines, following the Fmoc-tert-butyl strategy. The doubly protected precursor folded spontaneously at pH 7.2, at room temperature, releasing tert-butylmercaptan and forming two intramolecular disulfide bridges [43]. It is likely that the structure of the folded domain stabilized by two spontaneously formed disulfide bridges closely mimics that of the corresponding domain in the CS protein.

The folded peptide (designated CS 102) was shown to be immunogenic in mice and monkeys, and its murine homolog protected mice against against murine malaria infection. It generated strong immune response mediated by T-helper and cytotoxic lymphocytes, as well as antibodies that recognized the sporozoite in IFA [44].

Two phase Ia clinical trials were conducted with the C-terminal domain (amino acid 282-383) of the *Pf* CSP (CS102) to evaluate its safety, reactogenicity and immunogenicity in non-exposed adults and to determine the optimal antigen dose with adjuvant combination. The C-terminus was oxidized and folded as described above [43]. In the first trial, 2 doses of CSP were used (100 and 300 mg) with 2 adjuvants, alum and Montanide ISA 752. The lower dose of antigen together with Montanide showed better B and T cell immunogenicity than alum [45]. In the second trial, volunteers in 3 dose cohorts (10, 30 and 100 mg) were vaccinated with CS102 in combination with Montanide ISA 720 or GSK proprietary adjuvant system AS02A on day 0, 60, and 180 [46]. The 2 adjuvant formulations were well tolerated and safe. After the third injection, volunteers displayed marked specific anti-*Pf*CS102 and anti-sporozoite antibody responses and T cell proliferative responses with IFN-γ production. Five of 22 HLA-A2 and HLA-A3 volunteers developed CS102 specific IFN-γ secreting CD8+ T cell responses. The humoral and cellular responses were stable for 6 months after the third injection in respectively 32 and 27 of 34 volunteers. Also there was no substantial difference between 30 and 100 mg peptide doses. ASO2A formulations with doses of 30 or 100 mg induced one log_{10} fold higher antibody and IFN-γ responses than Montanide formulation.

It was concluded that 2 or 3 immunisations with a dose of 30 mg formulated with ASO2A was the most appropriate choice for subsequent clinical studies. Due to the GSK decision not to provide ASO2A for further CS102 clinical studies, a phase 2a clinical trial was conducted in Nijmegen, The Netherlands, using Montanide ISA 720. All 16 volunteers (10 received the vaccine formulation, 6 controls) were found infected after 9 days within an interval of 12 h following challenge with 5 live sporozoites (Genton B, *et al* submitted). Shortening of the polypeptide chain by trimming about 30 residues at the N terminus and replacing them with $(NVDPNANP)_3$-$(NANP)_3$-NA might result in a linear polypeptide construct folded at its N-terminus like the CS protein repeat domain.

Erythrocytic Stage Synthetic Malaria Vaccines

Erythrocytic stage vaccines are primarily aimed at reducing the level of blood infection and thus the severity of malaria symptoms. The major barriers to the development of these vaccines are the polymorphism and strain variability of many antigens, lack of immune correlates of protection and predictive animal models. In contrast to pre-erythrocytic vaccine candidates, assessement of efficacies of erythrocytic stage vaccines has to wait till natural challenge during field trials.

Erythrocytic synthetic vaccine candidates have been modelled on the sequences and structures of *Plasmodium falciparum* merozoite specific proteins such as MSP1, MSP2, MSP3, GLURP, AMA-1 . Spf 66 was the first such vaccine to be tested in humans [47].

Spf 66 is a high molecular weight polypeptide obtained by the oxidative polymerization of a linear synthetic peptide monomer of 45 amino acids containing cysteine residues at both N- and C- terminals: **CGDELEAETQNVYA**APNANP**YSLFQKEKMVLPNANP**PANKKNAG**C**. The monomer is constituted by two non-contiguous NANP units (in red) and three short peptide sequences supposely derived from three asexual blood-stage proteins of 83, 55 and 35 KDa, strung together in an arbitrary order. In fact, only the epitope marked in blue was later found in the *P. falciparum* genome. The resulting polyepitope polymer containing repeating cystine junctions

(GDELEAETQNVYAAPNANPYSLFQKEKMVLPNANPPANKKNAG**CysSSCys**)$_n$ was expected to induce an antibody response higher than that of the mixture of the individual merozoite peptides shown to induce partial or complete protection in *Aotus trivirgatus* monkeys experimentally infected with *Plasmodium falciparum* sporozoites.

Two distributions of molecular weights with average molecular weights of about 150 and 14 KDa were observed by SDS-PAGE, corresponding to linear polymers and to macrocyclic polypeptides with 2 to 4 monomer residues per cycle, respectively. The highly heterogeneous product was not fractionated or checked for the presence of free thiol groups.

An unavoidable outcome of the polymerization process is represented by the large number of sequential as well as structural neo-antigens at the 27 cystine junctions of the 150 KDa linear polypeptide. Each polymerization step can in fact generate four different neo-antigenic sequences at each -SS- bond as the result of head-to-head, head-to-tail, tail-to-head and tail-to-tail reactions:

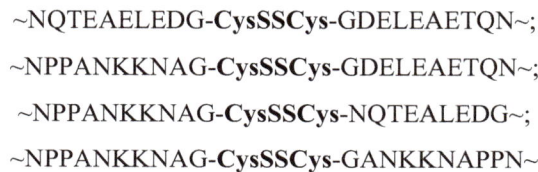

~NQTEAELEDG-**CysSSCys**-GDELEAETQN~;

~NPPANKKNAG-**CysSSCys**-GDELEAETQN~;

~NPPANKKNAG-**CysSSCys**-NQTEALEDG~;

~NPPANKKNAG-**CysSSCys**-GANKKNAPPN~

Due to the non-specificity of the oxidation reaction, the neo-antigens are also randomly distributed along the chain, further increasing the sequential heterogeneity of the individual chains. The reciprocal orientation of the epitopes could also have a profound effect on the specificity of the antibodies elicited and on the magnitude of the immune response [48].

The 3-dimensional structure of the neo-formed cystine residues may have important effects on the conformation of the flanking peptide sequences at each junction. The cystine disulfide bond may adopt either a left-handed spiral with the C^α-C^β bond vectors almost parallel or the right-handed hook with the C^α-C^β bond vectors approximately perpendicular to the -S-S- bond. Hence, the conformations of the cystine disulfides do influence the spatial orientation of the flanking peptides segments, introducing additional heterogeneity to the chain [49].

In proteins, a disulfide bond is very seldom formed between hydrogen-bonded residues on neighboring β strands, while it is quite common just past the ends of a β-strand pair. A disulfide bond cannot form between two cysteines in the same α-helix without extreme distortion. It is also surprisingly difficult and unusual to form an -S-S- bond between two α-helices. Thus, β-strand pairs can be induced to form at most of the 27 cystine junctions. The resulting conformations of the epitopes linked by the cystines in the linear polymer might then be quite different from those of the corresponding sequences in the native target proteins.

Thus, increasing the copy number of B-cell epitopes via oxidative polymerization of linear peptide monomers does not appear to be an advantage in terms of increasing antibody titres against the individual epitopes. On the contrary, the polymerization process produces several neo-antigenic sequences that greatly increase the number of linear and conformational determinants within the polypeptide formed. Apart from the presence of several neo-antigen sequences, very few peptide segments will be able to retain the conformational properties of the corresponding segments in the target protein. The same synthetic platform has been recently applied to the polymerization of MSP1 and AMA-1 peptide fragments, selected for their high-red-blood-cell binding ability and modified at some amino acid residues to provide protecting antibodies [50-53].

Prior to manufacturing and testing in monkeys, a careful assessment should be made of how disulfide bridges might affect the structure of the epitopes inserted into the polymeric constructs. A practical approach would be that of strictly controlling the degree of polymerization of the species obtained in the initial steps of the dithiol monomer oxidation. Terminating the polymerization at different times with NEM would easily provide peptide oligomers containing, on average, from 2 to 5 monomeric residues, useful for a precise conformational characterization by NMR and FTIR techniques.

SPf 66 initially showed promising results when tested in areas of low endemicity in South America and in children in a highly endemic area of Tanzania, delaying the onset of clinical malaria episodes [54-57]. Subsequent trials in infants in Gambia and Tanzania, children in Thailand and adults in Brazil failed to show any efficacy. The analysis of nine trials involving 9800 volunteers concluded that there was no evidence of efficacy for SPf 66 in Africa. The construct induced a modest reduction of malaria cases in South America [58].

MSP3 CANDIDATE

The conserved region of *Plasmodium falciparum* merozoite surface protein 3 (MSP3) 186-281 was prepared by a step-wise chemical synthesis as used for CS102. This fragment is predicted to be unstructured and found to have a random coil conformation by circular dichroism (G. Corradin, unpublished results). The GMP preparation was used in an open randomized two adjuvant (aluminum hydroxide and Montanide ISA 730) phase I malaria vaccine trial on 35 healthy volunteers [59]. No vaccine-related serious adverse events occurred throughout the trial. After the third injection of the long peptide antigen, volunteers displayed a marked specific anti-MSP3 antibody response, and anti-native MSP3 antibody response, a T-cell antigen-specific proliferative response and interferon γ production. The potential usefulness of this candidate vaccine is supported by the induction of a strong cytophilic antibody response (IgG1 or IgG3 anti-malaria antibodies). IgG1 or IgG3 are the antibodies found in the blood of protected individuals living in areas where malaria is endemic. Non-protected subjects produce mostly IgG2 and IgM antibodies [60]. MSP3 synthetic peptide induced long lasting immune response and showed strong biological activities against *Plasmodium falciparum* erythrocytic stages in ADCI (antibody-dependent cellular inhibition, [61]. This MSP3 construct is currently being evaluated in Phase IIb clinical trials and results should be available in the near future.

RECOMBINANT SUBUNIT VACCINE CANDIDATES

A list of recombinant subunit *P. falciparum* malaria vaccine candidates that are currently in advanced (Phase II or III) clinical development is given in Table 1[62]. The candidates are based on six parasite proteins (three selected as pre-erythrocytic stage and the other three from asexual blood stage). Table 1 contains fewer antigens than reported as being in clinical development in 2002 by Richie and Saul, since various blood stage antigens on their list have not advanced to Phase II trials, or have been dropped from their list after disappointing results in Phase I or II [63].

More recently, vaccine candidates based on some blood or liver stage antigens listed in Table 1 (MSP1, AMA1, LSA1) have also failed to provide any protective effect in efficacy trials (Phase IIa or IIb, see below). No blood-stage candidate has yet regularly induced biologically active growth-inhibitory antibodies (e.g. those showing good *in vitro* activity in GIA or ADCI assays) that could be correlated with any protective efficacy in these trials. Nevertheless, encouraging results have come from several clinical trials with the CSP-based RTS,S pre-erythrocytic vaccine. Suitably adjuvanted formulations of the RTS,S partially protected adults and children against clinical malaria (see below). However, to produce the RTS,S / AS candidate vaccine, at least 40 clinical trials of CSP-based vaccine candidates of all types – recombinant, synthetic peptide, DNA, virosome/virus-like particle or live-attenuated virus - have been undertaken over a period of over 20 years [64]. At least 10 different adjuvant formulations have also been tested with CSP-derived constructs.

Whether such an extensive clinical programme will need to be undertaken to optimise other vaccine candidates – especially for blood stage vaccines – is an open question. On the one hand, much has been learnt from the CSP programme, particularly about the importance of good adjuvant formulations. On the other hand, while the effectiveness of pre-erythrocytic candidates can easily be determined (ie absence of blood stage infection following challenge with infected mosquito bite), efficacies of blood stage candidates are much more difficult to ascertain as no functional assay has so far been found to objectively and reproducibly correlate with clinical protection in endemic areas. The fact also remains that RTS,S only offers partial protection and the impact on the overall malaria transmission and mortality in high transmission areas will most likely be modest thus warranting the continuous search for a more effective vaccine.

Table 1: Subunit Malaria Vaccine Candidates in Phase II or more advanced Clinical Development

Parasite Antigen / Stage	Vaccine (Parasite Strain)	Lead Developer / Collaboration	Expression System/Adjuvant	Development Phase
CSP / Sporozoite, Liver stage	RTS,S	GSK, MVI, WRAIR	*S. cerevisiae*, HBsAg particles coexpressing CSP / AS01- AS04	IIb / III
LSA1 / Liver stage	FMP011	WRAIR, GSK, MVI	*E. coli* / AS02 or AS01	I/IIa
LSA3 / Sporozoite, Liver stage	LSA3	Institut Pasteur, EMVI	*L. lactis* / alum, Montanide	I/IIa
MSP1 / Blood stage	MSP1-42 FMP-1 (3D7)	WRAIR, GSK	*E. coli* / AS02A	IIb
	MSP1-42 (3D7 & FVO)	NIAID	*E. coli* / alum, CPG7909	I
AMA1 / Blood stage	AMA1 FMP-2.1 (3D7)	WRAIR, GSK	*E.coli* / AS02A	IIb
	AMA1-C1 (3D7 & FVO)	NIAID	*P. pastoris* / alum, Montanide, CPG7909	IIb
	pfAMA-1 (FVO)	BPRC, EMVI	Recombinant protein / alum, Montanide, AS02A	Ib
MSP2 / Blood stage (See footnote)	Combination B (MSP1, MSP2 and RESA mix)	STI	*E. coli* / Montanide	IIb

- Adapted from Vekemans and Ballou [62] and information at the websites http://clinicaltrials.gov and http://www.who.int/vaccine_research/documents/Malaria%20Vaccine%20Rainbow%20Table_Clinical_Oct_2008.pdf

- Combination B is no longer in clinical development, but MSP2 constructs have entered clinical trials (see text)

- AMA: Apical membrane antigen; BPRC: Biomedical Primate Research Centre; CSP: Circumsporozoite surface protein; EMVI: European Malaria Vaccine Initiative; FMP: Falciparum malaria protein; GSK: GlaxoSmithKline; HBsAg: Hepatitis B surface antigen; LSA: Liver-stage antigen; MSP: Merozoite surface protein; MVI: Malaria Vaccine Initiative; NIAID: National Institute for Allergy and Infectious Diseases; pf: *Plasmodium falciparum*; RESA: Ring-stage infected erythrocyte surface antigen; STI: Swiss Tropical Institute; WRAIR: Walter Reed Army Institute of Research.

RTS,S AND THE CS PROTEIN

The RTS,S recombinant protein vaccine being developed by GSK is the product of an extensive and maturing programme [64]. RTS,S is a combination of two polypeptides – RTS (residues 207-395 of the CSP, essentially its repetitive and C-terminal regions, fused to the hepatitis B surface protein) and S (the hepatitis B surface protein alone) – self-assembled during synthesis in yeast to form a virus-like particle. Most of the clinical trials so far were carried out with RTS,S formulated with ASO2 adjuvant, which contains the immunostimulants MPL and QS21 in an oil-in-water emulsion.

In initial Phase I and IIa trials, RTS,S/AS02 was well-tolerated and completely protected about 40% of malaria-naïve volunteers against experimental sporozoite challenge, while delaying onset of parasitemia by two days or more in most of those who became infected. In Phase IIb trials in Gambian adults, RTS,S/AS02 reduced malaria infections by 34% to 47% (depending on the length of surveillance period and the number of injections received). In a larger, double-blind trial, the vaccine reduced first clinical malaria episodes in children (1-4 years old) in Mozambique by 35%, and severe malaria cases by about 50% [4]. This protective effect lasted over a year [65]. In later trials in infants [66,67], first or only malarial infections were reduced by about 65 % over the first three or six months after vaccination. In parallel, Phase IIa trials in the USA suggested that RTS,S formulated with another adjuvant, ASO1, might bemore effective than RTS,S/AS02. AS01 contains the same immunostimulants as AS02, but in a liposomal formulation. The safety and immunogenicity of RTS,S/AS01 in adults and children have been confirmed in Phase Ib trials in various areas of Africa. In a Phase IIb trial undertaken in East Africa [67,68], the efficacy of a pediatric RTS,S/AS01 formulation was somewhat higher (about 50%) than that previously reported for RTS,S/AS02 [65]. However, given the low number of clinical malaria cases reported and the declining rate of infection, the last results reported should be taken with caution [69].

Nevertheless, these results are clearly promising, although long-term studies under different malaria transmission intensities are needed to confirm the efficacies. But the duration of high level immune protection is uncertain and may depend on (among other factors) the persistence of low-level parasitemia in vaccinated individuals; as immunity was reported to wane more rapidly in vaccinated children who were treated when parasitemia was detected at regular examinations, than in those who were treated only if they presented with symptoms of malaria [70]. Another lingering question is the mechanism(s) of protection as the level of protection against clinical malaria in the children in Mozambique was observed not to fall in parallel with levels of antibody to the CSP. The role played by the ASO2 or AS01 adjuvant in the induction of protective immunity is also unknown [64]. Nevertheless, initial Phase IIb clinical trials suggest that an RTS,S-based formulation for infants can successfully be incorporated into the Expanded Programme for Immunisation with standard infant vaccines [67]. On the other hand, as discussed previously, addition of the variant repeat sequence (NVDPNANP)3 in the present RTS,S construct may potentially improve its efficacy. The results of proposed larger Phase III trials with RTS,S/AS01 will be awaited with interest.

LSA1

Recombinant liver stage antigen LSA1 is being developed by WRAIR, with the eventual aim of combining it with RTS,S. There is epidemiological evidence that immune responses to LSA1 correlate with protection against malaria [71]. The LSA1 vaccine candidate FMP011 is produced in *E. coli* and consists of the N-terminal (residues 28-154) and C-terminal (1630-1909) regions of the protein linked by two of the central 17-residue repeats [72]. When formulated with ASO1B, FMP011 was well-tolerated and induced LSA1-specific antibodies and CD4+ T cells in mice and rhesus monkeys [73,74]. However, no protection or delay in onset of parasitemia in vaccinated malaria-naïve volunteers was observed following experimental challenge in a Phase IIa trial [62,75], possibly as a result of insufficient induction of protective CD8+ cells.

MSP1

The large (195 kD) merozoite surface protein MSP1 has been of interest to vaccine developers for some time [62]. Aside from a conserved region near the N-terminus (see next section), most work has targeted the C-terminal 42 kD region ($MSP1_{42}$) of the membrane protein, which is cleaved during erythrocyte invasion leaving a 19kD fragment in a step that is important in the invasion process. While taking into account the genetic polymorphism of $MSP1_{42}$, at least two allelic forms are assumed to be required to achieve good vaccine coverage.

$MSP1_{42}$ from the 3D7 strain, named FMP-1, is being developed by WRAIR/GSK. The protein is expressed in *E. coli* [76]. Its AS02A formulation has been tested in a Phase Ia trial [77] in the USA and Phase Ib trials [78-81] in Kenya and Mali. The vaccine was well-tolerated and immunogenic but antibodies from volunteers immunised in the Phase Ia trial only showed small growth-inhibitory effect (15%) *in vitro*. However, no effect of the vaccine on malaria morbidity was seen in a Phase IIb trial in Kenyan children [81]. Besides the inherent problem of polymorphism associated with this molecule, the vaccine's failure could be attributed to the heterogeneity of the construct with numerous species as determined by SDS-PAGE. Different bands were recognized in Western blot by 2 monoclonal antibodies and the percentage of material recognized by the two antibodies used was not reported [76]. This lack of homogeneity and/ or native 3-dimensional conformation of $MSP1_{42}$ might have contributed to the failure to elicit strong GIA inhibitory antibodies in human volunteers [77].

A separate MSP1-based vaccine candidate with broader cross-reactivity against different MSP1 alleles, referred to FMP010, is also being developed by WRAIR/GSK. It recently entered Phase Ia trials in the USA in a formulation with AS01 adjuvant (http://clinicaltrials.gov/).

At NIAID, the $MSP1_{42}$ proteins from both 3D7 and FVO were expressed in *E. coli* and combined to give a vaccine candidate referred to as $MSP1_{42}$-C1. When formulated with alum and administered to volunteers in a Phase Ia trial, $MSP1_{42}$-C1 was well-tolerated and moderately immunogenic, but induced no growth-inhibitory effect that could be detected by an *in vitro* assay [82]. A separate trial is ongoing to determine whether including CpG 7909 in the formulation would improve the vaccine's immunogenicity (http://clinicaltrials.gov/).

At least two other vaccines containing MSP1-derived recombinant constructs have been tested in humans (see Section on MSP2/Combination B and reference 83). It is however disappointing that the use of adjuvants that are apparently stronger than Alhydrogel (eg Montanide ISA 720) has so far failed to induce high levels of growth-inhibitory antibodies in humans [83].

AMA1

The apical membrane antigen AMA-1 is a genetically polymorphic protein thought to be involved in the invasion of erythrocytes and perhaps also hepatocytes [84]. Prior to invasion, a short N-terminal peptide is cleaved from the 83 kDa protein to produce a of 66 kDa final product which is then exported to the merozoite surface. Correct refolding of much of the 66 kDa product is required to mimic the native protein. At least three different allelic forms of AMA1 are thought to be needed in a vaccine in order to generate functional immune response against most of its polymorphic variants [85].

In a Phase Ia trial of a combination of essentially full-length AMA-1 from parasite strains FVO and 3D7, expressed in *Pichia pastoris* and referred to AMA1-C1 [86], the vaccine was well-tolerated and induced specific antibodies in malaria-naïve volunteers. However, antibody levels were low and very high concentrations of purified IgG (5 or 10 mg/ml) were needed to demonstrate parasite growth inhibition in the GIA. In later Phase Ib trials of AMA-C1/Alhydrogel in Mali, immunogenicity remained a concern. In sera from adults, no growth-inhibitory antibodies were observed [87]; the antibody response in children aged 1 to 4 was also found to be short-lived [88]. In a larger Phase IIb trial, the vaccine induced no significant protective effect against malaria infection [89].

Addition of the adjuvant CpG 7909 to the AMA1-C1 / Alhydrogel formulation significantly improved its immunogenicity, including the ability to induce high titres of growth-inhibitory antibodies in malaria-naïve volunteers [90]. Phase Ib trials of the improved formulation in Malian adults and children are ongoing. A Phase Ia trial of AMA-C1 formulated in Montanide ISA 720 is also underway in the USA (http://clinicaltrials.gov/).

Two other recombinant AMA1 preparations are presently in clinical development. One, designated FMP2.1, is being developed by WRAIR and GSK. The AMA1 protein from 3D7 parasites was expressed in *E. coli* and formulated with AS02A. The vaccine proved safe and immunogenic in a Phase Ia trial [91] and in a Phase Ib trial performed in adults in Mali [92]. Sera from vaccinees in the Phase Ia trial were active in an *in vitro* growth inhibition assay (GIA). However, only very marginal activity in GIA (< 20 %) was observed in sera from vaccinees who received the higher vaccine dose (50 μg) in the Phase Ib trial; sera from those who received half the dose were not demonstrably active in this assay. A Phase IIa (experimental challenge) trial was carried out in the USA using FMP2.1 formulated with either AS02A or AS01 [93]. Although both formulations were immunogenic and induced growth-inhibitory antibodies (giving 30% inhibition of homologous parasite growth at 1:5 serum dilution), no protection or delay in prepatent period was observed after sporozoite challenge. However, a slight but significant reduction in parasitemia, assayed by quantitative PCR, was noted in the FMP2.1/AS02A group. The FMP2.1/AS02A formulation is currently being tested in a Phase I/IIb trial in Malian children (http://clinicaltrials.gov/).

The third AMA1 preparation to enter clinical trials is a construct from the FVO strain (AMA1-FVO (25-545) being developed at the BPRC in Holland. It was expressed in *P. pastoris*, [94], and tested in three formulations (Alum, ASO2 and Montanide ISA 720) in a Phase Ia trial in Nijmegen [95]. Highest antibody levels were induced by the AS02 formulation, but all formulations showed distinct reactogenicity profiles.

MSP2 AND COMBINATIONS A, B

Merozoite surface protein 2 is a genetically polymorphic antigen whose polymorphic variants fall into two families, MSP2-3D7 and MSP2-FC27. 'Combination A' was an alum-adjuvanted mixture of essentially full-length MSP2-3D7 and a recombinant CSP construct. In an early Phase I/IIa trial, it proved only moderately immunogenic and there was no evidence that it could protect against experimental challenge of malaria-naïve volunteers [96]. 'Combination B' was a mixture of MSP1 (a conserved amino-terminal region) with essentially full-length MSP2-3D7 and RESA (C terminal 771 amino acids) antigens, all expressed in *E. coli* and formulated with Montanide ISA 720. The individual proteins and the Combination were immunogenic, without significant antigenic competition (i.e. volunteers receiving a mixture of antigens had similar responses to those receiving the three antigens at separate injection sites). Again no protective effect against experimental challenge of malaria-naïve volunteers was observed in a Phase IIa trial [97].

Nevertheless, Phase Ib/IIb trials of the more immunogenic Combination B were undertaken in Papua New Guinea. In the Phase IIb trial, parasite levels were reduced by a significant 62% in vaccinated children, at least in the group not pre-treated with an anti-malarial drug. However, there was no reduction in episodes of clinical malaria [98,99]. This was later found to be because the vaccine reduced levels of parasites of the 3D7 type of MSP2 while favouring selection of parasites expressing MSP2-FC27 [100,101].

More recent work has therefore progressed towards the development of combination of the two allelic forms of MSP2, either as essentially full-length recombinant proteins or as synthetic peptides. The N-terminal section is involved in formation of fibrils in the full-length protein, followed by a long relatively unstructured region [102,103]. Data on phase Ia trial of combined recombinant proteins (MSP2-C1) are expected in 2010 (http://clinicaltrials.gov/).

LSA3

The gene for liver stage antigen LSA3 was isolated by differential screening of parasite cDNA using antibodies from sporozoite-immunised monkeys and humans. Preclinical development of LSA3 has included studies of synthetic peptides, lipid conjugates and recombinant protein expressed in *E. coli*. The recombinant protein partially protected chimpanzees from *P. falciparum* challenge [104], as did a more recent vaccination with LSA3 DNA [105]. In the latter study, chimpanzees were protected although antibodies to LSA3 protein were undetectable in their sera, which suggests an important role for cytotoxic T cells and/or cytokines in the protective response. A Phase Ia/IIa (safety/efficacy) study in volunteers injected with the recombinant protein is currently underway (http://clinicaltrials.gov/).

FUTURE PERSPECTIVES

If the results obtained in previous trials for RTS,S hold true in the phase III trials, a licensed malaria vaccine may be available in about 5 years or so. The efficacy however may be still limited and the overall impact on malaria transmission in the face of declining malaria-associated morbidity and mortality brought about by increasingly available alternative interventions is unknown. There is also need for more clarification on its mechanism(s) of protection and the exact duration of its sizeable efficacy. Further refinement of the formulation and more investments towards the discovery and evaluation of more efficacious vaccine candidates is thus required.

The selection of candidates to progress into the costly phase II field trials needs to follow a robust and rigorous process in order to avoid wastage of limited resources while providing opportunities for more candidates to get into phase Ia trial. So far it appears that progression into field trials is more often dictated by availability of funds and not necessarily due to fulfillment of promising criteria.

From our point of view the most important criteria are:

1. *in vitro* assessment of immune surrogates of protection associated with the selected immunogens;

2. association with protection;

3. lack or minimal presence of polymorphism and

4. elicitation of a 'protective' (biologically active) immune response in phase I human volunteers as judged by in vitro assays (GIA, ADCI).

Since these conditions are today only met by antigens associated with the erythrocytic stage or live attenuated sporozoites, a major antigen discovery effort should then be concentrated on the erythrocytic stage. Since protection at this stage is mediated by antibodies, it derives that particular attention must be given to the structural properties of the selected antigens. As discussed above, this process can be painstakingly long and not always satisfactory. To avoid such shortcoming and to speed up the discovery step, we concentrate our attention on relatively short structural protein motifs that would fold into the native structure once isolated: the coiled coil α-helical and the intrinsically unstructured domain [106, 107]. The former structure assumes an intertwined helix formed of 2 to 6 strands. The second structure is an ensemble of many short, difficult-to-define conformations in rapidly inter-converting equilibrium. Associated to the structural choice of antigens, we decided to base our down selection preferably on the ADCI. The reasons for this are simple and pragmatic. For antigen associated with GIA activity, assessment of the 3D structure of the antigen is essential, as a unique conformation of the antigen binding region is going to be involved in the interaction with red blood cell counter molecules. In addition, the binding region of the parasite molecule is also likely to be polymorphic in order to evade the immune defense mechanism of the host, as seen for MSP1, AMA1 and PfEMP1 antigens. Instead, in the case of antigens associated with ADCI activity, even though it is not clear what makes them active in ADCI, no relation with biological activity of the molecule is involved and no complex 3D structure recognized by the antibodies is needed (MSP3 constant unstructured segment, MSP2 unstructured dimorphic constant regions, P27A fragment from the novel protein PFF0165c [108] or simple α-helical coiled coil protein fragments). Present understanding of ADCI mechanism indicates that the only requirement needed to be satisfied is the presence of these molecules on the surface of invading merozoites and/or in their vicinity as soluble molecules released during schizont rupture [109]. It seems to us that ADCI based selection procedure gives fewer constraints in the search of new antigens. In fact, all the above-mentioned antigens are targets of an ADCI inhibitory antibody response, which is inactive in GIA [62, 103, 106, 108, 110].

In this regard, it will be interesting to follow the results of future planned clinical trials for AMA1 and MSP2. The former antigen formulated in alhydrogel plus CpG 7909 could elicit a GIA inhibitory response in Phase Ia volunteers [111]. The latter will be tested in a Phase Ia clinical trial as a combination of recombinant 3D7 and FC27 recombinant proteins formulated in ASO2A and alhydrogel.

For pre-erythrocytic stage vaccine candidates, a cut-off of about 50% protection in phase IIa trial will likely reduce number of failures and concomitant waste of resources in field trials.

The recent capacity to predict immunogenicity of vaccine candidates through the detection of naïve CD4 and CD8 T cell populations [112, 113] can potentially speed up antigen discovery. So also can the development of more potent adjuvants and formulations capable of inducing robust humoral and cellular immunity.

Overall, even though the past two decades of malaria vaccine development have been filled with lots of setbacks and modest achievements, the malaria community has learnt invaluable lessons on malaria vaccine development. The future lies in the formation of more effective partnerships and collaborations between the academia and the industry. Funding agencies also need to focus more on creation and standardization of functional assays capable of predicting protection and identification of new vaccine candidates rather than hurrying candidates into costly field trials.

REFERENCES

[1]   Snow RW, Guerra CA, Noor AM, Myint HY, Hay SI. The global distribution of clinical episodes of *Plasmodium falciparum* malaria. Nature 2005; 434: 214-7.
[2]   Greenwood B. Between hope and a hard place. Nature 2004; 430: 926-7.
[3]   Stoute A, Slaoui M, Heppner DG, *et al.* A preliminary evaluation of a recombinant circumsporozoite protein vaccine against *Plasmodium falciparum* malaria, RTS, S Malaria Vaccine Evaluation Group. N Engl J Med 1997; 336: 86-91.
[4]   Alonso PL, Sacarlal J, Aponte JJ, *et al.* Efficacy of the RTS, S/AS02A vaccine against *Plasmodium falciparum* infection and disease in young African children: randomized controlled trial. Lancet 2004; 364: 1411-20.
[5]   Gardner MJ, Hall N, Fung E, *et al.* Genome sequence of the human malaria parasite *Plasmodium falciparum*. Nature 2002; 419: 498-511.
[6]   Dame JB, Williams JL, McCutchan TF, *et al.* Structure of the gene encoding the immunodominant surface antigen on the sporozoite of the human malaria parasite *Plasmodium falciparum*. Science 1984: 225: 593-9.
[7]   Enea V, Ellis J, Zavala F, Arnot DE, Quakyi I, Nussenzweig RS. DNA cloning of *Plasmodium falciparum* circumsporozoite gene: Amino acid sequence of repetitive epitope. Science 1984; 225: 628-30.
[8]   Verdini AS and Pinori M. Composizione peptidica utile per la preparazione di vaccini per la malaria e di kits diagnostici per la determinazione di affezioni malariche. Italian Patent Application 21718 A/85, 25 Luglio 1985.
[9]   Gibson KD and Scheraga HA. Predicted conformations for the immunodominant region of the circumsporozoite protein of the human malaria parasite *Plasmodium falciparum*. Proc Natl Acad Sci USA 1986; 83: 5649-53.
[10]   Brooks BR, Pastor RW and Carson FW. Theoretically determined three-dimensional structure for the repeating tetrapeptide unit of the circumsporozoite coat protein of the malaria parasite *Plasmodium falciparum*. Proc Natl Acad Sci USA 1987; 84: 4470-74.
[11]   Herrington DA, Clyde DF, Losansky G, *et al.* Safety and immunogenicity in man of a synthetic peptide malaria vaccine against *Plasmodium falciparum* sporozoites. Nature 1987; 328: 257-9.
[12]   Nussenzweig V and Nussenzweig RS. Rationale for the development of an engineered sporozoite malaria vaccine. Adv Immunol 1989; 45: 283-334.
[13]   Etlinger HM, Gillessen D, Lahm HW, Matile H, Schönfeld HJ, Trzeciak A. Use of prior vaccinations for the development of new vaccines. Science 1990; 249: 423-5.
[14]   Ballou WR, Hoffman SL, Sherwood JA, *et al.* Safety and efficacy of a recombinant DNA *Plasmodium falciparum* sporozoite vaccine. Lancet 1987; 1: 1277-81.

[15]   Esposito G, Pessi A, Verdini AS. ^{1}H-NMR studies of synthetic polypeptide models of *Plasmodium falciparum* circumsporozoite protein tandemly repeated sequence. Biopolymers 1989; 28: 225-46.

[16]   Dyson HJ, Satterthwait AC, Lerner RA, Wright PE. Conformational preferences of synthetic peptides derived from the immunodominant site of the circumsporozoite protein of *Plasmodium falciparum* by ^{1}H-NMR. Biochemistry 1990; 29: 7828-37.

[17]   Satterthwait AC, Arrhenius T, Hagopian RA, Zavala F, Nussenzweig V, Lerner RA. The conformational restriction of synthetic peptides, including a malaria peptide, for use as immunogens. Phil Trans R Soc Lond B 1989; 323: 565-72.

[18]   Okitsu SL, Kienzl U, Moehle K, *et al.* Structure-activity-based design of a synthetic malaria peptide eliciting sporozoite inhibitory antibodies in a virosomal formulation. Chem Biol 2007; 14: 577-87.

[19]   Etlinger HM, Trzeciak A. Towards a synthetic malaria vaccine: cyclization of a peptide eliminates the production of parasite-unreactive antibody. Phil Trans R Soc Lond B 1993; 340: 69-72.

[20]   Monette M, Opella SJ, Greenwood J, Willis AE, Perham RN. Structure of a malaria parasite antigenic determinant displayed on filamentous bacteriophage determined by NMR spectroscopy: implication for the structure of continous peptide epitopes of proteins. Protein Sci 2001; 10: 1150-9.

[21]   Nanzer D, Torda A, Bisang C, Weber C, Robinson JA, van Gusteren WF. Dynamical studies of peptide motifs in the *Plasmodium falciparum* circumsporozoite surface protein by restrained and unrestrained MD simulations. J Mol Biol 1997; 267: 1012-25.

[22]   Bisang C, Weber C, Inglis I, Bosshard HR, Robinson JA. Stabilization of type I-β turn conformations in peptides containing the NPNA-repeat motif of the *Plasmodium falciparum* circumsporozoite protein by substituting proline for (S)-α-methylproline. J Am Chem Soc 1995; 117: 7904-15.

[23]   Bisang C, Jiang L, Freund E, *et al.* Synthesis, conformational properties and immunogenicity of a cyclic template-bound peptide mimetic containing an NPNA motif from the circumsporozoite protein of *Plasmodium falciparum*. J Am Chem Soc 1998; 120: 7439-49.

[24]   Moreno R, Jiang L, Moehle K, *et al.* Exploiting conformationally constrained peptidomimetics and an efficient human-compatible delivery system in synthetic vaccine design. Chembiochem 2001; 2: 838-43.

[25]   Zurbriggen R. Immunostimulating reconstituted influenza virosomes. Vaccine 2003; 21: 921-24.

[26]   Pfeiffer B, Peduzzi E, Moehle K, *et al.* A virosome-mimotope approach to synthetic vaccine design and optimization: synthesis, conformation, and immune recognition of a potential malaria-vaccine candidate. Angew Chem Int Ed 2003; 42: 2368-71.

[27]   Ghasparian A, Moelhe K, Linden A, Robinson JA. Crystal structure of an NPNA-repeat motif from the circumsporozoite protein of the malaria parasite *Plasmodium falciparum*. Chem Commun 2006; 174-6.

[28]   Genton B, Pluschke G, Degen L, *et al.* A randomized placebo-controlled Phase Ia malaria vaccine trial of two virosome-formulated synthetic peptides in healthy adult volunteers. PloS One 2007; 2: e 1018.

[29]   Okitsu SL, Silvie O, Westerfeld N, *et al.* A virosomal malaria peptide vaccine elicits a long-lasting sporozoite-inhibitory antibody response in a Phase 1a clinical trial. PloS One 2007; 2: e 1278.

[30]   Thompson FM, Porter DW, Okitsu SL, *et al.* Evidence of blood stage efficacy with virosomal malaria vaccine in a Phase IIa clinical trial. PloS One 2008; 3: e 1493.

[31]   Cavanagh DR, Remarque EJ, Sauerwein RW, Hermsen CC, Luty AJF. Influenza virosomes: a flu jab for malaria? Trends Parasitol 2008; 24: 382-5.

[32]   Verdini AS, Chiappinelli L, Zanobi A. Towards the elucidation of the mechanism of attachment and entry of malaria sporozoites into cells: synthetic polypeptides from the circumsporozoite protein of *Plasmodium falciparum* bind Ca^{2+} and interact with model phospholipid membranes. Biopolymers 1991; 31: 587-94.

[33]   Woody RW. Circular dichroism and conformations of unordered polypeptides. Adv Biophys Chem 1992; 2: 37-79.

[34]   Shi Z, Woody RW, Kallenbach NR. Is polyproline II a major backbone conformation in unfolded proteins? Adv Protein Chem 2002; 62: 163-240.

[35]   Rucker AL, Creamer TP. Polyproline II helical structure in protein unfolded states: Lysine peptides revisited. Protein Sci 2002; 11: 980-5.

[36]   Kajava AV, Steven AC. β-rolls, β-helices, and other β-solenoid proteins. Adv Protein Chem 2006; 73: 56-90.

[37]   Hennetin J, Jullian B, Steven AC, Kajava AV. Standard conformations of β-arches in β-solenoid proteins. J Mol Biol 2006; 358: 1094-1105.

[38]   Plassmeyer ML, Reiter K, Shimp Jr RL, *et al.* Structure of the Plasmodium falciparum Circumsporozoite Protein, a Leading Malaria Vaccine Candidate J Biol Chem 2009; 284. 26951-26963.

[39]   Coppi A, Pinzon-Ortiz C, Hutter C, Sinnis P. The Plasmodium circumsporozoite protein is proteolytically processed during cell invasion. J Exp Med 2005; 201: 27-33.

[40]   Del Giudice G, Tougne C, Renia L, *et al.* Characterization of murine monoclonal antibodies against a repetitive peptide from the circumsporozoite protein of the human malaria parasite, *Plasmodium falciparum*. Mol Immunol 1991; 28: 1003-9.

[41]   Padilla JE, Colovos C, Yeates TO. Nanohedra: using symmetry to design self-assembling protein cages, layers, crystals, and filaments. Proc Natl Acad Sci USA 2001; 98: 2217-21.

[42] Raman S, Machaidze G, Lustig A, Aebi U, Burkhardt P. Structure-based design of peptides that self-assemble into regular polyhedral nanoparticles. Nanomedicine: Nanotechol Biol Med 2006; 2: 95-102.

[43] Verdini A, Terenzi S, Brossard V, Roggero M, Corradin G. Oxidative folding of synthetic polypeptides S-protected as *tert*-buthylthio derivatives. J Peptide Sci 2008; 14: 1271-82.

[44] Roggero MA, Meraldi V, López JA, *et al.* The synthetic, oxidized C-terminal fragment of the *Plasmodium berghei* circumsporozoite protein elicits a high protective response. Eur J Immunol. 2000; 30:2679-85.

[45] López JA, Weilenman C, Audran R, *et al.* A synthetic malaria vaccine elicits a potent CD8(+) and CD4(+) T lymphocyte immune response in humans. Implications for vaccination strategies. Eur J Immunol 2001; 31:1989-98. Erratum in: Eur J Immunol 2001;31: 2839.

[46] Audran R, Lurati-Ruiz F, Genton B, *et al.* The synthetic *Plasmodium falciparum* circumsporozoite peptide PfCS102 as a malaria vaccine candidate: a randomized controlled phase I trial. PLoS One 2009; 4: e7304.

[47] Patarroyo ME, Romero P, Torres ML, *et al.* Induction of protective immunity against experimental infection with malaria using synthetic peptides. Nature 1987; 328: 629-32.

[48] Purcell AW, Zeng W, Mifsud NA, Ely LK, Macdonald WA, Jackson DC. Dissecting the role of peptides in immune response: Theory, Practice and the Application to vaccine design. J Peptide Sci 2003; 9: 255-81.

[49] Richardson JS and Richardson DC. Principles and patterns of protein conformation in prediction of protein structure and the principles of protein conformation. Fasman GD Ed. Plenum Press, New York and London, 1989 pp. 1-98.

[50] Cifuentes G, Patarroyo ME, Urquiza M, Ramirez LE, Reyes C, Rodriguez R. Distorting malaria peptide backbone structure to enable fitting into MHC class II molecules renders modified peptides immunogenic and protective. J Med Chem 2003; 46: 2250-53.

[51] Patarroyo ME, Cifuentes G, Vargas LE, Rosas J. Structural modifications enable conserved peptides to fit into MHC molecules thus inducing protection against malaria. ChemBioChem. 2004; 5: 1588-93.

[52] Patarroyo ME, Cifuentes G, Rodriguez R. Structural characterization of sporozoite components for a multistage, multi-epitope, anti-malarial vaccine. Int J Biochem Cell Biol 2008; 40: 543-57.

[53] Patarroyo ME, Patarroyo MA. Emerging rules for subunit-based, multiantigenic, multistage chemically synthesized vaccines. Acc Chem Res 2008; 41: 377-86.

[54] Valero MV, Amador LR, Galindo C, *et al.* Vaccination with Spf 66 a chemically synthesized vaccine, against *Plasmodium falciparum* malaria in Colombia. Lancet 1993; 341: 705-10.

[55] Alonso PL, Smith T, Armstrong Schellenberg JQM, *et al.* Randomized trial of efficacy of Spf 66 vaccine against *Plasmodium falciparum* malaria in children in South Tanzania. Lancet 1994; 344: 1175-81.

[56] Teucher T, Armstrong Schellenberg JQM, *et al.* Spf 66, a chemically synthesized subunit malaria vaccine, is safe and immunogenic in Tanzanians exposed to intense malaria transmission. Vaccine 1994; 12: 328-36.

[57] Alonso PL, Tanner M, Smith T, *et al.* A trial of the synthetic malaria vaccine Spf 66 in Tanzania: rationale and design. Vaccine 1993; 12: 181-6.

[58] Graves P, Gelband H. Vaccines for preventing malaria (Spf 66), Cochrane Database Syst Rev 2006; CD005966.

[59] Audran R, Cachat M, Lurati F, *et al.* Phase I Malaria Vaccine Trial With A Long Synthetic Peptide Derived From The MSP3 Antigen 3. Infect Immun 2005; 73: 8017-26.

[60] Bouharoun-Tayoun H, Druilhe P. *Plasmodium falciparum* malaria: evidence for an isotype imbalance which may be responsible for delayed acquisition of protective immunity. Infect Immun 1992; 60: 1473-81.

[61] Druilhe P, Spertini F, Soe S, *et al.* A malaria vaccine that elicits in humans antibodies able to kill *Plasmodium falciparum*. PLoS Med 2005, e344.

[62] Vekemans J, Ballou WR. *Plasmodium falciparum* malaria vaccines in development. Expert Rev Vaccines 2008; 7: 223-40.

[63] Richie and Saul A. Progress and challenge for malaria vaccine. Nature 2002; 415: 694-701.

[64] Bojang KA. RTS,S/AS02A for malaria. Expert Rev Vaccines 2006; 5: 611-5.

[65] Alonso PL, Sacarlal J, Aponte JJ, *et al.* Duration of protection with RTS,S/AS02A malaria vaccine in prevention of *Plasmodium falciparum* disease in Mozambican children: single-blind extended follow-up of a randomised controlled trial. Lancet 2005; 366: 2012-8.

[66] Aponte JJ, Aide P, Renom M, *et al.* Safety of the RTS,S/AS02D candidate malaria vaccine in infants living in a highly endemic area of Mozambique: a double blind randomised controlled phase I/IIb trial. Lancet 2007; 370: 1543-51.

[67] Abdulla S, Oberholzer R, Juma O, *et al.* Safety and immunogenicity of RTS,S/AS02D malaria vaccine in infants. N Engl J Med 2008; 359: 2533-44.

[68] Bejon P, Lusingu J, Olotu A, *et al.* Efficacy of RTS,S/AS01E vaccine against malaria in children 5 to 17 months of age. N Engl J Med 2008; 359: 2521-32.

[69] Gosling RD, Chadramohan D. RTS,S/AS01E vaccine against malaria. N Engl J Med 2009; 360: 12-13.

[70] Guinovart C, Aponte JJ, Sacarlal J, *et al.* Insights into long-lasting protection induced by RTS,S/AS02A malaria vaccine: further results from a phase IIb trial in Mozambican children PLoS One 2009; 4: e5165.

[71]   Kurtis JD, Hollingdale MR, Luty AJ, *et al*.. Pre-erythrocytic immunity to *Plasmodium falciparum*: the case for an LSA-1 vaccine. Trends Parasitol 2001; 17: 219-23.

[72]   Hillier CJ, Ware LA, Barbosa A,.*et al*. Process development and analysis of liver-stage antigen 1, a preerythrocyte-stage protein-based vaccine for *Plasmodium falciparum*. Infect Immun 2005; 73: 2109-15.

[73]   Pichyangkul S, Kum-Arb U, Yongvanitchit K,.*et al*. Preclinical evaluation of the safety and immunogenicity of a vaccine consisting of *Plasmodium falciparum* liver-stage antigen 1 with adjuvant AS01B administered alone or concurrently with the RTS,S/AS01B vaccine in rhesus primates. Infect Immun 2008; 76: 229-38.

[74]   Brando C, Ware LA, Freyberger H, *et al*.. Murine immune responses to liver-stage antigen 1 protein FMP011, a malaria vaccine candidate, delivered with adjuvant AS01B or AS02A. Infect Immun 2007; 75: 838-45.

[75]   75.Epstein JE, Giersing B, Mullen G, Moorthy V, Richie TL. Malaria vaccines: are we getting closer? Curr Opin Mol Ther 2007; 9: 12-24.

[76]   Angov E, Aufiero BM, Turgeon AM, *et al*. Development and pre-clinical analysis of a *Plasmodium falciparum* Merozoite Surface Protein-1(42) malaria vaccine. Mol Biochem Parasitol 2003; 128: 195-204.

[77]   Ockenhouse CF, Angov E, Kester KE, *et al*. Phase I safety and immunogenicity trial of FMP1/AS02A, a *Plasmodium falciparum* MSP-1 asexual blood stage vaccine. Vaccine 2006; 24: 3009-17.

[78]   Thera MA, Doumbo OK, Coulibaly D, *et al*. Safety and allele-specific immunogenicity of a malaria vaccine in Malian adults: results of a phase I randomized trial. PLoS Clin Trials 2006; 1: e34.

[79]   Withers MR, McKinney D, Ogutu BR, *et al*. Safety and reactogenicity of an MSP-1 malaria vaccine candidate: a randomized phase Ib dose-escalation trial in Kenyan children. PLoS Clin Trials 2006; 1: e32.

[80]   Stoute JA, Gombe J, Withers MR, *et al*. Phase 1 randomized double-blind safety and immunogenicity trial of *Plasmodium falciparum* malaria merozoite surface protein FMP1 vaccine, adjuvanted with AS02A, in adults in western Kenya. Vaccine 2007; 25:176-84.

[81]   Ogutu BR, Apollo OJ, McKinney D, *et al*. Blood stage malaria vaccine eliciting high antigen-specific antibody concentrations confers no protection to young children in Western Kenya. PLoS One 2009; 4: e4708.

[82]   Malkin E, Long CA, Stowers AW, *et al*. Phase 1 study of two merozoite surface protein 1 (MSP1(42)) vaccines for *Plasmodium falciparum* malaria. PLoS Clin Trials1989. 2007;2: e12.

[83]   83 Malkin E, Hu J, Li Z, *et al*. A phase 1 trial of PfCP2.9: an AMA1/MSP1 chimeric recombinant protein vaccine for *Plasmodium falciparum* malaria. Vaccine 2008; 26: 6864-73.

[84]   Silvie O, Franetich JF, Charrin S, *et al*. A role for apical membrane antigen 1 during invasion of hepatocytes by *Plasmodium falciparum* sporozoites. J Biol Chem 2004; 279: 9490-6.

[85]   Remarque EJ, Faber BW, Kocken CH, Thomas AW. Apical membrane antigen 1: a malaria vaccine candidate in review. Trends Parasitol 2008; 24: 74-84.

[86]   Malkin EM, Diemert DJ, McArthur JH, *et al*. Phase 1 clinical trial of apical membrane antigen 1: an asexual blood-stage vaccine for *Plasmodium falciparum* malaria. Infect Immun 2005; 73: 3677-85.

[87]   Dicko A, Diemert DJ, Sagara I, *et al*. Impact of a *Plasmodium falciparum* AMA1 vaccine on antibody responses in adult Malians. PLoS One 2007; 2: e1045.

[88]   Dicko A, Sagara I, Ellis RD, *et al*. Phase 1 study of a combination AMA1 blood stage malaria vaccine in Malian children. PLoS One 2008; 3: e1563.

[89]   Sagara I, Dicko A, Ellis RD, *et al*. A randomized controlled phase 2 trial of the blood stage AMA1-C1/Alhydrogelmalaria vaccine in children in Mali. Vaccine 2009; 27: 3090-8.

[90]   Ellis RD, Mullen GE, Pierce M, *et al*. A Phase 1 study of the blood-stage malaria vaccine candidate AMA1-C1/Alhydrogel((R)) with CPG 7909, using two different formulations and dosing intervals. Vaccine 2009; 27: 4104-9.

[91]   Polhemus ME, Magill AJ, Cummings JF, *et al*. Phase I dose escalation safety and immunogenicity trial of *Plasmodium falciparum* apical membrane protein (AMA-1) FMP2.1, adjuvanted with AS02A, in malaria-naïve adults at the Walter Reed Army Institute of Research. Vaccine 2007; 25: 4203-12.

[92]   Thera MA, Doumbo OK, Coulibaly D, *et al*. Safety and immunogenicity of an AMA-1 malaria vaccine in Malian adults: results of a phase 1 randomized controlled trial. PLoS One. 2008; 3: e1465.

[93]   Spring MD, Cummings JF, Ockenhouse CF, *et al*. Phase 1/2a study of the malaria vaccine candidate apical membrane antigen-1 (AMA-1) administered in adjuvant system AS01B or AS02A. PLoS One 2009; 4: e5254.

[94]   Kocken CH, Withers-Martinez C, Dubbeld MA, *et al*. High-level expression of the malaria blood-stage vaccine candidate *Plasmodium falciparum* apical membrane antigen 1 and induction of antibodies that inhibit erythrocyte invasion. Infect Immun 2002; 70: 4471-6.

[95]   Roestenberg M, Remarque E, de Jonge E, *et al*. Safety and immunogenicity of a recombinant *Plasmodium falciparum* AMA1 malaria vaccine adjuvanted with Alhydrogel, Montanide ISA 720 or AS02. PLoS One 2008; 3: e3960.

[96]   Sturchler D, Berger R, Rudin C, *et al*. Safety, immunogenicity, and pilot efficacy of *Plasmodium falciparum* sporozoite and asexual blood-stage combination vaccine in Swiss adults. Am J Trop Med Hyg 1995; 53: 423-31.

[97]   Saul A, Lawrence G, Smillie A, *et al*. Human phase I vaccine trials of 3 recombinant asexual stage malaria antigens with Montanide ISA720 adjuvant. Vaccine 1999; 17: 3145-59.

[98]   Genton B, Betuela I, Felger I, *et al*. A recombinant blood-stage malaria vaccine reduces *Plasmodium falciparum* density and exerts selective pressure on parasite populations in a phase 1-2b trial in Papua New Guinea. J Infect Dis 2002; 185: 820-7.

[99]   Graves P, Gelband H. Vaccines for preventing malaria (blood-stage). Cochrane Database Syst Rev 2006; (4): CD006199.

[100] Flück C, Smith T, Beck HP, *et al*. Strain-specific humoral response to a polymorphic malaria vaccine. Infect Immun 2004; 72: 6300-5.

[101] Flück C, Schöpflin S, Smith T, *et al*. Effect of the malaria vaccine Combination B on merozoite surface antigen 2 diversity. Infect Genet Evol 2007; 7: 44-51.

[102] Yang X, Adda CG, Keizer DW, *et al*. A partially structured region of a largely unstructured protein, *Plasmodium falciparum* merozoite surface protein 2 (MSP2), forms amyloid-like fibrils. J Pept Sci 2007; 13: 839-48.

[103] Zhang X, Perugini MA, Yao S, *et al*. Solution conformation, backbone dynamics and lipid interactions of the intrinsically unstructured malaria surface protein MSP2. J Mol Biol 2008; 379: 105-21.

[104] Daubersies P, Thomas AW, Millet P, *et al*. Protection against *Plasmodium falciparum* malaria in chimpanzees by immunization with the conserved pre-erythrocytic liver-stage antigen 3. Erratum in: Nat Med 2000; 6: 1412. Mohamed LB [corrected to BenMohamed L]. Comment in: Nat Med 2000; 6: 1218-9.

[105] Daubersies P, Ollomo B, Sauzet JP, *et al*. Genetic immunisation by liver stage antigen 3 protects chimpanzees against malaria despite low immune responses. PLoS One. 2008; 3: e2659.

[106] Villard V, Agak G, Frank G, *et al*. Rapid identification of malaria vaccine candidates based on alpha-helical coil protein motif. PLoS One. 2, e645.

[107] Corradin G, Villard V, Kajava A. Protein structure based strategies for antigen discovery and vaccine development against malaria and other pathogens. Endocr Metab Immune Disord Drug Targets 2007; **7**, 259-65.

[108] Olugbile S, Kulangara C, Bang G, *et al*. Vaccine potentials of an intrinsically unstructured fragment derived from the blood stage associated *P. falciparum* protein PFF0165c. Infect Immun 2009; 77, 5701-9.

[109] Jafarshad A, Dziegiel MH, Lundquist R, Nielsen LK, Singh S, Druilhe PL. A novel antibody-dependent cellular cytotoxicity mechanism involved in defense against malaria requires costimulation of monocytes FcgammaRII and FcgammaRIII. J Immunol 2007; 178: 3099-106.

[110] Flueck C, Frank G, Smith T, *et al*. Evaluation of two long synthetic merozoite surface protein 2 peptides as malaria vaccine candidates. Vaccine 2009; 27 :2653-61.

[111] Mullen GE, Ellis RD, Miura K, *et al*. Phase 1 trial of AMA1-C1/Alhydrogel plus CPG 7909: an asexual blood-stage vaccine for *Plasmodium falciparum* malaria. PLoS One 2008; 3: e2940.

[112] Moon JJ, Chu HH, Pepper M, McSorley SJ, Jameson SC, Kedl RM, Jenkins MK Naive CD4(+) T cell frequency varies for different epitopes and predicts repertoire diversity and response magnitude. Immunity 2007; 27: 179-80.

[113] Kotturi MF, Scott I, Wolfe T, *et al*. Naive precursor frequencies and MHC binding rather than the degree of epitope diversity shape CD8+ T cell immunodominance. J Immunol 2008; 181: 2124-33.

CHAPTER 4

Progress Toward the Development of a *Plasmodium Vivax* Malaria Vaccine

Sócrates Herrera* and Myriam Arévalo-Herrera

Centro Internacional de Vacunas, AA 26020, Cali, Colombia and Immunology Institute, Universidad del Valle, AA 25574, Cali, Colombia

Abstract: It is currently estimated that a total of 2.6 billion people live at a permanent risk of suffering malaria infection worldwide, and that 80-300 million experience *Plasmodium vivax* infections every year mostly in areas outside Africa. The increasing *P. vivax* drug resistance and recent reports of severe and lethal cases, the relapsing parasite behavior and the existence of *Plasmodium spp.* co-infections must prompt more investment and greater efforts for the development of a *P. vivax* vaccine. Because of funding shortage and technical difficulties, currently there are only two *P. vivax* vaccine candidates being tested in clinical trials and few others are being assessed in preclinical studies which contrast with the numerous *P. falciparum* vaccine candidates under evaluation. However, the recent availability of the *P. vivax* genome and ongoing proteomic analysis are likely to accelerate *P. vivax* vaccine development. Additionally, recent development of human sporozoite-challenge models would contribute to move clinical development forward and to identify mechanisms of immunity.

THE BURDEN OF *PLASMODIUM VIVAX* MALARIA

It is currently calculated that approximately 2.6 billion inhabitants from about 100 countries are exposed to infection by one or more of five malaria parasite species that could affect humans, resulting in 250-500 million malaria clinical cases every year. Therefore, malaria represents one of the major global public health problems that prevents social and economic development of vast areas of the tropical regions of the world [1, 2].

Although *P. falciparum* is the most abundant and virulent malaria species, *P. vivax,* which is the second most prevalent species, is also widely spread and coexists with *P. falciparum* in many endemic regions that include Southeast and East Asia, the Eastern Mediterranean region and Central and South America [3, 4]. Whereas in these regions *P. vivax* is highly prevalent, in the African continent it is limited to a few countries of the Eastern region of the continent where the population displays a higher prevalence of the Duffy (Fy) blood group than in sub-Saharan Africa [5, 6]. The Duffy blood group antigen (Fy) expressed on the erythrocytes surface has been shown to serve as a receptor for invasion by *P. vivax* [7].

It is estimated that *P. vivax* produces 80 to 300 million clinical cases per year [8], and although it is accepted that this species produces significantly less mortality than *P. falciparum*, it produces a very incapacitating disease with frequent development of parasite relapses. Recent studies have reported an increasing number of severe and complicated malaria cases resulting from *P. vivax* infections suggesting that this parasite may not be as benign as previously thought [9-11]. These epidemiological figures represent a great burden for tropical countries that translate into huge economic losses [12].

For the last six decades, malaria has been the target of intense campaigns aimed at eradicating parasite transmission through the application of vector control measures and the use of chemotherapy [13]. Although the areas with malaria transmission were reduced during the last decades, the number of cases has significantly increased worldwide during this period [3]. Countries located in the most northern and southern regions of the planet have eliminated malaria transmission whereas the number of malaria cases in tropical countries has increased [14], although the same control tools and strategies have been used in all regions. Most likely, measures such as sanitation and probably climate and other factors have contributed to malaria elimination in some areas but have made it difficult in others [3]. Among the most limiting factors making malaria eradication difficult are the emergence of mosquito strains resistant to insecticides [8] and the development and rapid spreading of parasite strains resistant to anti-malarial drugs [15]. In this regard, since a first report of *P. vivax* resistance to chloroquine in Papua New Guinea (PNG) in late 80s, an increasing number of reports of *P. vivax* resistance to first line anti-malarial drugs in Asia and Latin America have appeared [16, 17]. Moreover, the emergence of *P. vivax* strains with lower sensitivity to primaquine, the only drug currently available to prevent *P. vivax* relapses, has been reported [18]. Deterioration of social and economic conditions as well as demographic and political instability in some endemic countries

*Corresponding Author: Sócrates Herrera, Centro Internacional de Vacunas, Immunology Institute, Universidad del Valle, AA 25574, Cali, Colombia; Tel: (572) 557 4929; Fax: (572) 557 49 21; E-mail: sherrera@inmuno.org

Emilio Jirillo (Ed)
All rights reserved - © 2010 Bentham Science Publishers Ltd.

renders malaria control more difficult, by leading to disruption of health services and the reappearance of malaria outbreaks in regions where transmission had been eliminated.

Fortunately during the last two decades, there have been considerable efforts to develop new malaria control strategies. Recently, a significant increase in funding for malaria control has been experienced, reaching an estimated US$ 1.5 billion in 2008, with a significant amount directed to R&D, and around 60% spent on discovery and development of antimalarial drugs and vaccines. WHO/TDR and IVR programs have initiated intensive work to implement selective and sustainable prevention measures by strengthening local research capacities, and community participation in malaria endemic countries and it is estimated that the Global Fund and the Andean Health Organism programs have also increased global financing for intervention for HIV, TB and Malaria by USD 1.1 billion [19, 20].

RATIONALE FOR A *P. VIVAX* VACCINE

Although development of malaria vaccines has proven to be difficult, it is currently accepted that if developed they could represent a valuable complementary tool for future malaria elimination and eradication activities. Individuals permanently exposed to malaria in endemic regions eventually develop milder clinical manifestations or even asymptomatic infections, reflecting a significant degree of clinical immunity, that although does not completely prevent infection, significantly diminishes or abolishes the undesirable malaria symptoms. Although these asymptomatic infections may significantly contribute to perpetuate malaria transmission in endemic areas, clinical immunity of these communities greatly contributes to decrease the economical burden of the disease, and provides indirect evidence for malaria immune protection and therefore for the feasibility of developing a malaria vaccine [21, 22].

A number of other evidences from clinical studies suggest that a prophylactic malaria vaccine for humans is possible. Firstly, immunization of human malaria-naïve volunteers with malaria sporozoites attenuated by radiation exposure has been shown to confer sterile protection against experimental infection following laboratory-bred, sporozoite-infected mosquito bites [23, 24]. Secondly, naturally acquired immunity progressively builds up during the first two decades of life in children or in adult people permanently living in malaria endemic regions. This immunity primarily impacts the disease severity, and appears to be linked to continuous antigenic stimulation, waning rapidly in the absence of exposure [25, 26]. Thirdly, passive transfer of hyper-immune immuno-globulins from malaria-immune adults into malaria-naïve human volunteers has been shown to clear blood stage parasites [27]. Fourthly, malaria-naïve volunteers and subjects from malaria endemic communities may be partially protected by vaccination with the RTS,S vaccine, a recombinant *P. falciparum* vaccine candidate based on the circumsporozoite protein (CSP) [28-30].

Three parasite stages of the complex life cycle of *Plasmodium*, have been identified as potential targets for effective anti-parasite immune responses: the pre-erythrocytic phase of development which is the first one to occur in the human host and takes place without clinical manifestations would be ideal to block the infection and prevent the disease; the asexual phase that occurs only during parasite development in the blood circulation is associated with the clinical manifestations, therefore, vaccines targeting this phase would diminish or prevent the malaria clinical manifestations. Parasite sexual reproduction takes place into the mosquito midgut, then, vaccines targeting this phase would block parasite transmission from the malaria patient to the mosquito [31].

The proposed mechanisms for vaccine elicited immunity at the different stages include: 1) at the pre-erythrocytic stage, antibody-mediated blockage of hepatocyte invasion by sporozoites [32] and inhibition of development of liver stage schizonts; 2) at the asexual erythrocytic stage, antibody-mediated blockage of erythrocyte invasion by merozoites and arrest of development of blood stage schizonts by soluble immune mediators or antibodies [33]; and 3) during parasite sexual development, antibody-mediated blockage fertilization and further development in the mosquito midgut [34].

Because of the complex parasite life cycle and the co-existence of *falciparum* and *vivax* parasites in most malaria endemic regions around the world, it is accepted that a multi-antigen and multi-species vaccine should be developed for most endemic regions, as both parasite species display unique biological characteristics [34].

Besides the multiple parasite differences, due to the lack of *P. vivax in vitro* cultures and other technical limitations, most research towards developing a vaccine for this species has focused on orthologs of *P. falciparum* antigens. *P. vivax* antigens such as those corresponding to CSP, merozoite surface protein-1 (MSP-1), and from the 25 kD oocyst/ookinete surface protein (*Pv*s25) that are being developed as vaccines are based on studies on orthologs in *P. falciparum* [35]. However, the recent availability of the *P. vivax* genome and current possibilities for proteomic analyses are likely to accelerate *P. vivax* vaccine development [36]. In this regard, significant progress is presently being made by exploration of the *P. vivax* genome and proteome in search of antigens with vaccine potential. Development of high-throughput methods for *P. vivax* transfection and platforms for population diversity and genetic structure studies is currently ongoing [37, 38].

CURRENT STATUS OF *P. VIVAX* VACCINE DEVELOPMENT

The first evidence to support development of a protective malaria vaccine was obtained nearly four decades ago, when immunization experiments performed both in animals and human subjects using radiation attenuated malaria sporozoites provided sterile protection [39]. Additionally, these preliminary studies provided reagents to identify parasite components expressed during the pre-erythrocytic phase of development [24, 39] and both recombinant DNA technology and peptide synthesis have provided novel approaches to vaccine discovery and development for more than two decades. Using these means significant progress has been made in identifying parasite components that may be targets of protective immune response and therefore useful for vaccine development [40]. Currently more than 70 *P. falciparum* vaccine formulations composed of different antigens are under development and 23 of these are undergoing clinical testing [41, 42]. These include antigens that are expressed on sporozoite surface (CSP, SSP2/TRAP) [43], liver stages (LSA1, LSA3, EXP1), asexual blood stages (MSP-1, MSP-2, AMA-1), and sexual stages (*Pf*s25, *Pf*s45/48). The majority of these antigens have been identified by screening genomic and cDNA expression libraries with immune sera and monoclonal antibodies.

P. vivax vaccine development has been difficult due to both technical restrictions and the lack of funding support. Establishment of continuous *in vitro* culture systems has been a limiting factor for *in vitro* testing of potential vaccine candidates. *P. vivax* merozoites have a great selectivity for immature red cells (reticulocytes) that are scarce (<1%) in normal human blood and rapidly become mature erythrocytes in culture conditions; therefore until a permanent supply of reticulocytes e.g. from erythroid stem cells is developed, this technical restriction is likely to significantly limit *P. vivax* vaccine progress. However, as a consequence of the recent initiative to focus efforts on the goal of malaria elimination, the need for a vaccine for *P. vivax* malaria starts being recognized [44-46].

Despite these two major constraints, several *P. vivax* proteins homologous to known *P. falciparum* proteins from different stages of the parasite life cycle have been identified [34]. Two of these *P. vivax* proteins, the pre-erythrocytic CSP and the oocyst/ookinete *Pv*s25 proteins have been tested in Phase I clinical trials [47-49], whereas others have been tested in pre-clinical studies to evaluate their vaccine potential [50-57]. The current *P. vivax* vaccine candidates are outlined in Table 1.

PRE-ERYTHROCYTIC VACCINES

It is currently considered that malaria burden could be most efficiently reduced by vaccines that either prevent infection or prevent transmission; and a pre-erythrocytic vaccine has the potential to achieve both goals [58]. This vaccine would prevent sporozoites entry into hepatocytes and therefore inhibit their development into tissue schizonts, or alternatively, it could target antigens expressed during liver schizogony that are expected to induce cellular immune responses that inhibit intracellular parasite maturation. In both cases, the vaccine would arrest the infection before initiation of clinical symptoms and because no sexually differentiated parasites are developed, it would also prevent further parasite transmission to mosquito. Such a vaccine would also be ideal for *P. vivax* if it could inhibit the development of hypnozoites, the parasite forms that are responsible for the relapsing nature of the infection. Although sterile immunity has been achieved by vaccination of humans using *P. falciparum* [24] and *P. vivax* [23] radiation attenuated sporozoites, the mechanisms of protection are poorly understood. Currently, it is accepted that antibodies would mainly block sporozoite invasion and that cytokines may contribute to intracellular parasite killing, together leading to protection. It has been proposed that interleukin 12 (IL-12) produced by macrophages, dendritic cells, and Kupffer cells induces CD8+ T cells and natural killer (NK) cells to produce interferon-gamma (IFN-γ) that in turn activate hepatocytes to produce reactive metabolic intermediates, e.g. nitric oxide, that are toxic to intra-hepatic parasites [21, 59, 60]. Although multiple *P. falciparum* pre-erythrocytic vaccine candidates have been identified and are being tested in pre-clinical and clinical studies, only two *P. vivax* sporozoite antigens have been identified, namely, CSP and sporozoite surface protein 2 (SSP2/ TRAP).

Table 1: *Plasmodium vivax* vaccine candidates from the different parasite life cycle stages.

Parasite Stage	Antigen	Phase	Formulation	References
Sporozoite	CSP[a]-N	Phase I	Peptides in Montanide ISA 720/ISA 51	[47, 52, 72]
	CSP-R	Phase I		
	CSP-C	Phase I		
	SSP2/TRAP[b]	Preclinical	Peptide in Montanide ISA 720	[76]
Merozoite	MSP[c]-1p(19)	Preclinical (*Saimiri/Callithrix*)	Rec. protein in Alum/Freund	[100, 101]
	MSP-1p(42)	Preclinical (*Rhesus*)	Rec. protein in Montanide ISA 720	[104]
	MSP-1(200L)	Preclinical (*Aotus l.*)	Rec. protein in Montanide ISA 720	[79]
	MSP-3	Preclinical (*Saimiri*)	Rec. protein in Freund adjuvant	[50]
	MSP-9	Preclinical (mice)	Rec. protein in Montanide ISA 51	[84]
	PvRAP2	Preclinical (*Aotus n.*)	Rec. protein in Freund/Alum	[57]
	RBP-1/2	Preclinical (*Saimiri*)	Rec. protein	[50]
	DBP[d]-RII	Preclinical (*Aotus l., Rhesus*)	Rec. protein in Montanide/ Alum/ ASO2	[82, 93]
	AMA[e]-1	Preclinical (*Rhesus*)	Rec. protein in SBAS2	[108]
Sexual stages	Pvs25	Phase I	Rec. protein in Alum/ Montanide ISA 51	[48, 49]
	Pvs28	Preclinical (mice)	Rec. protein in Alum	[116]
Combined antigens	CSP, SSP2, AMA-1, MSP-1	Preclinical	DNA	[56]
	CSP, MSP-1, AMA-1, Pvs24	Preclinical (mice)	Peptides in CpG ODN	[54]
	DBP-RII, MSP-1p(19)	Preclinical (mice)	Rec. proteins in Montanide ISA 720	[55]
	MSP-1 p(19)/p(42)	Preclinical (mice)	Rec. proteins in Montanide/ASO2A	[102]

[a]**CSP**: Circumsporozoite Protein, [b]**SSP2/TRAP**: Sporozoite Surface Protein 2/Thrombospondin Related Adhesive Protein, [c]**MSP**: Merozoite Surface Protein, [d]**DBP**: Duffy Binding Protein, [e]**AMA**: Apical Membrane Antigen

P. Vivax Circumsporozoite Protein

The *P. vivax* CSP is one of the most extensively studied antigens and is considered to be a leading malaria vaccine candidate. It is composed of an immuno-dominant central repeat domain displaying either of the dimorphic forms denoted VK210 and VK-247 [61, 62]. In addition, non-repetitive flanking amino (N) and carboxyl (C) regions contain highly conserved sequences, namely, Region I (85-89aa) and Region II-plus (338-355aa). Antibodies targeting Region II-plus block hepatocyte invasion by sporozoites [63, 64]. A *P. vivax* recombinant CSP (rPvCS-1) demonstrated to induce high neutralizing antibody responses in mice [65] and was proposed as vaccine candidate. However, two clinical trials carried out subsequently with this recombinant protein, did not induce significant immune responses to justify further development [66, 67]. More recently another chimeric recombinant *P. vivax* CSP containing a central repeat region composed of both VK210 and VK247 was produced in *E. coli* and different formulations in Montanide ISA 720, Montanide ISA 51 and incomplete Freund's adjuvants were highly immunogenic in BALB/c mice [68].

During the same period, important efforts were concentrated on the immune characterization of CSP, with the aim of rationally designing a vaccine [52]. After identifying multiple B, T-helper and CD8+ T cell epitopes [69-71], three long synthetic peptides (LSP) corresponding to the N-terminal and C-terminal regions as well as to the central repeat domain (peptide R) were produced and tested for antigenicity in humans and immunogenicity in animals [72]. The latter studies carried out in *Aotus* monkeys, indicated that the three LSP formulated in Freund's adjuvant and Montanide ISA 720, induced vigorous humoral responses with antibodies recognizing not only the native protein on sporozoites but also displaying the same fine specificity as that induced by natural exposure of humans to malaria. Peptides also stimulated *in vitro* production of IFN-γ by *Aotus* peripheral blood mononuclear cells (PBMC) [73].

Given the consistently high immunogenicity of CSP in non-human primates, as well as its recognition by sera and immune cells from naturally exposed individuals [72], CSP was taken up for clinical development. Two Phase I clinical trials have been conducted by the Malaria Vaccine and Drug Development Center (MVDC) in Cali, Colombia to evaluate safety and immunogenicity of the vaccine. In the first trial a total of 69 malaria-naïve volunteers were vaccinated three times with escalating doses of 10, 30, and 100 µg of the *P. vivax* CS-derived N, R and C polypeptides formulated in Montanide ISA 720 [47]. The vaccines were well tolerated and no serious adverse events were reported. Peptides N and R elicited stronger humoral responses than peptide C. Antibodies to the three peptides recognized *P. vivax* sporozoites in immunofluorescence antibody tests (IFAT) and PBMCs from most immunized volunteers also produced IFN-γ upon *in vitro* peptide stimulation [47].

Although in the preclinical studies both BALB/c mice and *Aotus* monkeys indicated that the vaccine was immunogenic, interestingly mice developed the highest specific IgG antibody titer to the C peptide, whereas monkeys responded preferentially to the N peptide in response to the same vaccine formulation. In a second Phase I clinical trial using combinations of the three LSPs formulated in Montanide ISA 720 and in Montanide ISA 51 indicated that vaccination was safe, well tolerated and adverse events reported were similar to those described previously [47, 74]. After three vaccination doses, sero-conversion occurred in >90% of the vaccinees and antibodies that lasted for about a year recognized the sporozoite protein in immunofluorescence assays and were able to partially block sporozoite invasion into hepatoma cell lines *in vitro*. Volunteers presented better antibody response to vaccines formulated in Montanide ISA 51 and all three peptides stimulated the production of IFN-γ both in the animal models and in human. Both adjuvants stimulated the production of high antibody levels that lasted for up to 1 year. These results encourage further testing of the vaccine protective efficacy in Phase II trials.

Sporozoite Surface Protein 2 (SSP2/TRAP)

The *Pv*SSP2/*Pv*TRAP protein belongs to the trans-membrane TRAP/MIC2 protein family that is present in the micronemes and on the surface of both sporozoites and liver-stage parasites, and mediates adhesion to host cells and tissue surfaces, directing parasite motility and cell invasion [65]. *P. vivax* SSP2/TRAP contains a single copy of the cell adhesive motif CSVTCG that is highly conserved among all malaria CSP and one copy of a thrombospondin-like sulfatide-binding domain used by the sporozoite for hepatocyte invasion [75]. The vaccine potential of *P. vivax* SSP2/TRAP has been tested in mice and monkeys, inducing high levels of specific antibodies [56]. More recently, a synthetic peptide-derived from a conserved region of the TRAP protein located in N-terminal region (209-256aa), and formulated in Montanide ISA 720, proved to be immunogenic and provided partial protection against challenge of *Aotus* monkeys with *P. vivax* sporozoites [76].

ASEXUAL BLOOD STAGE VACCINES

Asexual blood stage vaccines are aimed at preventing clinical manifestation and severity of malaria infection, therefore reducing mortality and morbidity. During the erythrocytic stage of *P. vivax* merozoites released from liver schizonts, invade reticulocytes where they multiply by schizogeny to yield 20-30 new merozoites. Because invasion by *P. vivax* merozoites is restricted to reticulocytes, peak parasitemia is usually lower than 1%, however, the intensity of clinical symptoms can be highly incapacitating. Similar to *P. falciparum,* clinical manifestations induced by *P. vivax* infection decrease after repeated exposure to infection in endemic areas due to development of protective immune responses that control parasitemia and protect against clinical disease [12]. The mechanisms of protection include inhibition of invasion by antibodies against merozoite proteins, enhancement of phagocytosis by antibodies that recognize merozoite surface, antibody-dependent cellular inhibition; antibody-dependent neutralization of malarial toxins produced during schizont rupture [77] and release of cytokines such as IFN-γ [78].

Multiple asexual *P. vivax* parasite antigens have been identified and immunologically characterized. Although the Duffy binding protein (DBP) and merozoite surface protein 1 (MSP-1) have received the most attention [79-82] several other antigens from the asexual blood stages (MSP-3, MSP-4, MSP-5, MSP-9, RBP, *Pv*RAP2) have been identified, expressed as recombinant products [83, 84] and partially characterized [50, 57, 85] for function and individual or combine vaccine potential [54, 55].

Duffy Binding Protein

P. vivax merozoites require interaction with the Duffy blood group antigen for reticulocyte invasion. As a result, individuals who lack the Duffy antigen are protected from blood stage infection by *P. vivax*. The parasite ligand, located within the micronemes of *Plasmodium* merozoites [7], which bind the Duffy antigen are functionally conserved and belong to a family of Erythrocyte Binding Proteins (EBP) that includes *P. vivax* and *P. knowlesi* DBPs [86]. The binding domains which are located in region II, a N-terminal cysteine-rich region, is polymorphic suggesting that it is under immune pressure [87], however, sequence analysis demonstrates that the receptor binding residues within *Pv*RII are highly conserved [88].

Because *P. knowlesi* and *P. vivax* DBPs share homology that is greater than 70%, the three dimensional structure of the *P. knowlesi* region II, can be used to model the structure of *Pv*RII [89]. Serological studies in children in Mugil, a *P. vivax* endemic region of Papua New Guinea [90] appear to confirm the prediction based on the structural model. In this study, most children had high antibody titers against *Pv*RII, some of which had high titer binding inhibitory antibodies. The sera from these children blocked binding of 5 *Pv*RII polymorphic domains with similar efficiency, indicating that these binding inhibitory antibodies are strain transcending and were associated with protection against *P. vivax* infection [91]. Immunization with recombinant *Pv*RII elicits high titer binding inhibitory antibodies that block the binding of *Pv*RII with erythrocytes [81]. The binding inhibitory titers of vaccine elicited antibodies are significantly higher than naturally acquired antibodies providing support for the development of a vaccine based on *Pv*RII. Methods to produce recombinant *Pv*RII for use in clinical trials have been developed [81, 92] and pre-clinical studies to identify an optimum adjuvant formulation for clinical development are currently underway.

Immunization of *Aotus* monkeys with the *Pv*RII formulated in Freund's adjuvant and in Montanide ISA 720 indicated high immunogenicity [82]. Freund's formulation yielded higher ELISA antibody titers and offered partial protection against intravenous challenge of animals with *P. vivax* asexual blood forms. Animals immunized with *Pv*RII vaccine had a longer prepatent period and lower parasitemias compared to control animals. Although the Montanide ISA 720 formulation was immunogenic, it did not induce any protection [82]. Strong and sustained antibody responses were obtained in *Rhesus* monkeys immunized with this protein formulated with Alum, AS02 or Montanide ISA 720 [93].

Merozoite Surface Protein 1 (MSP-1)

MSP-1 is expressed abundantly on the merozoite surface and is the target of naturally acquired antibody responses following exposure to infection [94]. Immunization with MSP-1 has been shown to provide protection in animal models [95, 96].

P. vivax MSP-1 (*Pv*200) is a polymorphic protein that consists of several conserved and dimorphic domains designated interspecies conserved blocks (ICBs) [97]. Several studies have demonstrated the high antigenicity of different regions of this protein in Brazil (*Pv*MSP-1 N- and C-Terminal regions) [98, 99], and Colombia (*Pv*200L) [79]. These studies, together with the diverse protective efficacy observed in preclinical vaccine trials using *P. falciparum* recombinant MSP-1$_{42}$ and MSP-1$_{19}$ proteins, stimulated the study of *P. vivax* MSP-1$_{19}$ in *Saimiri boliviensis* [79, 100-104], and the same MSP-1 fragment from *P. cynomolgy* in *Macaca sinica*. Partial protection was observed in the first study and effective protection was achieved in the second trial [80, 105]. A *P. vivax* MSP-1 fragment *Pv*200L defined by homology to *Pf*190L was produced as a recombinant protein in *E. coli* and was found to be highly immunogenic in BALB/c mice and *Aotus* monkeys [79]. Primates immunized with recombinant *Pv*200L formulated in Montanide ISA 720 showed strong antibody responses that recognized parasite antigens in western blot and immunofluorescence assays. Immunized animals were partially protected against *P. vivax* infectious challenge as determined by lower parasitemia, reduced anemia and spontaneous parasite clearance [79]. Further studies are required to assess which MSP-1 fragment has greater vaccine potential.

Apical Membrane Antigen 1 (AMA-1)

AMA-1 in micronemes and translocates to the surface of merozoites during invasion of erythrocytes. It is expressed as an 83 kDa product in *P. falciparum* or as a 66 kDa in all other species studied with considerable conservation of primary and predicted secondary amino-acid structures [33]. AMA-1 plays a role in apical reorientation of merozoites following initial attachment during invasion. By proteomic analysis the protein was also found to be expressed in sporozoites, and together with TRAP, appears to be involved in hepatocyte invasion [106]. *Pv*AMA-1 is recognized by sera from naturally-exposed individuals [107]. Monoclonal antibodies raised against PF83/AMA-1 inhibits erythrocyte invasion by *P. falciparum in vitro*. Primate experiments using *P. knowlesi* AMA-1 and *P. fragile* AMA-1 have indicated protective efficacy [33]. The *P. vivax* AMA-1 gene has been used to construct a nucleic acid vaccine that proved to be immunogenic in mice [56] and a recombinant *P. vivax* AMA-1 protein produced in *Pichia pastoris* has proven to be highly immunogenic in *Rhesus* monkeys [108]. Recently it was shown that the *Pv*AMA-1 protein can play a role in the innate immune response by altering maturation of dendritic cells [109].

TRANSMISSION BLOCKING VACCINES

Malaria transmission blocking (TB) vaccines target the sexual stages of the parasite in the mosquito to reduce malaria transmission. Both antibodies and cytokines have been shown to block the fertilization process and parasite development in the mosquito, consequently preventing further transmission among humans [110]. Proteins that are expressed either by parasite sexual-stages or by oocysts/ookinetes to mediate functional roles such as penetration of the mosquito midgut are currently being evaluated [111, 112] for the development of TB vaccines. This is likely to be an effective strategy in the control of malaria in areas of low transmission intensity where it would prevent transmission from new foci of infection in the community and would control the escape of parasite mutants from vaccines that target other stages of the parasite life cycle.

P. vivax Pvs25 and Pvs28

These two proteins are ookinete surface antigens that are highly conserved in field isolates from different continents [113]. However, recent studies have reported sequence polymorphisms in these proteins in *P. vivax* field isolates from Iran [114]. These proteins are composed of four tandem epidermal growth factor (EGF)-like domains, putatively anchored to the parasite surface by a glycosyl-phosphatidyl-inositol moiety [115]. Both *Pvs*25 and *Pvs*28 expressed as recombinant proteins in *Saccharomyces cerevisae* are highly immunogenic and induced blocking antibodies in mice and monkeys [116]. Recombinant *Pvs*25 protein produced under Good Manufacturing Practice (GMP) has been tested in *Aotus* monkeys. *Pvs*25 formulated in Montanide ISA 720 induced specific antibodies that were evident 30 days after first immunization, peaked on day 150 and remained detectable for almost a year. Antibodies against *Pvs*25 displayed significant transmission blocking activity in artificial membrane feeding assays performed with *Anopheles albimanus* fed with *P. vivax* infected human blood. *Aotus* monkeys were additionally exposed to infection with *P. vivax* blood stages and, as expected, no boosting on the antibody titers was observed apart from the development of mature gametocytes, indirectly confirming that *Pvs*25 expression is restricted to ookinete/oocysts stages [117].

Phase I clinical trials have been carried out using *Pvs*25 formulated in Aluminum hydroxide and Montanide ISA 51. A dose escalating trial was conducted in using a total of 30 volunteers using a recombinant *Pvs*25H expressed in *S. cerevisiae*, formulated with Alhydrogel®. Volunteers were immunized intramuscularly on days 0, 28, and 180 in an open label study. No vaccine-related serious adverse events were observed and this formulation induced antibodies that peaked after the third dose and remained detectable in most volunteers for a year after first vaccination. Antibodies to recombinant *Pvs*25H protein induced TB activity in an antibody concentration-dependent manner as determined in membrane feeding assays [48]. The second trial was conducted in 72 healthy volunteers to evaluate the safety and immunogenicity of recombinant *Pfs*25 and *Pvs*25 vaccine candidates formulated in Montanide ISA 51. Although significant anti-*Pfs*25 antibody responses with blocking activity were obtained, this trial was stopped due to serious adverse events [49]. Efforts are being focused on the development of safe and immunogenic formulations with these transmission blocking vaccine candidates.

PERSPECTIVES FOR *P. VIVAX* PHASE II VACCINE TRIALS

As *P. vivax* vaccine candidates enter clinical development, one will need efficient methods to test the protective efficacy of vaccines that are found to be safe and immunogenic in Phase I clinical trials. For that purpose, efforts have been invested to develop a Phase IIa sporozoite challenge model in Colombia in which immunized human volunteers could be challenged with live *P. vivax* sporozoites [118]. Two clinical trials have been recently conducted in malaria-naïve volunteers to test the safety and reproducibility of the challenge method. In a first trial a total of 18 volunteers were challenged with live, mature *P. vivax* sporozoites produced by experimental infection of *An. albimanus* fed with blood from acutely infected patients [118, 119]. Together in the two trials, sporozoites from four different parasite isolates were tested at doses ranging from two to ten mosquito bites. Thirty four out of the 35 volunteers challenged, developed patent parasitemia with mean pre-patent periods of 11 to 14 days and volunteers were immediately provided standard anti-malarial treatment. All treated individuals cleared their blood-stage infections within 1-2 days of anti-malarial treatment [118, 119]. The fact that human malaria-naïve volunteers can be safely and reproducibly infected by bites of as low as two *P. vivax* infected *An. albimanus* mosquitoes provides the conditions to proceed to Phase IIa vaccine trials with pre-erythrocytic vaccine candidates. Additionally, the availability of this challenge system in malaria endemic countries would allow the establishment of small size Phase IIb trials under laboratory conditions, involving volunteers previously exposed to malaria. This would represent valuable proof-of-principle for further Phase IIb and Phase III trials. This sporozoite challenge method also provides a unique possibility to assess asexual blood stages antigens expressed on merozoites, because liver-derived merozoites express at least some of the antigens (e.g. *Pv*RII-DBP, MSP-1) expressed during blood schizogony and challenge by mosquito bite is the most natural system for *Plasmodium*. Optimal use of such models can greatly help accelerate clinical development of vaccines for *P. vivax* malaria.

Irradiated Sporozoites Vaccine

Vaccination with radiation attenuated *Plasmodium* sporozoites results in sterile immunity in more than 90% of human volunteers and therefore is considered the malaria vaccine gold standard. Studies using *P. falciparum* irradiated sporozoites for immunization have provided great experience with this vaccination system and also allowed the identification of protective immune responses elicited and enabled selection of several candidate antigens for malaria vaccine development [120]. This has encouraged development of a non-replicating, metabolically active, radiation-attenuated, cryopreserved *P. falciparum* vaccine [121]. Although, only a few volunteers have been vaccinated with *P. vivax* irradiated sporozoites, at least 1 volunteer, has been similarly protected by this system [24]. The lack of *P. vivax in vitro* cultures currently prevents attempts to manufacture a *P. vivax* attenuated vaccine under proper GMP, however, this system is currently being developed in Colombia with the support of the US National Institutes of Health as a means to study immune responses with the goal of identifying immune correlates of protection and novel parasite antigens for vaccine development.

CONCLUSIONS

Development of a *P. vivax* vaccine certainly lags behind that of *P. falciparum*, but considering the limited investment and the technical restrictions described, considerable progress has been made. Two vaccine candidates: CSP and *Pv*s25 have already been tested in Phase I trials and two antigens from asexual blood stages DBP and MSP-1 are likely to reach clinical testing within the next two years. In addition, a growing number of antigens are being added to the list of potential candidates. Availability of *P. vivax* genome information provides the foundation for rapidly increase the number of genes/antigens selected *in vitro* and eligible to be further developed as vaccine candidates.

Because most malaria endemic regions of the world have endemic *P. vivax* transmission, prompt and greater investment in *P. vivax* vaccine development is urgently required, so that communities exposed to both parasites could be adequately protected by a functional multi-species vaccine. There is no doubt that endemic communities from Africa, where *P. falciparum* is highly prevalent, will benefit from elimination of the malaria burden; however, a species mono-specific vaccine may create unpredictable epidemiological changes in other regions where *P. vivax* and other malaria species are simultaneously transmitted.

ACKNOWLEDGMENTS

Part of the work described here has been or is currently being supported by the Colombian Research Council (Colciencias), the Colombian Ministry of Social Protection, WHO/TDR and WHO/IVR Programmes, the European INCO-DC programme, US NIAID/NHLBI/NIH, Department of Biotechnology (DBT), Government of India, Indo-US Vaccine Action Program and PATH Malaria Vaccine Initiative. We are very grateful to the members of Malaria Vaccine and Drug Development Center (MVDC), Immunology Institute of Universidad del Valle, Cali, Colombia, and the Biochemistry Department of the Lausanne University, Lausanne, Switzerland for their contribution in the studies described herein. We are indebted to the malaria-endemic communities of the Colombian Pacific coast who have contributed for years to our studies as well as with volunteers that have participated in the *P. vivax* vaccine and sporozoite challenge trials.

REFERENCES

[1]   WHO. World Malaria Report. Geneva: World Health Organization 2008.
[2]   Hay SI, Guerra CA, Tatem AJ, *et al*. The global distribution and population at risk of malaria: past, present, and future. Lancet Infect Dis 2004; 4: 327-36.
[3]   Feachem R, Group TME. Shrinking the Malaria Map: A guide on Malaria Elimination for Policy Makers: University of California, San Francisco 2009.
[4]   Gusmao R. Overview of malaria control in the Americas. Parassitologia 1999; 41: 355-60.
[5]   Miller LH, Mason SJ, Clyde DF, *et al*. The resistance factor to *Plasmodium vivax* in blacks. The Duffy-blood-group genotype, FyFy. N Engl J Med 1976; 295: 302-4.
[6]   Langhi DM, Jr., Bordin JO. Duffy blood group and malaria. Hematology 2006; 11: 389-98.

[7]   Chitnis CE. Molecular insights into receptors used by malaria parasites for erythrocyte invasion. Curr Opin Hematol 2001; 8: 85-91.

[8]   Sina B. Focus on *Plasmodium vivax*. Trends Parasitol 2002; 18: 287-9.

[9]   Kochar DK, Das A, Kochar SK, Saxena V, *et al.* Severe *Plasmodium vivax* malaria: a report on serial cases from Bikaner in northwestern India. Am J Trop Med Hyg 2009; 80: 194-8.

[10]   Sharma A, Khanduri U. How benign is benign tertian malaria? J Vector Borne Dis 2009; 46: 141-4.

[11]   Lacerda MV, Hipolito JR, Passos LN. Chronic *Plasmodium vivax* infection in a patient with splenomegaly and severe thrombocytopenia. Rev Soc Bras Med Trop 2008; 41: 522-3.

[12]   Mendis K, Sina BJ, Marchesini P, *et al.* The neglected burden of *Plasmodium vivax* malaria. Am J Trop Med Hyg 2001; 64: 97-106.

[13]   WHO. WHO Expert Commitee on Malaria--Twentieth Report. World Health Organization. Geneva, 2000; Technical No. 892.

[14]   Limongi JE, Chaves KM, Paula MB, et al. Malaria outbreaks in a non-endemic area of Brazil, 2005. Rev Soc Bras Med Trop 2008; 41: 232-37.

[15]   Baird JK. Chloroquine resistance in *Plasmodium vivax*. Antimicrob Agents Chemother 2004; 48: 4075-83.

[16]   Pukrittayakamee S, Chotivanich K, Chantra A, *et al.* Activities of artesunate and primaquine against asexual- and sexual-stage parasites in *falciparum* malaria. Antimicrob Agents Chemother 2004; 48: 1329-34.

[17]   Tjitra E, Anstey NM, Sugiarto P, *et al.* Multidrug-resistant *Plasmodium vivax* associated with severe and fatal malaria: a prospective study in Papua, Indonesia. PLoS Med 2008; 5: e128.

[18]   Arias AE, Corredor A. Low response of Colombian strains of *Plasmodium vivax* to classical antimalarial therapy. Trop Med Parasitol 1989; 40: 21-3.

[19]   Roll Back Malaria. Global malaria action plan. Available at: http://wwwrbmwhoint/gmap/indexhtml; 2008.

[20]   Grabowsky M. The billion-dollar malaria moment. Nature 2008; 451: 1051-2.

[21]   Riley EM, Wahl S, Perkins DJ, *et al.* Regulating immunity to malaria. Parasite Immunol 2006; 28: 35-49.

[22]   Cucunuba ZM, Guerra AP, Rahirant SJ, *et al.* Asymptomatic *Plasmodium* spp. infection in Tierralta, Colombia. Mem Inst Oswaldo Cruz 2008; 103: 668-73.

[23]   Clyde DF. Immunization of man against *falciparum* and *vivax* malaria by use of attenuated sporozoites. Am J Trop Med Hyg 1975; 24: 397-401.

[24]   Clyde DF. Immunity to *falciparum* and *vivax* malaria induced by irradiated sporozoites: a review of the University of Maryland studies, 1971-75. Bull World Health Organ 1990; 68 Suppl: 9-12.

[25]   Artavanis-Tsakonas K, Tongren JE, Riley EM. The war between the malaria parasite and the immune system: immunity, immunoregulation and immunopathology. Clin Exp Immunol 2003; 133: 145-52.

[26]   Doolan DL, Dobano C, Baird JK. Acquired immunity to malaria. Clin Microbiol Rev 2009; 22: 13-36, Table of Contents.

[27]   McGregor IA. The passive transfer of human malarial immunity. Am J Trop Med Hyg 1964; 13: SUPPL 237-9.

[28]   Cohen J. Malaria vaccine development: trials, tribulations and reasons for hope. Hum Vaccin 2009; 5: 2-5.

[29]   Polhemus ME, Remich SA, Ogutu BR, *et al.* Evaluation of RTS,S/AS02A and RTS,S/AS01B in adults in a high malaria transmission area. PLoS One 2009; 4: e6465.

[30]   Ballou WR. The development of the RTS,S malaria vaccine candidate: challenges and lessons. Parasite Immunol 2009; 31: 492-500.

[31]   Hoffman S, Miller L. Perspectives on malaria vaccine development. In: Hoffman S, editor. Malaria vaccine development. Washington DC.: ASM Press 1996.p.p. 1-13.

[32]   Hollingdale MR. Anti-sporozoite antibodies. Bull World Health Organ 1990; 68 Suppl: 47-51.

[33]   Holder A. Preventing the merozoite invasion of erythrocyte. In: Hoffman S, editor. Malaria Vaccine development A multi-immune response approach. Washington DC.: ASM Press. 1996. p.p 77-104.

[34]   Arevalo-Herrera M, Chitnis C, Herrera S. Current status of *Plasmodium vivax* vaccine. Hum Vaccin 2010; 6: 124-32.

[35]   Carlton JM, Escalante AA, Neafsey D, *et al.* Comparative evolutionary genomics of human malaria parasites. Trends Parasitol 2008; 24: 545-50.

[36]   Carlton J, Silva J, Hall N. The genome of model malaria parasites, and comparative genomics. Curr Issues Mol Biol 2005; 7: 23-37.

[37]   Serruto D, Rappuoli R. Post-genomic vaccine development. FEBS Lett 2006; 580: 2985-92.

[38]   List EO, Berryman DE, Bower B, *et al.* The use of proteomics to study infectious diseases. Infect Disord Drug Targets 2008; 8: 31-45.

[39]   Nussenzweig R, Vanderberg J, Most H. Protective immunity produced by the injection of x-irradiated sporozoites of *Plasmodium berghei*. IV. Dose response, specificity and humoral immunity. Mil Med 1969; 134: 1176-82.

[40]   Tediosi F, Maire N, Penny M, *et al.* Simulation of the cost-effectiveness of malaria vaccines. Malar J 2009; 8: 127.

[41]   WHO/IVR.   Portafolio   of   candidates   malaria   vaccines   currently   in   development. http://wwwcolumbiaedu/itc/hs/medical/pathophys/id/2005/LarussaMalariaTablepdf 2005; March 2005.

[42]   Moorthy VS, Diggs C, Ferro S, *et al.* Report of a consultation on the optimization of clinical challenge trials for evaluation of candidate blood stage malaria vaccines, 18-19 March 2009, Bethesda, MD, USA. Vaccine 2009; 27: 5719-25.

[43]   Nussenzweig V, Nussenzweig RS. Rationale for the development of an engineered sporozoite malaria vaccine. Adv Immunol 1989; 45: 283-334.

[44]   Brown GV, Moorthy VS, Reed Z, *et al.* Priorities in research and development of vaccines against *Plasmodium vivax* malaria. Vaccine 2009.

[45]   Mueller I, Moorthy VS, Brown GV, *et al.* Guidance on the evaluation of *Plasmodium vivax* vaccines in populations exposed to natural infection. Vaccine 2009; 27: 5633-43.

[46]   Mueller I, Galinski MR, Baird JK, *et al.* Key gaps in the knowledge of *Plasmodium vivax*, a neglected human malaria parasite. Lancet Infect Dis 2009; 9: 555-66.

[47]   Herrera S, Bonelo A, Perlaza BL, *et al.* Safety and elicitation of humoral and cellular responses in colombian malaria-naïve volunteers by a *Plasmodium vivax* circumsporozoite protein-derived synthetic vaccine. Am J Trop Med Hyg 2005; 73: 3-9.

[48]   Malkin EM, Durbin AP, Diemert DJ, *et al.* Phase 1 vaccine trial of *Pv*s25H: a transmission blocking vaccine for *Plasmodium vivax* malaria. Vaccine 2005; 23: 3131-8.

[49]   Wu Y, Ellis RD, Shaffer D, *et al.* Phase 1 trial of malaria transmission blocking vaccine candidates *Pf*s25 and *Pv*s25 formulated with montanide ISA 51. PLoS One 2008; 3: e2636.

[50]   Galinski MR, Barnwell JW. *Plasmodium vivax*: who cares? Malar J 2008; 7 Suppl 1: S9.

[51]   Herrera S, Corradin G, Arevalo-Herrera M. An update on the search for a *Plasmodium vivax* vaccine. Trends Parasitol 2007; 23: 122-8.

[52]   Arevalo-Herrera M, Herrera S. *Plasmodium vivax* malaria vaccine development. Mol Immunol 2001; 38: 443-55.

[53]   Herrera S, Perlaza BL, Bonelo A, *et al.* Aotus monkeys: their great value for anti-malaria vaccines and drug testing. Int J Parasitol 2002; 32: 1625-35.

[54]   Bhat AA, Seth RK, Babu J, *et al.* Induction of mucosal and systemic humoral immune responses in murine system by intranasal immunization with peptide antigens of *P. vivax* and CpG oligodeoxynucleotide (ODN) in microparticle delivery. Int Immunopharmacol 2009; 9: 1197-208.

[55]   Devi YS, Mukherjee P, Yazdani SS, *et al.* Immunogenicity of *Plasmodium vivax* combination subunit vaccine formulated with human compatible adjuvants in mice. Vaccine 2007; 25: 5166-74.

[56]   Rogers WO, Gowda K, Hoffman SL. Construction and immunogenicity of DNA vaccine plasmids encoding four *Plasmodium vivax* candidate vaccine antigens. Vaccine 1999; 17: 3136-44.

[57]   Rojas-Caraballo J, Mongui A, Giraldo MA, *et al.* Immunogenicity and protection-inducing ability of recombinant *Plasmodium vivax* rhoptry-associated protein 2 in Aotus monkeys: a potential vaccine candidate. Vaccine 2009; 27: 2870-6.

[58]   Speake C, Duffy PE. Antigens for pre-erythrocytic malaria vaccines: building on success. Parasite Immunol 2009; 31: 539-46.

[59]   Hollingdale MR, Nardin EH, Tharavanij S, *et al.* Inhibition of entry of *Plasmodium falciparum* and *P. vivax* sporozoites into cultured cells; an in vitro assay of protective antibodies. J Immunol 1984; 132: 909-13.

[60]   Doolan DL, Hoffman SL. The complexity of protective immunity against liver-stage malaria. J Immunol 2000; 165: 1453-62.

[61]   Kain KC, Brown AE, Webster HK, *et al.* Circumsporozoite genotyping of global isolates of *Plasmodium vivax* from dried blood specimens. J Clin Microbiol 1992; 30: 1863-6.

[62]   Gonzalez JM, Hurtado S, Arevalo-Herrera M, *et al.*Variants of the *Plasmodium vivax* circumsporozoite protein (VK210 and VK247) in Colombian isolates. Mem Inst Oswaldo Cruz 2001; 96: 709-12.

[63]   Tewari R, Spaccapelo R, Bistoni F, *et al.* Function of region I and II adhesive motifs of *Plasmodium falciparum* circumsporozoite protein in sporozoite motility and infectivity. J Biol Chem 2002; 277: 47613-8.

[64]   Coppi A, Pinzon-Ortiz C, Hutter C, *et al.* The *Plasmodium* circumsporozoite protein is proteolytically processed during cell invasion. J Exp Med 2005; 201: 27-33.

[65]   Yuda M, Ishino T. Liver invasion by malarial parasites: how do malarial parasites break through the host barrier? Cell Microbiol 2004; 6: 1119-25.

[66]   Herrington DA, Nardin EH, Losonsky G, *et al.* Safety and immunogenicity of a recombinant sporozoite malaria vaccine against *Plasmodium vivax*. Am J Trop Med Hyg 1991; 45: 695-701.

[67]   Fries LF, Gordon DM, Schneider I, *et al.* Safety, immunogenicity, and efficacy of a *Plasmodium falciparum* vaccine comprising a circumsporozoite protein repeat region peptide conjugated to Pseudomonas aeruginosa toxin A. Infect Immun 1992; 60: 1834-9.

[68]   Bell BA, Wood JF, Bansal R, *et al.* Process development for the production of an E. coli produced clinical grade recombinant malaria vaccine for *Plasmodium vivax*. Vaccine 2009; 27: 1448-53.

[69]   Arevalo-Herrera M, Roggero MA, Gonzalez JM, *et al.* Mapping and comparison of the B-cell epitopes recognized on the *Plasmodium vivax* circumsporozoite protein by immune Colombians and immunized Aotus monkeys. Ann Trop Med Parasitol 1998; 92: 539-51.

[70]   Herrera S, Escobar P, de Plata C, *et al.* Human recognition of T cell epitopes on the *Plasmodium vivax* circumsporozoite protein. J Immunol 1992; 148: 3986-90.

[71]   Arevalo-Herrera M, Valencia AZ, Vergara J, *et al.* Identification of HLA-A2 restricted CD8(+) T-lymphocyte responses to *Plasmodium vivax* circumsporozoite protein in individuals naturally exposed to malaria. Parasite Immunol 2002; 24: 161-9.

[72]   Herrera S, Bonelo A, Perlaza BL, *et al.* Use of long synthetic peptides to study the antigenicity and immunogenicity of the *P. vivax* circumsporozoite protein. Int J for Parasitol 2004; 34: 1535-46.

[73]   Arevalo-Herrera M, Soto L, Perlaza BL, *et al.* Antibody-mediated and cellular immune responses induced in naïve volunteers by vaccination with long synthetic peptides derived from the *Plasmodium vivax* circumsporozoite protein. Am J Trop Med Hyg 2009; In press.

[74]   Herrera S, Fernández O, Vera O, *et al.* Phase I Safety and Immunogenicity Trial of *Plasmodium vivax* CS Derived Long Synthetic Peptides Adjuvanted with Montanide ISA 720 or ISA 51. Am J Trop Med Hyg 2009; In Press.

[75]   Frevert U, Sinnis P, Cerami C, *et al.* Malaria circumsporozoite protein binds to heparan sulfate proteoglycans associated with the surface membrane of hepatocytes. J Exp Med 1993; 177: 1287-98.

[76]   Castellanos A, Arevalo-Herrera M, Restrepo N, *et al. Plasmodium vivax* thrombospondin related adhesion protein: immunogenicity and protective efficacy in rodents and Aotus monkeys. Mem Inst Oswaldo Cruz 2007; 102: 411-6.

[77]   Karunaweera ND, Wijesekera SK, Wanasekera D, *et al.* The paroxysm of *Plasmodium vivax* malaria. Trends Parasitol 2003; 19: 188-93.

[78]   Herrera MA, Rosero F, Herrera S, *et al.* Protection against malaria in Aotus monkeys immunized with a recombinant blood-stage antigen fused to a universal T-cell epitope: correlation of serum gamma interferon levels with protection. Infect Immun 1992; 60: 154-8.

[79]   Valderrama-Aguirre A, Quintero G, Gomez A, *et al.* Antigenicity, immunogenicity, and protective efficacy of *Plasmodium vivax* MSP-1 PV200l: a potential malaria vaccine subunit. Am J Trop Med Hyg 2005; 73: 16-24.

[80]   Perera KL, Handunnetti SM, Holm I, *et al.* Baculovirus merozoite surface protein 1 C-terminal recombinant antigens are highly protective in a natural primate model for human *Plasmodium vivax* malaria. Infect Immun 1998; 66: 1500-6.

[81]   Yazdani SS, Shakri AR, Mukherjee P, *et al.* Evaluation of immune responses elicited in mice against a recombinant malaria vaccine based on *Plasmodium vivax* Duffy binding protein. Vaccine 2004; 22: 3727-37.

[82]   Arevalo-Herrera M, Castellanos A, Yazdani SS, *et al.* Immunogenicity and protective efficacy of recombinant vaccine based on the receptor-binding domain of the *Plasmodium vivax* Duffy binding protein in Aotus monkeys. Am J Trop Med Hyg 2005; 73: 25-31.

[83]   Barnwell JW, Galinski MR, DeSimone SG, *et al. Plasmodium vivax, P. cynomolgi,* and *P. knowlesi*: identification of homologue proteins associated with the surface of merozoites. Exp Parasitol 1999; 91: 238-49.

[84]   Oliveira-Ferreira J, Vargas-Serrato E, Barnwell JW, *et al.* Immunogenicity of *Plasmodium vivax* merozoite surface protein-9 recombinant proteins expressed in *E. coli.* Vaccine 2004; 22: 2023-30.

[85]   Galinski MR, Xu M, Barnwell JW. *Plasmodium vivax* reticulocyte binding protein-2 (*Pv*RBP-2) shares structural features with *Pv*RBP-1 and the *Plasmodium* yoelii 235 kDa rhoptry protein family. Mol Biochem Parasitol 2000; 108: 257-62.

[86]   Adams JH, Hudson DE, Torii M, *et al.* The Duffy receptor family of *Plasmodium* knowlesi is located within the micronemes of invasive malaria merozoites. Cell 1990; 63: 141-53.

[87]   Cole-Tobian J, King C. Diversity and natural selection in *Plasmodium vivax* Duffy binding protein gene. Mol Biochem parasitol 2003; 127: 121-32.

[88]   VanBuskirk KM, Sevova E, Adams JH. Conserved residues in the *Plasmodium vivax* Duffy-binding protein ligand domain are critical for erythrocyte receptor recognition. Proc Natl Acad Sci U S A 2004; 101: 15754-9.

[89]   Singh S, Pandey K, Chattopadhayay R, *et al.* Biochemical, biophysical, and functional characterization of bacterially expressed and refolded receptor binding domain of *Plasmodium vivax* duffy-binding protein. J Biol Chem 2001; 276: 17111-6.

[90]   King CL, Michon P, Shakri AR, *et al.* Naturally acquired Duffy-binding protein-specific binding inhibitory antibodies confer protection from blood-stage *Plasmodium vivax* infection. Proc Natl Acad Sci U S A 2008; 105: 8363-8.

[91]   Cole-Tobian JL, Michon P, Biasor M, *et al.* Strain-specific duffy binding protein antibodies correlate with protection against infection with homologous compared to heterologous p*lasmodium vivax* strains in papua new guinean children. Infect Immun 2009.

[92]   Yazdani SS, Shakri AR, Pattnaik P, *et al.* Improvement in yield and purity of a recombinant malaria vaccine candidate based on the receptor-binding domain of *Plasmodium vivax* duffy binding protein by codon optimization. Biotechnol Lett 2006; 28: 1109-14.

[93]   Moreno A, Caro-Aguilar I, Yazdani SS, *et al.* Preclinical assessment of the receptor-binding domain of *Plasmodium vivax* Duffy-binding protein as a vaccine candidate in rhesus macaques. Vaccine 2008; 26: 4338-44.

[94]   Riley EM, Allen SJ, Wheeler JG, *et al.* Naturally acquired cellular and humoral immune responses to the major merozoite surface antigen (*Pf*MSP-1) of *Plasmodium falciparum* are associated with reduced malaria morbidity. Parasite Immunol 1992; 14: 321-37.

[95]   Siddiqui WA, Tam LQ, Kramer KJ, *et al.* Merozoite surface coat precursor protein completely protects Aotus monkeys against *Plasmodium falciparum* malaria. Proc Natl Acad Sci U S A 1987; 84: 3014-8.

[96] Lyon JA, Angov E, *et al.* Protection induced by *Plasmodium falciparum* MSP-1(42) is strain-specific, antigen and adjuvant dependent, and correlates with antibody responses. PLoS One 2008; 3: e2830.

[97] del Portillo HA, Longacre S, Khouri E, *et al.* Primary structure of the merozoite surface antigen 1 of *Plasmodium vivax* reveals sequences conserved between different *Plasmodium* species. Proc Natl Acad Sci U S A 1991; 88: 4030-4.

[98] Soares IS, Levitus G, Souza JM, *et al.* Acquired immune responses to the N- and C-terminal regions of *Plasmodium vivax* merozoite surface protein 1 in individuals exposed to malaria. Infect Immun 1997; 65: 1606-14.

[99] Yeom JS, Kim ES, Lim KJ, *et al.* Naturally acquired IgM antibody response to the C-terminal region of the merozoite surface protein 1 of *Plasmodium vivax* in Korea: use for serodiagnosis of *vivax* malaria. J Parasitol 2008; 94: 1410-4.

[100] Stowers AW, Cioce V, Shimp RL, *et al.* Efficacy of two alternate vaccines based on *Plasmodium falciparum* merozoite surface protein 1 in an Aotus challenge trial. Infect Immun 2001; 69: 1536-46.

[101] Collins WE, Kaslow DC, Sullivan JS, *et al.* Testing the efficacy of a recombinant merozoite surface protein (MSP-1(19) of *Plasmodium vivax* in Saimiri boliviensis monkeys. Am J Trop Med Hyg 1999; 60: 350-6.

[102] Sachdeva S, Ahmad G, Malhotra P, *et al.* Comparison of immunogenicities of recombinant *Plasmodium vivax* merozoite surface protein 1 19- and 42-kiloDalton fragments expressed in *Escherichia coli*. Infect Immun 2004; 72: 5775-82.

[103] Rosa DS, Iwai LK, Tzelepis F, *et al.* Immunogenicity of a recombinant protein containing the *Plasmodium vivax* vaccine candidate MSP-1(19) and two human CD4+ T-cell epitopes administered to non-human primates (*Callithrix jacchus*). Microbes Infect 2006; 8: 2130-7.

[104] Kaushal DC, Kaushal NA, Narula A, *et al.* Biochemical and immunological characterization of E. coli expressed 42 kDa fragment of *Plasmodium vivax* and *P. cynomolgi bastianelli* merozoite surface protein-1. Indian J Biochem Biophys 2007; 44: 429-36.

[105] Genton B, Al-Yaman F, Anders R, *et al.* Safety and immunogenicity of a three-component blood-stage malaria vaccine in adults living in an endemic area of Papua New Guinea. Vaccine 2000; 18: 2504-11.

[106] Oaks SC, Mitchell S, Pearson GW, *et al.* Malaria, obstacles and opportunities. Institute of Medicine. National Academy Press, Washington, DC 1991.

[107] Rodrigues MH, Rodrigues KM, Oliveira TR, *et al.* Antibody response of naturally infected individuals to recombinant *Plasmodium vivax* apical membrane antigen-1. Int J Parasitol 2005; 35: 185-92.

[108] Kocken CH, Dubbeld MA, Van Der Wel A, *et al.* High-level expression of *Plasmodium vivax* apical membrane antigen 1 (AMA-1) in Pichia pastoris: strong immunogenicity in Macaca mulatta immunized with *P. vivax* AMA-1 and adjuvant SBAS2. Infect Immun 1999; 67: 43-9.

[109] Bueno LL, Fujiwara RT, Soares IS, *et al.* Direct effect of *Plasmodium vivax* recombinant vaccine candidates AMA-1 and MSP-119 on the innate immune response. Vaccine 2008; 26: 1204-13.

[110] Tsuboi T, Tachibana M, Kaneko O, *et al.* Transmission-blocking vaccine of *vivax* malaria. Parasitol Int 2003; 52: 1-11.

[111] Chowdhury DR, Angov E, Kariuki T, *et al.* A potent malaria transmission blocking vaccine based on codon harmonized full length *Pf*s48/45 expressed in *Escherichia coli*. PLoS One 2009; 4: e6352.

[112] Takeo S, Hisamori D, Matsuda S, *et al.* Enzymatic characterization of the *Plasmodium vivax* chitinase, a potential malaria transmission-blocking target. Parasitol Int 2009; 58: 243-8.

[113] Tsuboi T, Kaslow DC, Gozar MM, *et al.* Sequence polymorphism in two novel *Plasmodium vivax* ookinete surface proteins, *Pv*s25 and *Pv*s28, that are malaria transmission-blocking vaccine candidates. Mol Med 1998; 4: 772-82.

[114] Zakeri S, Raeisi A, Afsharpad M, *et al.* Molecular characterization of *Plasmodium vivax* clinical isolates in Pakistan and Iran using pvmsp-1, pvmsp-3alpha and pvcsp genes as molecular markers. Parasitol Int 2009.

[115] Kaslow DC, Quakyi IA, *et al.* A vaccine candidate from the sexual stage of human malaria that contains EGF-like domains. Nature 1988; 333: 74-6.

[116] Hisaeda H, Stowers AW, Tsuboi T, *et al.* Antibodies to malaria vaccine candidates *Pv*s25 and *Pv*s28 completely block the ability of *Plasmodium vivax* to infect mosquitoes. Infect Immun 2000; 68: 6618-23.

[117] Arevalo-Herrera M, Solarte Y, Yasnot MF, *et al.* Induction of transmission-blocking immunity in Aotus monkeys by vaccination with a *Plasmodium vivax* clinical grade PVS25 recombinant protein. Am J Trop Med Hyg 2005; 73: 32-7.

[118] Herrera S, Fernandez O, Manzano MR, *et al.* Successful sporozoite challenge model in human volunteers with *Plasmodium vivax* strain derived from human donors. Am J Trop Med Hyg 2009; 81: 740-6.

[119] Herrera S, Solarte Y, Jordán-Villegas A, *et al.* Consistent Safety and Infectivity in Sporozoite Challenge Model of *Plasmodium vivax* in Malaria-Naïve Human volunteers. Am J Trop Med Hyg 2009; In Press.

[120] Sharma S, Pathak S. Malaria vaccine: a current perspective. J Vector Borne Dis 2008; 45: 1-20.

[121] Luke TC, Hoffman SL. Rationale and plans for developing a non-replicating, metabolically active, radiation-attenuated *Plasmodium falciparum* sporozoite vaccine. J Exp Biol 2003; 206: 3803-8.

CHAPTER 5

Entamoeba histolytica: Host Defense and Immune Responses

Leanne Mortimer and Kris Chadee*

Department of Microbiology and Infectious Diseases, Faculty of Medicine, University of Calgary, Calgary, Alberta Canada

Abstract: Amebiasis caused by the enteric protozoan parasite *Entamoeba histolytica* is among the three top causes of death from parasitic infections worldwide, as a result of amebic colitis (dysentery) and liver or brain abscess. The protective host factors as well as those that contribute to the onset of pathology remain poorly understood. *E. histolytica* uses a variety of strategies to suppress local and systemic host immune responses, thus allowing the parasite to persist in immunocompetent hosts. During invasive disease there is a marked down-regulation of macrophage functions rendering the cells incapable of antigen presentation and unresponsive to cytokine stimulation. Furthermore, during infections there are decreased levels of helper CD4+ T cells that are unable to proliferate with a corresponding increased level of CD8+ T cells. Not only are cell-mediated immune responses impaired during amebic infection, but humoral defenses also fail to eliminate the parasite. The relative ineffectiveness of anti-amebic antibodies during a primary infection is correlated with cysteine proteases secreted by the parasites, which can degrade human intestinal IgA and cleave the heavy chains of IgG. Moreover, *E. histolytica* trophozoites can internalize and degrade immunoglobulin fragments bound on their surface. As the complexity of the interactions between *E. histolytica* and the host is increasingly understood, it provides the tools required for the development of successful vaccines against amebiasis.

INTRODUCTION

Entamoeba histolytica is the causative agent of amebiasis, which manifests as amebic colitis and amebic liver abscess. Amebiasis is endemic in developing parts of the world. Infection begins in the gastrointestinal tract after ingestion of infective cysts through contaminated food or water (Fig. **1**). Upon excystation, trophozoites colonize in the colon where they actively feed upon the resident microflora and luminal contents of the gut. This stage can become invasive and can cause massive tissue destruction within the host. However, 99% of infections remain asymptomatic and the parasite remains in the gut lumen as a harmless commensal. For reasons not fully understood, in 1% of infected individuals the parasite becomes invasive, resulting in 100 million cases of amebiasis and 100,000 deaths per year. This ranks amebiasis only second to malaria in mortality caused by a protozoan parasite [1].

E. histolytica is widespread geographically, though, the prevalence of infection and disease is highest in tropical climates. In developing tropical countries, it is not uncommon to find infection with *E. histolytica* in 10% to 50% of the population. In Mexico, serological studies suggest more than 8% of the population have had amebiasis and a study in Egypt found that 38% of patients reporting to a clinic for acute diarrhea were suffering from amebic colitis [2, 3]. Adequate water sanitation would be the best way to prevent infections by this parasite and other water-borne pathogens. Unfortunately, as the populations in developing countries remain at risk for infection, there is a need for other protective measures.

At present, drugs are available for effective treatment of amebiasis. Unfortunately, therapeutics are expensive and often inaccessible to those requiring them. Moreover, they do very little to prevent diarrheal and dysenteric illnesses caused by *E. histolytica*, which account for the majority of deaths inflicted by this parasite. To compound the issue, even though acquired immune responses develop as a result of infection, recent evidence suggests that effective immunological memory may be short lived [4, 5]. Thus, individuals (especially children) remain susceptible to re-infection and re-invasion.

In light of these facts, there is strong precedence for the development of an amebiasis vaccine. In fact, eradication of *E. histolytica* through vaccination is thought achievable for several reasons. First, *E. histolytica* has a simple two stage life cycle and expresses immunogenic molecules that are antigenically stable and there is good evidence for protective immunity. Second, *E. histolytica* has straightforward transmission dynamics; it does not use vectors for transmission between hosts and there are no significant animal reservoirs harboring *E. histolytica*.

PATHOGENESIS OF AMEBIASIS

There are two categories of invasive amebiasis based on whether infections remain in the intestine or whether they disseminate to extraintestinal sites. In intestinal infections, diarrhea and/or dysentery are the most common forms. Usually the parasite is cleared at this stage.

*Corresponding Author: Kris Chadee, Department of Microbiology and Infectious Diseases, Faculty of Medicine, University of Calgary, Calgary, Alberta Canada; Email: kchadee@ucalgary.ca

Emilio Jirillo (Ed)
All rights reserved - © 2010 Bentham Science Publishers Ltd.

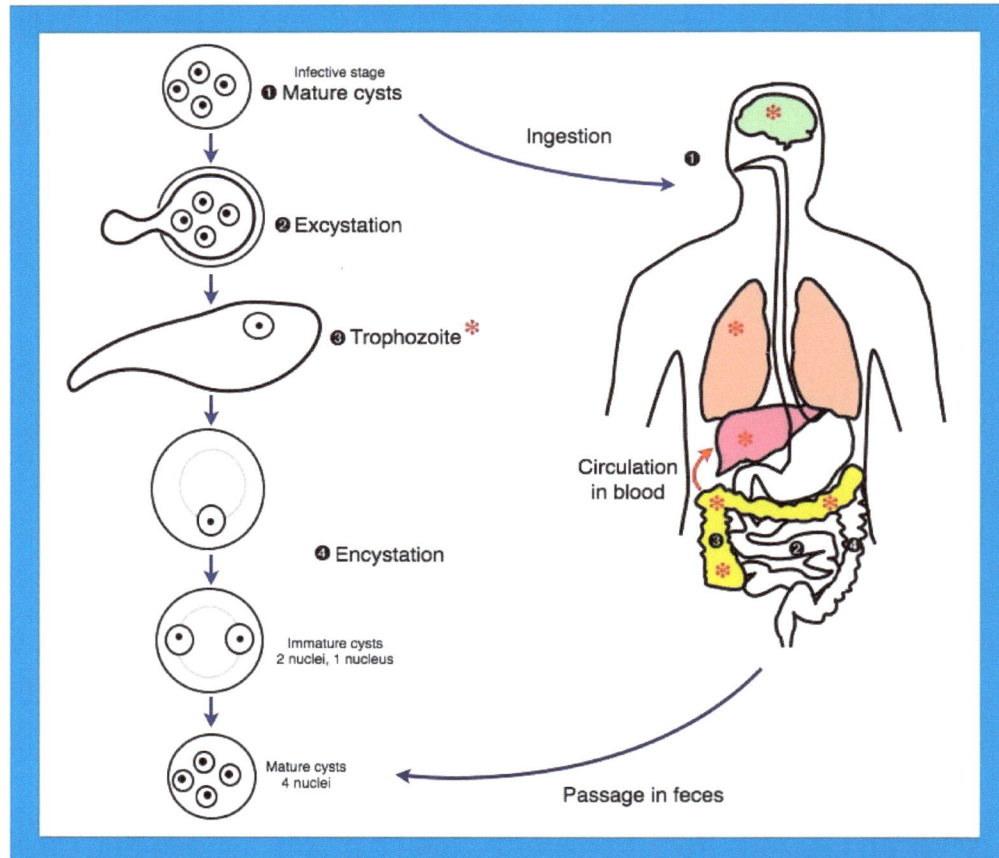

Figure 1: 2 Mature cysts are ingested through contaminated food or water and pass to the lower small intestine where they excyst. 3. Trophozoites are released and migrate to the large intestine. Here trophozoites colonize in or on the protective mucus layer where they feed on intestinal luminal contents and multiply by binary fission. However, for unknown reasons they can become invasive and invade the tissues causing cause intestinal disease. In the colon, trophozoites can enter mesenteric capillary beds and/or lymphatic vessels where they are carried via the hepatic portal circulation to the liver and then onto other extraintestinal sites such as the lungs and brain. 4. In the descending colon trophozoites encyst and the cysts are passed out in stool, which can survive in the external environment for days to weeks and remain infective. When an infective cyst is ingested, the life cycle continues.

However, in some instances amebic infections persist and trophozoites invade deeper tissues causing colonic ulcerations. In a small percentage of cases, ulcers develop very rapidly throughout large areas of the colon. Termed fulminant colitis, this form of intestinal amebiasis is very severe and requires a partial or complete removal of the colon. Apart from amebic colitis, other intestinal pathologies that may develop are: amebic appendicitis, ameboma and toxic megacolon.

Extraintestinal amebic infections most frequently develop in the liver (small numbers of cases in the brain and lungs have been reported). These infections result from the entrance and survival of trophozoites in the mesenteric blood vessels and their subsequent dissemination through the portal system to the liver. Once in the liver they can cause extensive tissue damage and abscess formation.

Intestinal Pathogenesis

In 1970 Prathap and Gilman [6] published what now serves as the classical description of *E. histolytica* invasion through the colon. These authors described five types of lesions from human biopsies that mark the progress of tissue destruction. Combined with descriptions from similar studies, development of intestinal amebiasis at the microscopic level is well understood.

In the early and intermediate stages of invasion the host mounts a robust inflammatory response. Initially, the epithelium remains intact and trophozoites are restricted to the gut lumen. There is a mild to moderate inflammation and infiltration of neutrophils below the epithelium, and within nearby lymphoid follicles there are increased numbers of proliferating lymphocytes in contact with histiocytic cells. The histiocytes are antigen-presenting cells loaded with amebic antigens. They interact with T cells to drive adaptive immune responses. At this point, goblet cells in the epithelium respond to amoeba by increasing the production and secretion of mucus [6].

As the invasion progresses, goblet cells become devoid of mucus containing vesicles and cease mucus secretion. Secretions from amoeba are thought to cause excessive local irritation of the epithelium that exhausts mucus production. As a result, the parasite erodes the remaining protective mucus layer and directly exposes epithelial cells. Large numbers of trophozoites are seen to aggregate into exposed sites and aggressively lyse the epithelium. However, the initial mucosal invasion may occur via a more passive process. In a gerbil model tracking the onset of intestinal amebiasis, amoebae were seen adhering to epithelial cells without inflicting damage [7]. The first breakage, which appeared as microerosions in the epithelium, may instead have been caused by an accumulation of underlying inflammatory fluid. The authors suggest the parasites enter internal tissues opportunistically via pre-existing breaks in the epithelium [7]. Regardless, once beyond the epithelial barrier, trophozoites move into the mucosa and engorge on host tissue. At this stage, there is an abundant infiltration of neutrophils, macrophages, eosinophils, plasma cells and lymphocytes into the area. However, these inflammatory cells appear to pose little threat to combating the invading trophozoites and are rapidly lysed by amoeba [6].

In the late stages of invasion, trophozoites reach the submucosa and migrate laterally, creating the classic flask-shaped ulcer of amebic colitis. In the center of amebic ulcers are dense necrotic cores abundant in neutrophils, but devoid of trophozoites. Trophozoites are present around advancing edges of ulcers, which are areas that contain few inflammatory cells. Interestingly, trophozoites can also be found in adjacent undamaged tissue [6]. In fact, at this stage of invasion, compared to the extent of tissue destruction there is relatively little inflammation both in and around the ulcer [8]. When trophozoites reach the submucosa they can enter mesenteric capillary beds and be carried via the portal vein to the liver.

Liver Abscess Pathogenesis

In humans, the early development of amebic liver abscess (ALA) is not well known. Moreover, there is a wide discrepancy of findings in human cases that may reflect observations taken at different stages of disease or the presence of other disease conditions [9]. In this regard, ALA in Mongolian gerbils (one of several rodent species used to study ALA) is thought to progress similar to humans, as the two species pathophysiologies correspond closely. In gerbil, liver infections are instigated by intrahepatic or intraportal injection of virulent trophozoites [9]. Within the first few days of infection, there is an acute inflammatory reaction accompanied by a massive infiltration of polymorphonuclear leukocytes (PMNs). Neutrophils are the predominant cell type in this first wave of cells. The lesion then progresses rapidly to form granulomas (Fig. **2**). This is marked by a second wave of infiltrating cells predominated by macrophages which deposit a fibrous layer around the site of infection. Macrophages infiltrate the fibrin layer and histiocytes populate the inner side. While this event corresponds to a reduced number of PMNs around the infection, the remaining neutrophils and mast cells are joined by plasma cells in the periphery of the lesion. In the center of the lesion, amoebae create a dense necrotic mass. They aggregate on the inner side of the granuloma wall where they lyse its components and any cells they encounter. This enables the parasites to disseminate to adjacent areas, and in this manner the lesion continues to grow and multiple granulomas is formed. As the infection progresses lymphocytes become the predominant immune cells surrounding the granulomas. Eventually the granulomas coalesce into a single mass enclosed by a thick wall [9].

Throughout the infection, the liver undergoes modifications in areas adjacent to the infection. Initially, the alterations are minimal, but as the granulomas enlarge surrounding cells become flattened, hepatocytes degenerate, neutrophils infiltrate areas around blood vessels, and lymphocytes flux into the portal area. The most severe changes take place at the height of abscess growth; there is a dense portal infiltrates, portal fibrosis, proliferation of the bile duct epithelium and extensive hepatocyte degeneration. In later stages, when the granulomas have coalesced, the surrounding tissue reverts to normal and appears to reflect the chronic stage of human ALA [9].

Though *E. histolytica* infections are well characterized at the microscopic level, the molecular interactions between the host and parasite, which determine the outcome of infection, are only partially resolved. The essential players are the components of the host immune system and the trophozoite. Their interactions can be placed into two major phases, those comprising the innate immune defenses and those of the adaptive immune response. In a small percentage of cases, the parasite successfully subverts both phases of the host's immune response and chronic disease ensues.

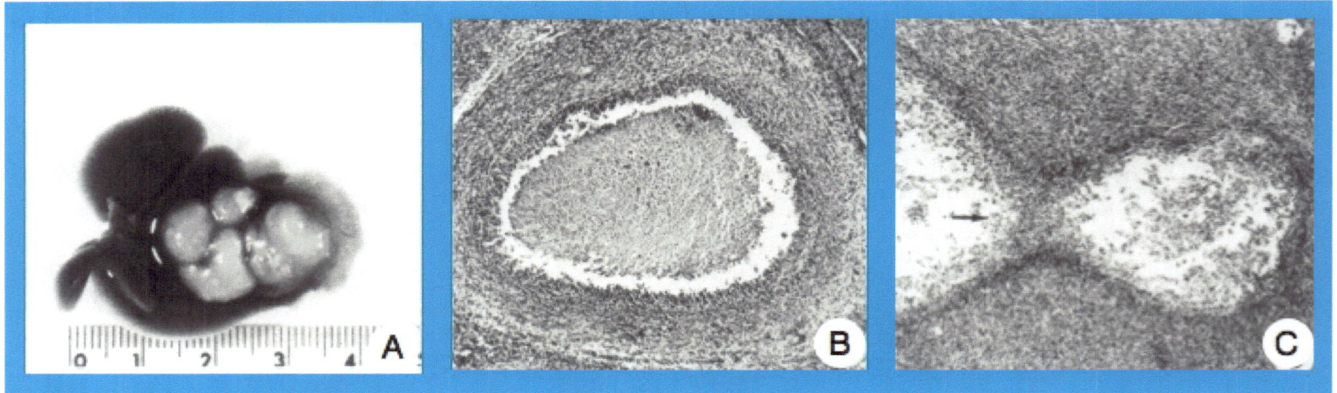

Figure 2: Amebic liver abscess in the gerbil. A) Amebic liver abscess 30 days after inoculation. The scale bar is in centimeters. B) Organized granuloma with a thick fibrous wall and a necrotic center 10 days after inoculation. C) Budding of granuloma with trophozoite movement (arrow) in the direction of the bud . Reprinted from Am J Pathol 1984, 117:71-80 with permission from the American Society for Investigative Pathology [9].

E. HISTOLYTICA AND INNATE HOST DEFENSES

Innate immunity refers to the first line of host defense and involves mechanisms that are constitutively active and ones that become activated within hours of pathogen exposure. When trophozoites are released into the gut, they encounter both the innate and the specific gut associated lymphoid immune system.

Interactions within the Mucus Layer

E. histolytica establishes itself in or on the mucus layer by binding with its surface adhesin, the Galactose/N-acetyl Galactosamine inhibitable lectin (Gal-lectin), to mucin oligosaccharides. Colonic mucins are the structural component of the mucus gel that are produced and secreted by goblet cells. Their peptide cores are linked via O-glycosidic bonds to sugar moieties that are rich in galactose (Gal) and N-acetyl galactosamine (GalNAc) [10]. The Gal-lectin binds with high affinity to Gal and GalNAc residues through its cysteine rich carbohydrate recognition domain, which enables the parasite to efficiently colonize the mucus layer as well as bind to bacteria and host cells [11-14]. Gal-lectin is a heterodimer composed of a 170 kDa heavy subunit and a 30 to 35 kDa light subunit [15]. It has many functions that are central to the pathogenicity of *E. histolytica*.

i. Effects of the Resident Gut Flora

Under non-pathogenic conditions trophozoites remain in the mucus layer feeding upon the resident microflora and luminal contents without causing harm. In some instances however, trophozoites cause focal erosions in the mucus barrier and come in direct contact with epithelial cells. What triggers the transition from a commensal to a pathogenic state is unknown (Fig. 3).

Interaction with the resident microflora is one possible cause. Monoxenic cultures of *E. histolytica* have shown strains of *Escherichia coli* can alter amoeba level of virulence and adhesion to target cells [16-19]. However, there are conflicting findings, as in some circumstances virulence decreases whereas in others it increases. In the case of non-pathogenic *E. coli*, the bacterial effects on virulence seem to depend on the length of co-culture and the serotype. One study investigated the effects of two *E. coli* serotypes, normally present in the human colon, which utilize different mechanisms of adherence to amoeba. One serotype interacted with the parasite by engaging Gal-lectin with its lipopolysaccharide and Gal and GalNAc residues, while the other bound mannose residues on amoeba surfaces with its type I pilus lectin. Amoebae were monoxenically cultured with bacteria for various lengths of time. Similar to what previous studies had shown, short-term associations with either serotype raised amebic virulence. It is thought that amoeba use ingested bacteria to scavenge oxidized molecules and possibly use bacterial catalase to detoxify hydrogen peroxide [16]. These metabolic changes are believed to increase amoeba ability to withstand the oxygenated environment bathing host cells. However, a longer-term association with *E. coli* interacting via the Gal-lectin temporarily lowered virulence. This was associated with reduced expression of the Gal-lectin light subunit.

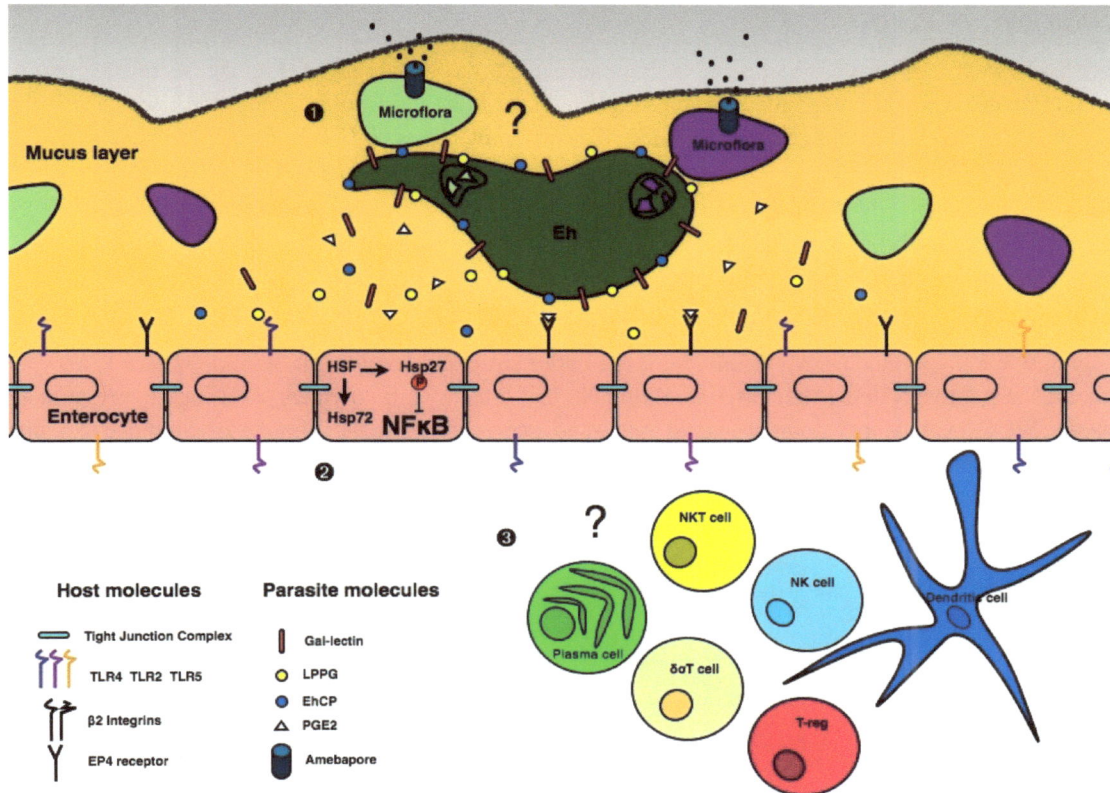

Figure 3: 1) Under non-pathogenic conditions, trophozoites adhere to the mucus layer via binding of the Gal-lectin to mucin oligosaccharides where they feed upon the resident microflora and luminal gut contents. Interactions with the microflora are thought to trigger *E. histolytica* to switch from gut commensal to pathogen. **2)** *E. histolytica* secreted products induce cytoprotective responses in the epithelium by upregulating expression of HSF-1, which in turn upregulates Hsp72 and Hsp27 expression. Hsp27 is phosphorylated and inhibits activation of NFκB, and thereby dampens NFκB-driven inflammation. Hsp72 has anti-apoptotic effects and promotes enterocyte survival. **3)** The role host immune cells play in shaping the outcome of infection are currently unknown. Only recently, have we begun to appreciate the complex interplay between enterocytes, immune cells of hematopoietic origin and the resident flora that together maintain gut homeostasis. Undoubtedly, these contribute to the regulation or disregulation of an *E. histolytica* infection.

Altered virulence and Gal-lectin expression were not observed with the mannose-binding *E. coli*. Interestingly, after an extended period of time amoeba cultured with Gal-lectin-binding *E. coli* regained their original level of virulence, which corresponded to restored expression of the Gal-lectin light subunit [18]. The molecular pathways leading to altered Gal-lectin expression and possibly functions have not been identified.

As mixed intestinal infections are common in areas endemic to *E. histolytica*, the effects of enteropathogens on amebic virulence have been recently explored [19]. It was shown that when amoeba phagocytose enteropathogenic *E. coli* or *Shigella dysenteriae*, they inflict more damage on epithelial cells than when amoeba phagocytose non-pathogenic *E. coli* or amoeba cultured alone. Their increased pathogenicity was correlated with elevated expression of the Gal-lectin and increased activity of the parasite's cysteine proteases (another major group of virulence factors). The molecular mechanisms responsible for this induction are not known. Interestingly, this study also showed that pathogenic bacteria induce responses in the colonic epithelium that would facilitate invasion by *E. histolytica* [19]. For example, these bacteria cause enterocytes to release interleukin (IL)-8, which is proposed to be a chemoattractant for amoeba. Thus, during a mixed infection pathogenic bacteria could induce trophozoite migration and contact with the epithelium. These bacteria also open epithelial cell tight junctions, and this could allow secreted parasite molecules that would otherwise remain in the lumen to cross into the internal environment. It was also shown that epithelium exposed first to bacteria and then to amoeba that had not phagocytosed bacteria was more susceptible to damage by amoeba. Moreover, amoeba adhered to the epithelium exposed to pathogenic bacteria more efficiently [19]. Although these studies have not revealed the mechanisms by which amoeba and enteric bacteria communicate, they have provided some insight into how amoeba and microorganisms in the gut might interact in their natural habitat to influence the outcome of disease.

ii. Manipulation of the Mucus Gel

E. histolytica has a wealth of virulent components that can deplete the mucus layer (Fig. **4**). Secreted products from the parasite contain potent mucus secretagogues that cause goblet cells to hyper-produce mucin [20], which *in vivo* can cause mucin depletion. The degree of mucus secretion elicited from different strains of *E. histolytica* correlates with their levels of virulence, which suggests that virulent amoeba use this strategy for invasion. One possible parasite secretagogue is prostaglandin E2 (PGE_2). Binding of PGE_2 to EP4 receptors on human colonic cells stimulated mucin exocytosis [21] and interestingly, *E. histolytica* has a novel COX-like enzyme that uses arachidonic acid to synthesize PGE_2 [22].

Trophozoites also degrade mucus directly. Their secretions contain abundant glycosidases that are capable of cleaving the oligosaccharides that protect the protein backbone of mucin [23]. In addition, they secrete cysteine proteases that proteolytically cleave colonic mucins. MUC2 mucin is the major structural component of colonic mucus, and *E. histolytica* cysteine proteases target the cysteine rich C-terminal domain that links mucin polymers. Cleavage by cysteine proteases at two sites in the MUC2 C-terminal domain causes mucus to depolymerize [24]. Thus, the combined actions of mucus secretagogues, glycosidases and cysteine proteases enables the parasite to subvert the mucus layer, allowing the parasite to come in direct contact with intestinal epithelial cells.

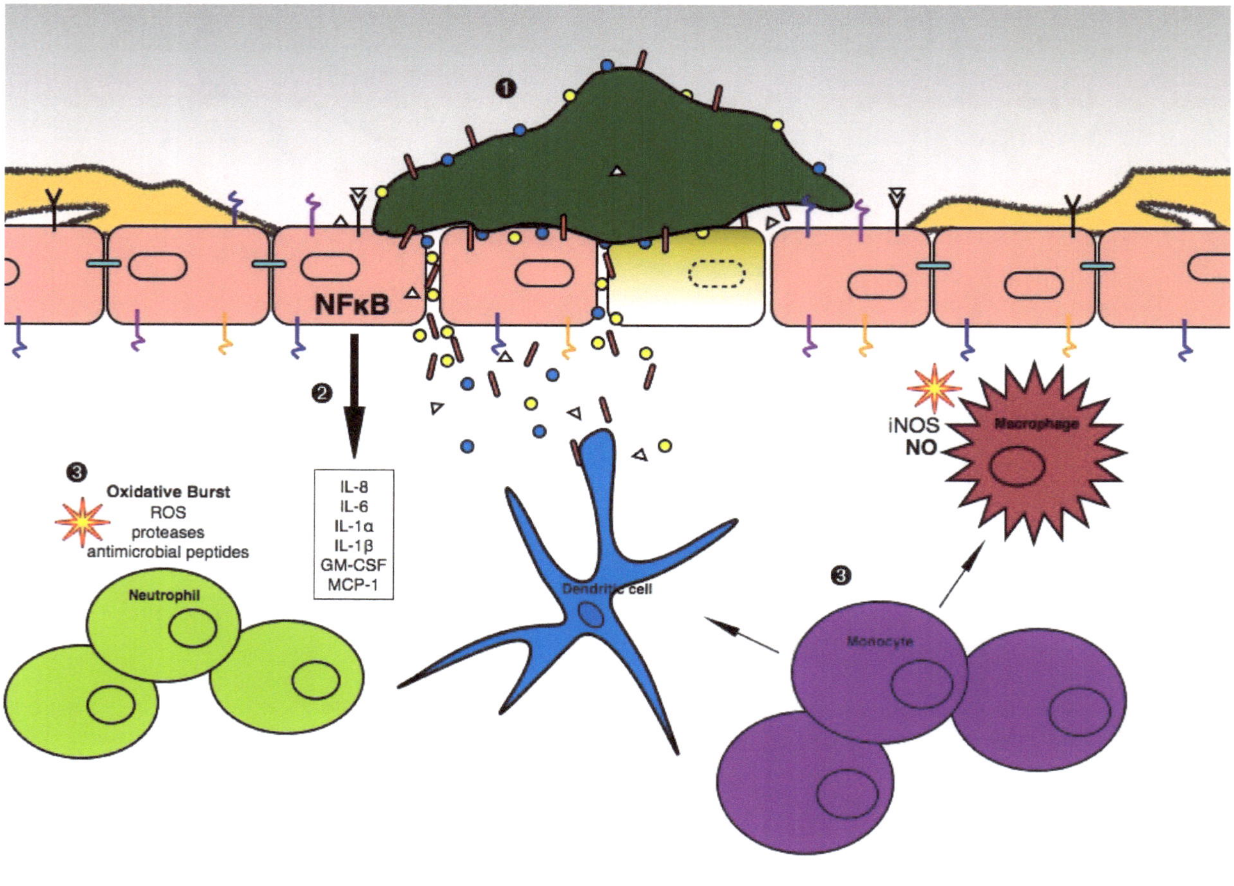

Figure 4: 1) Under pathogenic conditions, *E. histolytica* degrades and depletes the mucus layer. Parasite cysteine proteases cleave MUC2 causing the mucus gel to depolymerize. Upon contact with the epithelium, *E. histolytica* disrupts tight junctions, transfers molecules to the internal milieu, and induces enterocytes to undergo apoptosis/necrosis. **2)** Enterocytes recognize invasion via pathogen recognition receptors and other surface receptors, which initiate a robust NFκB-driven inflammatory response. Inflammatory enterocytes release cytokines and chemokines that attract neutrophils, monocytes and other immune cells to the site of invasion. **3)** Neutrophils are the first immune effectors to arrive; they release reactive oxygen intermediates (ROS), proteases and antimicrobial peptides. When monocytes arrive they can differentiate into naive dendritic cells, which sample parasite antigens and traffic to lymphoid tissue to coordinate an adaptive immune response, or they can become macrophages that release nitric oxide (NO) via inducible nitric oxide synthase (iNOS).

Interactions with the Intestinal Epithelium

After trophozoites compromise the mucus layer, they can interact directly with epithelial cells, which are not passive to invasion. The epithelium is a critical player in mucosal immunity; it forms not only a physical barrier, but also executes immunoregulatory functions via the secretion of cytokines, chemokines and anti-microbial peptides which modulate both hematopoietic and non-hematopoietic (canonical and non-canonical immune) cells.

i. Inflammatory Response

Studies *in vitro* and *in vivo* have shown colonic epithelial cells respond to *E. histolytica* by increasing expression and secretion of multiple pro-inflammatory mediators including IL-8, IL-1α, IL-1β, IL-6, growth regulated protein-α (CXCL1), monocyte chemoattractant protein-1 (MCP-1) and granulocyte macrophage colony stimulating factor (Fig. **4**) [25-29]. Furthermore, these events are not exclusively contact dependent. Experiments where live amoeba were prevented from contacting the epithelium, demonstrated that epithelial cells activate inflammatory pathways in response to constitutively secreted parasite molecules. For example, secreted amoeba molecules induce alternative activation of Nuclear Factor-kappa B (NF-κB) in epithelial cells, which leads to production of MCP-1, a potent chemoattractant for monocytes and macrophages [29]. Similarly, PGE_2 that are synthesized and secreted by amoeba, trigger IL-8 release from colonic epithelial cells via binding to their EP4 receptors [26].

However, the interaction between the epithelium and *E. histolytica* appears to be more complex than clear-cut activation of inflammation. For example, *E. histolytica* secreted products also induce a cytoprotective and an anti-inflammatory response in colonic epithelial cells by activating host stress response pathways (Fig. **3**). *E. histolytica* secreted products cause up-regulation of heat-shock protein (Hsp)72 and Hsp27 and induce Hsp27 phosphorylation. Amoeba-induced phosphorylation of Hsp27 causes it to associate with and inhibit IκBα kinase activity. This in turn prevents nuclear translocation of NF-κB subunit p65 and prevents activation of an NF-κB-mediated inflammatory response [30].

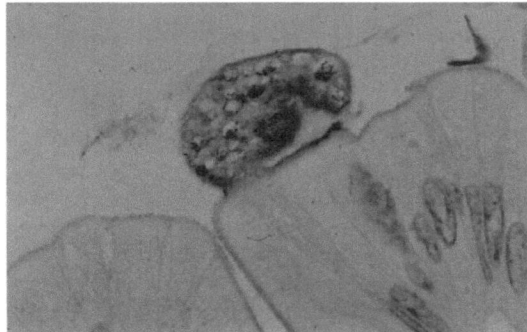

Figure 5: A trophozoite binding and effacing colonic epithelial cells. Reprinted from J Innate Immun 2009, 1: cover with permission from S. Karger AG, Basel [38].

Cellular adhesion is vital to *E. histolytica* pathogenicity, as much of its capacity to destroy tissues while simultaneously avoiding immune responses is mediated through direct interactions with host cells (Fig. **5**). When trophozoites contact epithelial monolayers they disrupt the molecular organization of tight junctions and cause an increase in paracellular permeability [27, 31]. This event is linked to transfer of *E. histolytica* molecules across the epithelium and into the internal milieu. Live amoebae are known to translocate two molecules, Gal-lectin and lipophosphopeptidogylcan (LPPG), upon contact [32, 33]. LPPG like Gal-lectin is abundant on the trophozoite surface and mediates cell adherence. *In vitro*, trophozoites transfer LPPG to the apical surface of epithelial monolayers prior to both tight junction opening and Gal-lectin transfer. Then, following the disruption of tight junctions, both Gal-lectin and LPPG are moved to the basolateral side of the epithelium [33]. The functional significance of these events is unknown, but they are thought to alter the tissue environment in a way that enables the parasite to survive.

Central to the immunoregulatory function of epithelium are the pathogen recognition receptors (PRR) that recognize a broad array of molecular patterns shared by pathogens. When PRR are engaged they launch immune and inflammatory responses and function as an important link between innate and adaptive immune responses. Toll-like receptors (TLR) are a class of PRR belonging to a superfamily called the IL-1 Receptor/TLR superfamily. TLRs are transmembrane signaling proteins that function through adaptor proteins such as MyD88, TRIF and TIRAP. Upon binding their cognate ligands TLRs activate two major signaling pathways, NF-κB and Mitogen-Activated Protein Kinases (MAPK). In this regard, *E. histolytica* LPPG binds TLR2 and TLR4 and activates NF-κB mediated release of IL-10, IL-12, TNF-α and IL-8 in human monocytes [34]. Thus, LPPG has the capacity to stimulate a pro-inflammatory response. Interestingly, extended incubation of human monocytes with LPPG also down-regulated TLR-2 gene expression, indicating that LPPG may also be immunosuppressive [34].

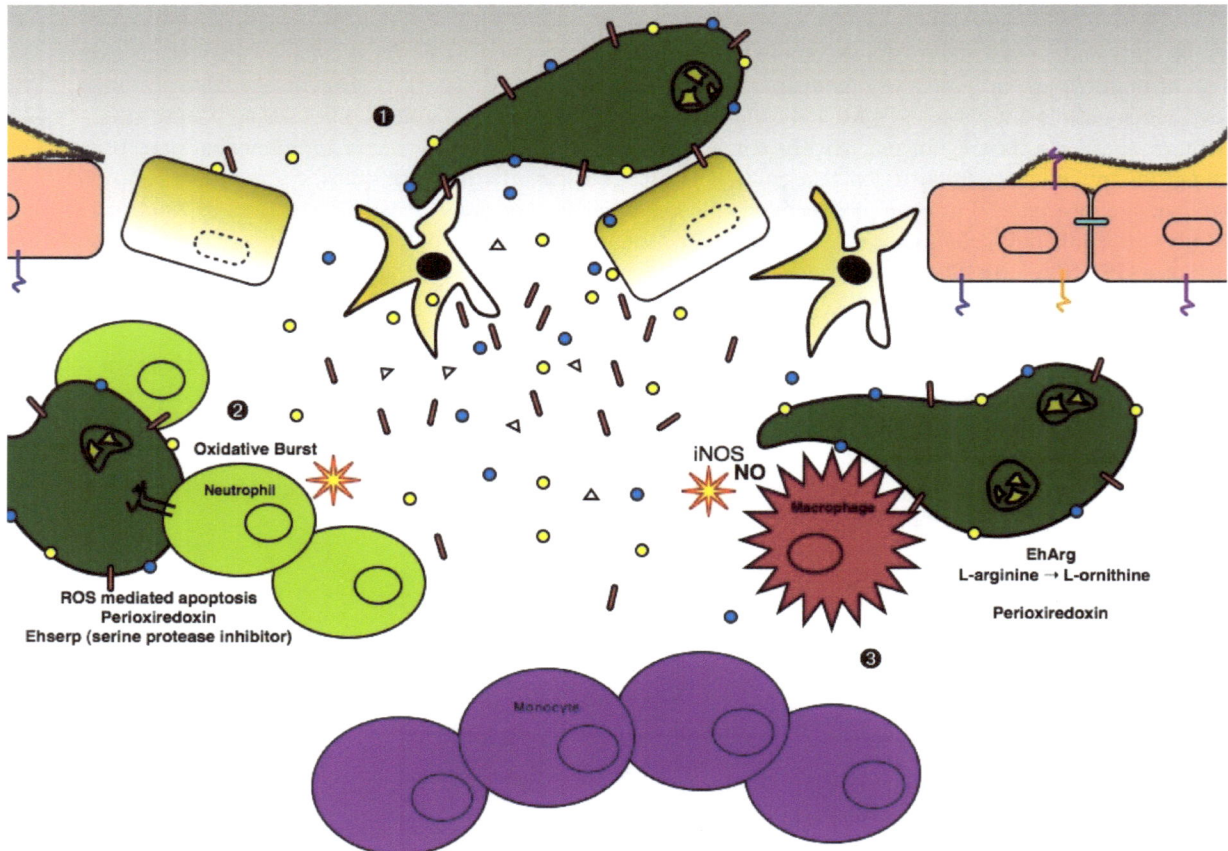

Figure 6: 1) As trophozoites advance into internal tissues they kill cells via apoptosis which they rapidly phagocytose. This is thought to reduce inflammation and allow the parasite to evade the immune response. **2)** Neutrophils release their amebicidal oxidative burst into infected tissues. However, *E. histolytica* possesses a surface perioxiredoxin that detoxifies ROS and secretes a serine protease inhibitor, Ehserp, which inactivates neutrophil protease cathepsin G. Trophozoites also induce neutrophil apoptosis via engagement of their β2 integrins which leads to activation of NADPH oxidase and ROS-mediated apoptosis. **3)** IFN-γ activated macrophages that release NO and other oxygen free radicals can efficiently kill trophozoites. However, *E. histolytica* counteracts the NO defense by secreting products that down-regulate macrophage iNOS expression and by consuming L-arginine, a precursor of NO, via its arginase, which converts L-arginine to L-ornithine.

As TLR-2 and TLR-4 are expressed on the intestinal epithelium, LPPG may also modulate epithelial cell responses.

Similarly, soluble Gal-lectin elicits immune responses in various cell types. Purified Gal-lectin triggers a transient rise in intracellular calcium levels and activates MAPK signaling that leads to nuclear translocation of NF-κB and transcription of pro-inflammatory genes [35, 36]. Epitopes on Gal-lectin that mediate adherence and activation of pro-inflammatory signaling pathways have been mapped [37], however specific PRRs interacting with Gal-lectin have not been reported.

ii. Apoptosis/Necrosis and Phagocytosis

The final interaction between *E. histolytica* and the intestinal epithelium is parasite-induced apoptosis and/or necrosis (Fig. 6). *In vitro*, amoebae destroy a variety of cell types through contact-dependent mechanisms. Killing requires that amoebae are alive, as secreted products and lysed amoeba are not inherently cytotoxic [39]. Following cell death amoeba quickly phagocytoses the cellular corpses [40]. The rapid clearance of host cells facilitates invasion by, 1) providing amoeba with a rich source of food and, 2) dampening activation of the host immune system.

Within 30 seconds of contact, amoeba induces a rapid irreversible rise in their target cell intracellular calcium concentration. After this encounter cell death occurs within 15 minutes [41]. Interestingly, purified Gal-lectin causes the same elevation of intracellular calcium concentration and inhibition of Gal-lectin after amoebae adhere to cells blocks cytotoxicity. This suggests that Gal-lectin acts not only as an adherence factor, but actively triggers cytotoxic events via engagement of a host cell receptor [42]. Multiple studies have shown *E. histolytica* activates a non-classical pathway of apoptosis, in that it does not signal through Fas receptors or activate the upstream activators of apoptosis, pro-caspases 8 and 9. Instead, amoebae activate the apoptotic pathway downstream at pro-caspase 3 [43, 44]. They do this through an unknown mechanism.

E. histolytica apoptosis/necrosis and phagocytosis are two linked and highly ordered events. For example, apoptosis exposes ligands such as phosphatidylserine on host cell surfaces that the parasite uses for ingestion [40]. Phagocytosis by *E. histolytica* is mediated by multiple adhesion molecules and to this extent serine rich *E. histolytica* protein (SREHP), phagosome associated transmembrane kinase, a 220 kDa lectin-like protein, a 112 kDa surface adhesin composed of a cysteine protease and adherence protein, and Gal-lectin have all been implicated [13, 42, 45, 46, 57]. Phagocytosis is also coordinated by a number of intracellular signaling components and the actin cytoskeleton. In eukaryotes, the Ras-related superfamily of small GTPases is typically involved in these processes. These proteins associate with and regulate the function of other proteins by cycling between GDP-bound inactive and GTP-bound active forms. Rab GTPases function in vesicle trafficking, and multiple *E. histolytica* Rab-like GTPases have been localized to developing phagosomes including: EhRabB, EhRab5 and EhRab7-like GTPases [48-51]. Rac GTPases activate actin polymerization and in *E. histolytica* EhRacA and EhPAK are critical regulators of this process. Constitutive activation of these two proteins disrupts amoeba phagocytosis [52, 53].

In some instances *E. histolytica* appears to trigger necrosis rather than apoptosis. This is likely mediated via a family of pore-forming peptides, called amebapores. These parasite-derived proteins insert themselves into plasma membranes and form channels through which water, ions and small molecules can pass [54- 56]. *In vitro*, that amebapores cause cell lysis without inducing classic signs of apoptosis, suggests they cause necrotic cell death. Indeed, necrotic destruction of the intestinal epithelium may account for a portion of the pro-inflammatory molecules released during early the stages of invasion. In epithelial monolayers, trophozoites trigger cytolytic release of pro-inflammatory peptides, including pre-IL-1α and pre-IL-1β [25]. Active IL-1α and IL-1β are thought to act as endogenous danger signals released by dying cells [57-59]. It was recently demonstrated that IL-1α is a critical factor provoking inflammation caused by necrotic cells [60]. Interestingly, *E. histolytica* cysteine proteases cleave pre-IL-1β into its bioactive form [61]. While IL-1α and IL-1β amplify the release of multiple pro-inflammatory cytokines that attract and activate lymphocytes that are important for clearing the infection, several of these cytokines such as IL-1β, TNF-α and IL-8 are also trophozoite chemoattractants [19, 62, 63]. Therefore, the intestinal epithelium inflammatory response could exacerbate an infection by recruiting trophozoites deeper into the submucosa to exacerbate the invasion process.

iii. An Important Role for IL-10 at the Mucosal Barrier?

The relationship between amoeba and host appears to be very complex. Efforts to date have not revealed why most people maintain commensal infections and why, during invasion, most only succumb to acute illness. On the flip side, it is not known why *E. histolytica* in some situations gets beyond the innate mucosal defenses and establishes chronic disease. It is evident that both host and parasite factors play a role. Alterations in the hematopoietic and non-hematopoietic compartments could predispose the host to invasion.

A determining factor may be the level of IL-10 at the mucosal barrier. IL-10 is crucial for the maintenance of gut homeostasis. A recently developed model of mouse amebic colitis has shown that the constitutive effects of IL-10 produced by hematopoietic cells are necessary for innate resistance to amebic invasion [64]. In mouse, some strains are variably susceptible (C3H and CBA) to amebic colitis while others are completely resistant (C57BL/6). After intracecal injection, C57BL/6 mice eliminate trophozoites within hours and there is no indication that they respond to the parasite, as they have no inflammation nor epithelial breakdown, and no change in gene expression. Furthermore, C57BL/6 knockouts of innate pro-inflammatory pathways remain completely resistant [65, 66]. However, C57BL/6 IL-10$^{-/-}$ mice are extremely susceptible to amebic colitis. Through chimera studies, it was shown that IL-10 exerts its protective effects on the non-hematopoietic compartment, while the source of IL-10 required for this innate resistance comes from hematopoietic cells [64]. IL-10 has multiple roles in intestinal homeostasis; it dampens pro-inflammatory NF-κB signaling in intestinal epithelial cells, affects MUC2 production, suppresses immune cell activation and has an anti-apoptotic effect on the epithelium [67-70]. Likely, IL-10 contributes to C57BL/6 resistance in multiple ways. In terms of human *E. histolytica* infections, an IL-10 deficiency could weaken the mucus layer allowing the parasite to contact an epithelium that is already pre-disposed to developing an inflammatory response, which could in turn promote parasite invasion.

Interactions with Innate Effector Hematopoietic Cells

i. Neutrophils

When *E. histolytica* invades either the colon or the liver, neutrophils are the first cells to arrive [6, 7, 9]. Neutrophils are highly equipped for killing microorganisms via their oxidative burst. When activated, they produce reactive oxygen species (ROS) within their phagosomes. They also recruit proteases, anti-microbial peptides and permeability-increasing proteins to their phagosomes and release them into infected tissue.

Whether neutrophils can kill *E. histolytica* during an infection however, remains controversial. *In vitro*, interferon (IFN)-γ activated neutrophils kill trophozoites via contact and contact-independent manners [71]. However, amoebae are also extremely efficient at killing neutrophils. Virulent strains can defeat human neutrophils *in vitro* at a ratio of 1 amoeba to 3,000 neutrophils, and even low-virulence strains can do this at a 400 to 1 ratio of neutrophils to amoeba [8, 72].

Several mechanisms account for this remarkable ability (Fig. 6). Firstly, trophozoites possess machinery that incapacitates neutrophil defenses. They express an iron containing superoxide dismutase that is induced by superoxide anions to produce hydrogen peroxide (H_2O_2) [73]. The parasite possesses a bifunctional NADPH: flavin oxidoreductase that also converts superoxide to H_2O_2 [74, 75]. *E. histolytica* then uses its thiol-rich 29 kDa surface perioxiredoxin to detoxify cytotoxic H_2O_2 [76, 77]. The surface perioxiredoxin appears to be a crucial factor protecting *E. histolytica* against oxidative killing as early studies found H_2O_2 to be the main reactive oxygen species that kills amoeba and highly virulent strains are less susceptible to H_2O_2 [78, 79]. The importance of perioxiredoxin is also suggested by its presence in the outer surface of *E. histolytica*, which differs from the closely related but non-pathogenic species, *E. dispar*. *E. dispar* is highly sensitive to H_2O_2 and expresses perioxiredoxin intracellularly. Also, *E. histolytica* expression of perioxiredoxin is 50 fold higher than *E. dispar* [76]. Amoebae further dismantle the neutrophil defense by secreting a serine protease inhibitor, Ehserp, which inactivates neutrophil protease cathepsin G [80].

The definitive action that enables amoeba to overcome neutrophils is they kill them via apoptosis. They do this through engagement of β2 integrins on neutrophil surfaces. This leads to activation of NADPH oxidase and ROS-mediated apoptosis [81]. Trophozoites then phagocytose the dying neutrophils, which further reduces inflammation and allows the parasite to evade the immune response [81, 82]. However, evidence from *in vivo* studies argues that neutrophils contribute significantly to controlling *E. histolytica*. A mouse model of amebic colitis suggests neutrophils eliminate amoeba during initial stages of invasion [65]. The CBA strain exhibits partial resistance to *E. histolytica* induced colitis after intracecal inoculation. If a CBA mouse clears the parasite it does so within 24-96 hours of exposure, which indicates their immunity relies on innate mechanisms. When CBA mice are depleted of neutrophils however, they become highly susceptible to amebic colitis, demonstrating that neutrophils are actively involved in early clearance of *E. histolytica* [65]. Other studies have shown that neutrophils limit liver abscess development in animal models of ALA [83, 84]. Together, these data suggest neutrophils have two roles in combating amebiasis: 1) they prevent the establishment of invasive infections and, 2) they limit disease once infection occurs.

In naturally occurring human infections, whether neutrophils are able to contain invasive *E. histolytica* could depend on a number of factors. For example, their effectiveness may depend on how many neutrophils infiltrate the site of infection compared to amoeba, or whether neutrophils are properly activated to kill. As most cases of intestinal amebiasis pass quickly and progress no further than dysentery/diarrhea and neutrophils are the first inflammatory cells following invasion, one could speculate that in most circumstances neutrophils sufficiently control invasive amebic infections. However, other innate immune cells —such as NK cells, NKT cells, δγT cells and mast cells— are likely to be involved and how they influence the outcome of is infection is largely unexplored.

ii. Macrophages

Macrophages cooperate alongside neutrophils in innate host defense and in adaptive immunity when CD4[+] effector T cells activate them. Activated inflammatory macrophages produce copious amounts of NO which plays a critical role in killing trophozoites and inhibiting the activity of destructive *E. histolytica* cysteine proteases [85]. *In vitro*, IFN-γ or TNF-α stimulated macrophages release NO and efficiently kill trophozoites [86]. *In vivo*, NO has shown to be an important component of host protection. For example, in a murine model of amebic liver abscess, mice with a targeted deletion in the gene encoding inducible nitric oxide synthase (iNOS) developed significantly larger abscesses than their wild type counterparts [87].

However, chronic amebiasis is associated with defects in cell mediated immunity [88, 89], especially impaired macrophage functions. Macrophages isolated from rodent amebic liver lesions are refractive to IFN-γ and LPS activation; they do not produce inflammatory cytokines and they are unable to kill amoeba. This immunosuppression of macrophage functions is local because macrophages at distant sites in these animals are unaffected [90-92].

E. histolytica has several mechanisms that deactivate macrophages. Trophozoites secrete proteins that decrease macrophage iNOS expression, which reduces macrophage NO production and amebicidal activity [91]. The parasite also inhibits NO production by consuming L-arginine, a metabolic precursor of NO that is present in the environment. *E. histolytica* possesses an arginase, EhArg that hydrolyzes L-arginine to L-ornithine and urea. Arginine metabolism is required by *E. histolytica* for growth. However, the activity of EhArg concomitantly inhibits macrophage NO synthesis [93]. Furthermore, because amoebae cause macrophages to become unresponsive to IFN-γ, their expression of TNF-α, which is induced by IFN-γ, is prevented. Amoebae also interfere with TNF-α production by increasing macrophage PGE$_2$ biosynthesis [90]. IFN-γ and TNF-α synergize to activate cytotoxic pathways including NO production, and IFN-γ also activates MHC class II transcription. Thus, macrophages deactivated by amoeba are ineffective at T cell antigen presentation and are unable to mount a cytotoxic response.

Evasion of Complement

To establish an invasive infection, trophozoites must avoid the host complement system. Complement is activated by proteolysis of zymogens present in serum. This produces an enzyme cascade that results in non-specific binding of complement components to pathogen surfaces. Two primary functions of complement are lysis of foreign cells by the membrane attack complex C5b-9 and opsonization of pathogen surfaces, which helps other immune mechanisms target pathogens.

Interestingly, an *E. histolytica* cysteine protease directly activates complement by cleaving the alpha chain of C3 and turning it into functional C3b [94,95]. However, *E. histolytica* is highly capable of resisting complement. The pathogenic laboratory strain, HM1-IMSS, when cultured in human serum becomes insensitive to complement-mediated killing and trophozoites from colitis and amebic liver abscess patients have this resistance [96-99].

Several mechanisms appear to explain the parasite's ability to evade complement. The first involves Gal-lectin and a recently identified 21 kDa surface protein that possess epitopes of the complement inhibitory protein, CD59. In humans, CD59 is present on cell surfaces to prevent complement-mediated lysis of 'self' cells by preventing formation of the membrane attack complex C5b-9. Like CD59, Gal-lectin inhibits assembly of C5b-9 complexes, and the 21 kDa surface protein likely has the same activity [100, 101]. Another reason for *E. histolytica* resistance to complement may be the thick glycolax, formed by membrane bound LPPG and lipophosphoglycan (LPG), creates an impenetrable barrier to complement proteins [102]. Recently, it was shown that interference of GPI anchor synthesis, which attaches LPPG and LPG to the membrane, greatly reduces their expression and concomitantly renders trophozoites sensitive to complement [103]. In addition, that the LPPG/LPG glycolax on the closely related non-pathogenic and complement susceptible species, *E. dispar*, is much thinner suggests LPPG and LPG play a role in resisting complement [104].

Another interesting feature is that the *E. histolytica* cysteine protease responsible for activating C3, also cleaves and inactivates C3a, the anaphylatoxin generated from cleavage of C3. It also cleaves and inactivates C5a [105]. C3a and C5a are potent activators of inflammatory responses. Together, they induce an influx and activation of inflammatory cells [106]. C3a and C5a increase vascular permeability and smooth muscle contraction. They trigger release of histamine from mast cells, lysosomal enzymes from leukocytes, and pro-inflammatory cytokines such as IL-6 and TNF-α from B-cells and monocytes [107, 108]. They also attract neutrophils, monocytes, eosinophils, mast cells, basophils, activated B-cells and T-cells [107, 108]. Thus, amoeba can diminish inflammatory responses once complement is activated by inactivating anaphylatoxins. This may account for the lack of inflammatory cells observed in amebic ulcers and liver abscesses [105].

Recently, it was shown that differences exist in male versus female complement activity against *E. histolytica*, which may explain the prevalence of invasive amebiasis in adult males. Sera from women not previously exposed to *E. histolytica* were significantly more efficient at killing trophozoites than sera from unexposed men. The phenomenon was reliant on functional complement, however the mechanism and molecules responsible for these differences remains to be clarified

[109]. In men, the rates of amebic liver abscess and amebic dysentery is five to seven times higher than in women, even though male versus female rates of gut colonization do not appear to differ [110]. As evasion of complement is essential for trophozoite survival inside host tissue, gender differences in complement activity appear to be a reason why amebiasis predominates in males.

E. HISTOLYTICA AND ADAPTIVE HOST DEFENSES

Immunosuppression

In the intestinal biopsies described by Prathap and Gilman proliferating lymphoid aggregates were seen in contact with antigen presenting cells [6]. These images illustrated that amoebae induce expansion of lymphocyte populations in the adaptive immune response. However, human and animal studies have shown host immunosuppression occurs in chronic invasive amebiasis. Peculiarly, recently recovered ALA patients have decreased proliferative responses to the T cell mitogen concanavalin A (ConA) [88]. Though total T cell counts in these individuals are normal, their $CD4^+:CD8^-$ ratio is markedly lowered. A reduced number of $CD4^+$ cells and an increased number of $CD8^+$ cells accounts for this phenomenon. The $CD4^+:CD8^+$ ratio was found to correlate positively with ConA-induced proliferative responses. Most patients at one-year post recovery had regained a normal T cell ratio and proliferative response. This type of immunosuppression is also recapitulated in ALA in animal models of the disease. Serum from infected gerbils suppressed naive T cell proliferative responses to Con A via an IL-2 dependent mechanism [89]. In this instance, the suppressive effect was independent of PGE_2 (which is induced by amoeba in macrophages and mediates macrophage suppression). Although, this does not rule out a role for PGE_2 and other molecules like IL-10 in suppressing T cell proliferation, because lymphocytes from infected gerbils were also inherently defective at proliferating. When lymphocytes from infected gerbils were cultured in the presence of uninfected control serum and stimulated with Con A, their response was 73% to 93% less than uninfected cells, depending on the day after infection [89].

Th1 Versus Th2 Responses

There are multiple lines of evidence indicating chronic amebiasis is perpetuated by an anti-protective Th2 response and that Th1 immunity is required to control this stage of amebiasis (Fig. 7). Human data show that recovery from ALA is associated with cell-mediated immunity. For example, lymphocytes from cured ALA patients that are stimulated with purified amebic proteins produce IFN-γ and demonstrate amebicidal activity [111]. Furthermore, a similar Th1 response in gerbils immunized against Gal-lectin protects them from developing liver abscesses upon challenge with *E. histolytica* [36, 112-114].

The Th1/Th2 paradigm of resistance and susceptibility is also strongly reinforced by animal models of amebiasis. A murine amebic colitis model has shown that non-protective immune responses against *E. histolytica* are associated with a mixed Th2 and Th17 profile [115]. Infected animals develop chronic non-healing infections and intestinal inflammation. They have highly elevated levels of signature Th2 and Th17 cytokines (IL-4, IL-13, IL-5 and IL-17, IL-23, respectively). They also highly express Arginase-1 compared to iNOS. Levels of Arginase-1 and iNOS are used to measure proportions of alternatively and classically activated macrophages, respectively. Thus, alternatively activated macrophages, which are anti-inflammatory and promote wound repair processes, dominate in this model of amebic colitis. Blockade of IL-4 by way of IL-4 neutralizing monoclonal antibodies, reverses Th2 responses in these animals and allows a Th1 response to develop. As a result, copious amounts of IFN-γ are produced, the Arginase-1 to iNOS ratio is reversed, and infections are cleared. These results are consistent with a similar study showing that depletion of $CD4^+$ cells mitigates intestinal disease, which correlates with a reversal in Th2 cytokine expression [116].

The Th1 cytokine, IFN-γ, is paramount to controlling amebic infections. In the model described above, mice administered both IL-4 and IFN-γ neutralizing antibodies do not clear their intestinal infections [115]. ALA models also show that IFN-γ plays an important role in host protection. Mice with disruptions in their IFN-γ receptor develop larger liver abscesses [84]. Furthermore, in mouse males are more susceptible to ALA than females, as they develop larger abscesses and take longer to clear their infections. Interestingly, males produce higher amounts of IL-4, while females produce higher levels of IFN-γ, and females treated with IFN-γ neutralizing antibodies become more susceptible to ALA [117].

In addition, several other lines of evidence implicate a central role for IFN-γ in host protection. As previously discussed, macrophages that are activated *in vitro* by IFN-γ are highly amebicidal. Vaccine models have demonstrated protective immunity is associated with antigen-specific IFN-γ responses [112, 113, 114, 36]. Moreover, epidemiological data from a large-scale study of children in Bangladesh showed a correlation between high parasite-specific IFN-γ production by peripheral blood mononuclear cells and lower susceptibility to future amebic dysentery and diarrhea [118].

Collectively, these findings indicate that during chronic amebic infections, defective CD4$^+$ Th2 responses occur which allow *E. histolytica* to persist in internal tissues, and adaptive responses that drive high IFN-γ production are protective against chronic and acute amebic illnesses.

Humoral Immunity

i. Anti-Gal-Lectin Antibody Response

Invasive amebiasis elicits a humoral immune response to a number of amebic antigens. In humans, anti-Gal-lectin responses are the best characterized. Gal-lectin antibodies are detectable in sera and mucosal secretions of ALA and amebic colitis patients, and in mucosal secretions of asymptomatic cyst passers [119-123]. As Gal-lectin plays a primary role in trophozoite adherence to the mucus layer and host cells, antibodies against it are thought to provide protection largely by preventing trophozoite attachment. However, the answer appears to be two sided.

A prospective study of children living in an urban slum of Dhaka, Bangladesh showed that children with stool IgA that recognizes the Gal-lectin carbohydrate recognition domain (CRD) are protected from developing new *E. histolytica* infections [4, 5, 123].

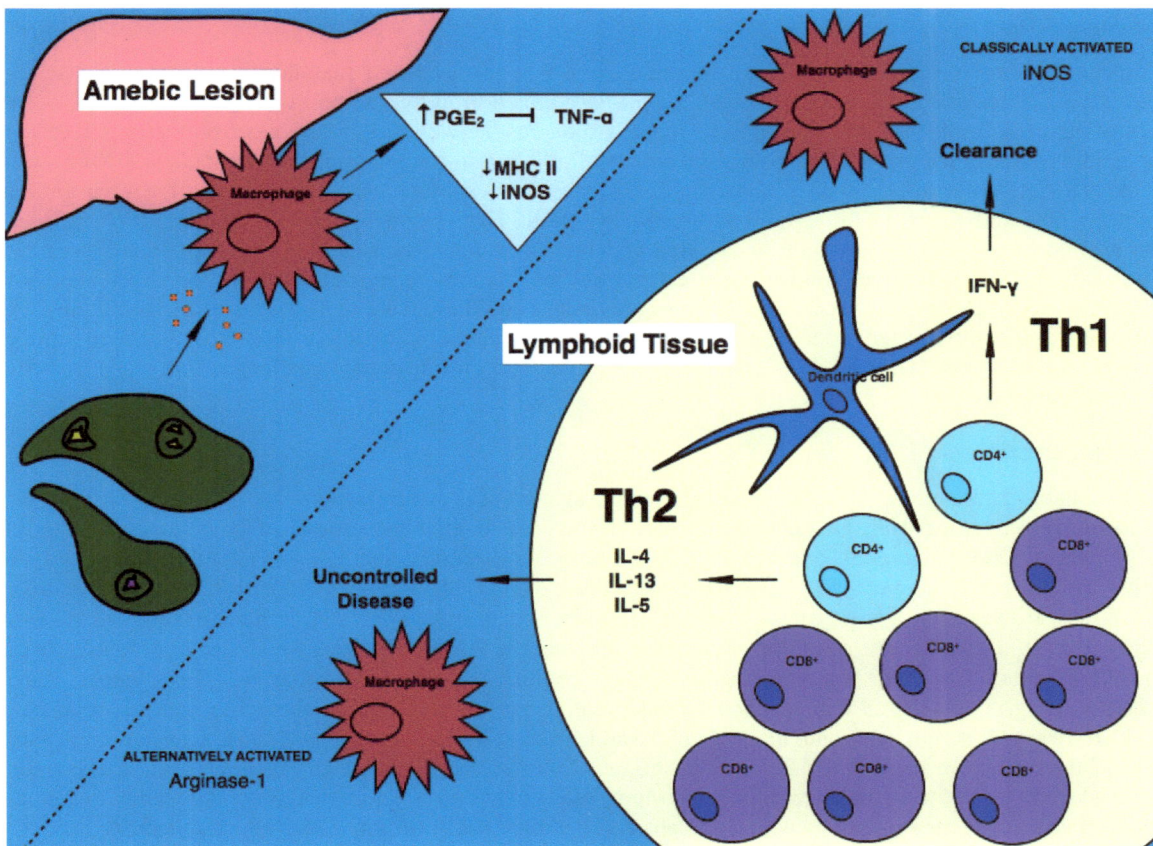

Figure 7: The adaptive immune responses towards *Entamoeba histolytica*. Evidence from humans and animal models of the disease suggest that Th1 responses control disease and lead to cure, while Th2 responses do not control disease and allow chronic infections to develop and persist in the host. In amebic lesions *E. histolytica* locally impairs macrophage function; they are unresponsive to stimulation, unable to produce nitric oxide, are not amebicidal and are ineffective at antigen presentation. Prostaglandin E$_2$ biosynthesis (PGE$_2$) is up regulated in macrophages by amoeba. PGE$_2$ mediates a number of suppressive effects in these cells, such as inhibition of TNF-α expression. TNF-α synergizes with IFN-γ to activate cytotoxic pathways including NO production. IFN-γ also activates MHC class II transcription. Thus, macrophages deactivated by amoeba are ineffective at T cell antigen presentation and are unable to mount a cytotoxic response.

This is consistent with the data from animal models where antisera from immunized animals inhibit trophozoite cell binding, and passive immunization with immune sera against the CRD protects against ALA [124-126].

However, this study also found that children with serum IgG responses that lack anti-CRD antibodies have an increased risk to *E. histolytica*, as they get new infections more frequently, are more likely to develop amebic diarrhea/dysentery and take longer to clear their infections [4]. Humoral immunity in this higher risk group has been suggested to reflect the development of an anti-protective Th2 response. These children produce IgG4 isotypes, which in humans are induced by Th2 cytokine IL-4, and this isotype is not found in children that produce anti-CRD IgG. It is interesting to note that not all children mount an IgG response to *E. histolytica*. In fact, there is good evidence for a genetic association of this trait, as the IgG response shows familial aggregation and most children that are IgG negative do not become IgG positive [4].

Other studies have shown that sera from ALA patients with high titers of anti-Gal-lectin antibodies differ markedly in their effects on trophozoite adherence. Some produce sera that inhibit trophozoite adherence while others produce sera that significantly enhances adherence [122]. Epitopes on Gal-lectin that increase adherence to both host cells and mucus have been mapped [125]. Thus, during the course of a natural infection an individual can generate either protective or anti-protective humoral responses to Gal-lectin. It has not been determined whether the host genotype influences which epitopes on Gal-lectin are recognized. But, it is possible that MHC restriction plays a role. In support of this idea, the MHC class II allele DQB1*0601 is associated with resistance to *E. histolytica* [127]. As the role of MHC class II molecules is to present foreign peptides to CD4$^+$ T cells, an individual's repertoire of MHC class II alleles is likely to influence their response to infection by determining which epitopes are recognized by CD4$^+$ T cells.

ii. Immunological Memory

Immunological memory is the capacity of the immune system to produce and maintain memory cells that respond to subsequent infections faster and more robustly than the primary infection. Acquired immunity to *E. histolytica* develops and plays an important role in how humans respond to repeat exposures. However, it is less clear how long effective memory responses endure. After four years of monitoring the cohort of children in Bangladesh, it was concluded that protective IgA responses to the CRD of Gal-lectin were short lived [5]. However, another group has shown intestinal anti-Gal-lectin antibodies to persist and fluctuate throughout a three-year period. They compared the IgA dynamics of recovered ALA patients to asymptomatic individuals living in an area endemic to *E. histolytica*. Both groups continued to produce fecal IgA. However, the ALA group maintained a greater level of immune responsiveness to repeat challenge than the asymptomatic group. ALA subjects produced more antibody peaks and these were of higher magnitude and longer duration. Furthermore, a significantly larger proportion of the ALA group remained completely free of *E. histolytica* infections. It was proposed that recovered ALA subjects mount a more robust response to repeat challenges that leads to a more rapid clearance of the parasite [121].

iii. IgA and IgG Degradation

IgA is the dominant immunoglobulin of the mucosal immune system. It is mostly exported across mucosal surfaces where it functions to neutralize toxins from pathogenic microorganisms and to limit the growth of commensals in the gut lumen [128]. In humans, *E. histolytica* elicits a secretory IgA response. As discussed above, anti-Gal-lectin secretory IgA in stool is protective against new infections [5, 123]. *In vitro*, human salivary IgA blocks amoeba cell adherence to epithelial monolayers [129]. However, amoeba cysteine proteases degrade human IgA [130, 131]. In humans there are two subclasses of IgA, termed IgA1 and IgA2. The main difference between them is that IgA2 is more resistant to proteases because of a 13 amino acid deletion in the hinge region that contains the recognition site for IgA1 proteases [128]. Amoebae are capable of degrading both IgA1 and IgA2 with surface bound cysteine proteases [131]. In the same manner, amoeba cysteine proteases also degrade serum immunoglobulin, IgG, and render it non-functional [132]. Cleavage of anti-amoeba immunoglobulin may reduce the affinity for amebic antigens, interfere with antigen disposal, or could mask amoeba from the immune system by coating their immunogenic molecules with Fab fragments [133]. The latter is an interesting possibility, as it suggests a mechanism by which amoeba could slip by the host immune system undetected.

Vaccine Development

Several factors regarding *E. histolytica* biology make development of an amebiasis vaccine feasible. First, for a parasite *E. histolytica* has a comparatively simple two-stage life history, the cyst and the trophozoite, of which only the trophozoite needs to be targeted by vaccination. Second, trophozoites express several immunogenic molecules that elicit protective immune responses. And third, one of these immunogenic molecules is known to be antigenically stable, even across diverse geographic isolates.

That being said, for a vaccine to be effective several requirements must be met. A vaccine must: induce the appropriate type of immune response that will provide protection against the pathogen of interest, produce a robust and long-lasting immunity, and provide protection against different strains of the pathogen.

Given the central role of Gal-lectin in pathogenesis, and that it is both strongly immunogenic and highly conserved, the native molecule or selected portions of it are excellent candidates for a vaccine (Table **1**). In the first Gal-lectin vaccine study, the purified molecule was emulsified in Freund's adjuvant and injected into gerbils. Upon intrahepatic challenge, 67% of animals were completely protected from ALA. However, immunized animals that were not protected developed larger abscesses than unimmunized controls [134]. This exacerbation of disease in some animals showed the anti-Gal-lectin immune response could be deleterious and emphasized the importance of isolating epitopes that elicit protective responses.

For this reason, subsequent studies have mainly used recombinant versions of the Gal-lectin cysteine rich region (Fig. **8**). Vaccination with this portion of the molecule in Freund's adjuvant has achieved between 62% and 81% protection without potentiating abscess development in unprotected animals [125, 135, 136]. It was later found that the N-terminal domain of Gal-lectin contains epitopes that elicit anti-protective humoral responses [125].

The basis for protection is that Gal-lectin can stimulate a cell-mediated immune response. Splenocytes from immunized animals respond to parasite challenge by producing Th1 cytokines and have amebicidal activity [112]. On macrophages, the cysteine rich region activates cytokines, IL-12 and TNF-α, which drive Th1 responses [37, 137]. In monocyte-derived dendritic cells, Gal-lectin causes activation and maturation, which is critical for induction of a T cell response. After stimulation with Gal-lectin, dendritic cell co-stimulatory markers and IL-12 are up regulated and adoptive transfer of Gal-lectin treated dendritic cells into naive mice initiates a Gal-lectin-specific Th1 response [36].

Inclusion of the right adjuvant(s) for a vaccine is equally important as the selection of antigens. Adjuvants are molecules or compounds that boost the potency and longevity of the immune response towards specific antigens. They can also be used to manipulate the type of immune response elicited by an antigen. IL-12 and IFN-γ play major roles in directing Th1 responses and adjuvants that can enhance their production will be important components of an amebiasis vaccine. Early studies showed Gal-lectin induced strong protective immune responses. However, these investigations used adjuvants that are unsuitable for human use due to their high toxicity. This has lead to testing of other types of vaccines that can safely augment immune responses.

Table 1: Amebiasis vaccines tested in animal models. aa: amino acid; CP: cysteine poor; CR: cysteine rich; Gal-lectin: galactose Hgl: Heavy Gal-lectin chain; Ig: immunoglobulin; MLIF: monocyte locomotion inhibitory factor; PR: pseudorepeat; SREHP: serine rich Entamoeba histolytica protein.

Vaccine candidate	Animal model	Adjuvant	Vaccination route	Efficacy	Responses	Reference
Native Gal-lectin	Gerbil	Freund's	Intraperitoneal Subcutaneous	67% protected	Ig directed against Hgl only Unprotected animals developed larger abscesses	[134]
Gal-lectin heavy subunit domains CR: aa 799-939, 939-1053 PR: aa 436- 624 CP: aa1-436	Gerbil	Freund's	Intraperitoneal	CR: aa 799-939 11% protected; aa 939-1053 62% protected PR: 38% protected CP: 0% protected, larger abscesses	CR: sera inhibit amoeba adherence strong lymphocyte proliferation PR: sera weakly inhibit amoeba adherence strong lymphocyte proliferation CP: sera weakly inhibit amoeba adherence weak lymphocyte proliferation	[125]
Native Gal-lectin	Gerbil	CpGODN	Intranasal Intraperitoneal	100% protected	Strong lymphocyte proliferation Humoral immunity Th1 and Th2 cytokines	[114]
Native Gal-lectin	Gerbil	EhDNA	Intramuscular	100% protected	Activation of innate pro-inflammatory immunity EhDNA stimulates macrophage expression of TNF-α, and iNOS via TLR9	[141]
DNA encoding Gal-lectin heavy subunit aa 894–1081	Mouse	Plasmid	Intradermal	Not assessed	Strong lymphocyte proliferation Humoral Th1 type immunity High levels of IgG2a	[139]
Gal-lectin heavy subunit peptides from the CR domain corresponding to epitopes recognized by human intestinal IgA	Baboon	Cholera toxin	Intranasal	Not assessed	Humoral immunity Anti-Gal-lectin serum IgG, serum IgA and intestinal IgA	[143]

SREHP fused to maltose binding protein	Gerbil	Freund's	Intranperitoneal Intradermal	Intranperitoneal: 64% protected Intradermal: 100% protected	Humoral immunity Anti-SREHP Ig	[147]
SREHP	Gerbil	Live attenuated *S. typhimurium*	Oral	78% protected	Humoral immunity Anti-SREHP serum IgG, serum IgA and mucosal IgA	[149]
DNA encoding SREHP fused to maltose binding protein	Mouse Gerbil	Plasmid	Intramuscular	Mouse: 80% completely protected reduced abscess size in other animals Gerbil: 40% completely protected reduced abscess size in other animals	Humoral immunity Strong lymphocyte proliferation	[148]
MLIF polymer	Gerbil	None	intramuscular	Short-term: 100% survival Long-term: no protection	No humoral immunity detected Weak lymphocyte proliferation	[145]

DNA vaccination has been one approach. DNA vaccines are new types of vaccines that introduce antigens from the pathogen of interest via a plasmid or an attenuated virus encoding the corresponding genes. Upon transfection of host cells, vector genes are expressed and the encoded antigens are endogenously produced by transfected cells

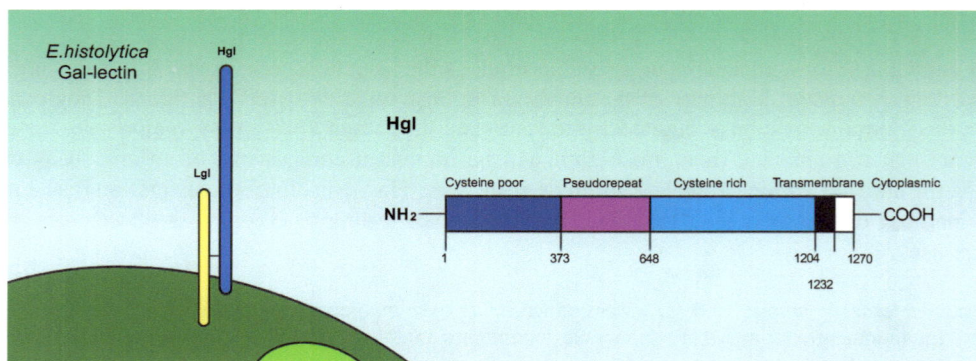

Figure 8: *E. histolytica* Gal-lectin. The Gal-lectin is a heterodimer composed of a 170-kDa heavy chain (Hgl) and a 35/31-kDa light chain (Lgl). The heavy chain is immunogenic and highly conserved. The light subunit is not immunogenic. Structural domains of the Gal-lectin heavy chain are shown. The N-terminal, cysteine poor domain contains anti-protective epitopes, while protective epitopes are present in the cysteine rich and pseudorepeat domains. The cysteine rich domain also contains the carbohydrate recognition domain.

[138]. An exciting feature is that cytokine genes can be incorporated into these vectors, and thereby enable a direct control over the immune response. In this regard, a codon-optimized DNA vaccine encoding a portion of the Gal-lectin has been produced and tested in mice. Because *E. histolytica* has an A:T rich genome whereas mammalian genomes are G:C rich, the sequence encoding the Gal-lectin was re-written to account for the codon bias in rodents. The rodent-optimized gene was highly expressed and stimulated Gal-lectin specific T cells and the production of Th1 antibodies [139].

Another alternative has been to incorporate unmethylated CpG motifs into the vaccine. In mammalian DNA, a cytosine followed by a guanine is usually methylated. However, in bacteria these sites are unmethylated and the innate immune system has evolved to recognize unmethylated CpG dinucleotides as pathogen associated molecular patterns (PAMPs) through TLR9. Synthetic oligodeoxynucleotides containing unmethylated CpGs are a novel class of adjuvants that safely activate Th1 responses [140]. Both systemic and mucosal immunization of gerbils with the Gal-lectin plus CpG oligodeoxynucleotides induced 100% protection against ALA. Serum IgG and stool IgA from immunized animals inhibited trophozoite adherence between 70% and 80%, which is higher than what other vaccination regimes have achieved. Furthermore, immunized animals mounted a robust IFN-γ response, indicating development of protective Th1 immunity. However, they also significantly expressed IL-4, a hallmark of an anti-protective Th2 immune response [113, 114]. It is possible that in this context, IL-4 is beneficial to the extent that it enhances secretory IgA production.

Interestingly, *E. histolytica* DNA also contains PAMPs that activate TLR9. Combined immunization of *E. histolytica* DNA and Gal-lectin protected gerbils 100% from ALA, and activated cytokine responses similar to those induced by CpG oligodeoxynucleotides regimes [141]. This suggests that *E. histolytica* DNA would be another useful component of a vaccine.

When a vaccine has high efficacy in animals, testing can move to human trials. However, one of the drawbacks with the rodent models is that they do not naturally develop amebiasis and therefore they may not sufficiently predict vaccine efficacy in humans. One solution is to use a primate model. Recently, a Gal-lectin-based vaccine has been tested in baboons, which in the wild become naturally infected with *E. histolytica* [142]. Peptides corresponding to Gal-lectin epitopes recognized by immune human secretory IgA were administered with cholera toxin B. The vaccination stimulated strong intestinal IgA responses and serum and fecal antibodies that inhibited amebic cell adherence [143]. However, challenge infections remain to be tested.

Besides the Gal-lectin, several other candidate molecules have been tested for a vaccine. An intriguing candidate is monocyte locomotion inhibitory factor (MLIF). MLIF is a small anti-inflammatory pentapeptide (Met-Gln-Cys-Asn-Ser) produced by *E. histolytica*. Like its name suggests, it inhibits monocyte movement. It also inhibits leukocyte respiratory burst and NO production and reduces pro-inflammatory chemokine expression [144]. MLIF is cleaved from a larger parent protein whose identity remains illusive and there have been uncertainties regarding MLIF expression *in vivo*. However, immunization against MLIF conferred gerbils with sustained protection from ALA. Interestingly, cellular responses to MLIF appeared weak and humoral responses were undetectable, which leaves unanswered questions regarding how MLIF stimulates protection [145].

Another highly promising candidate is the serine rich protein, SREHP. It is both immunogenic and highly expressed on trophozoite surfaces. SREHP appears to participate in phagocytosis and adherence, but its functions are largely unexplored. Multiple studies have shown immunization against this molecule generates protection. Passive immunization with SREHP antibodies protected SCID mice from ALA, parenteral immunization with recombinant SREHP fused to maltose-binding protein generated protection in 64% to 100% of gerbils, and a SREHP DNA vaccine demonstrated similar levels of protection [146-148]. Mucosal immunization with attenuated bacterial strains expressing SREHP has also been explored [149, 150]. The bacterial delivery vehicle has several advantages. First, attenuated bacteria stimulate a potent immune response directly in the gastrointestinal tract, which could be more effective than parenteral immunization at generating secretory IgA. Therefore, colonization and invasion may be better prevented. Second, the live-attenuated bacterium establishes a non-invasive gut infection, which can promote long-lasting immunological memory. Third, these vaccines have the potential to provide dual protection against enteric pathogens, as the vectors themselves are immunogenic. To this end, attenuated *Salmonella typhimurium* and *Vibrio cholerae* have been used and both induced a strong mucosal and systemic antibody response directed at both SREHP and the vector [149, 150]. Intrahepatic challenge was evaluated with *S. typhimurium* and 78% of animals were completely protected [149].

CONCLUSIONS AND FUTURE DIRECTIONS

Evidence suggests both the innate and adaptive arms of the immune response can clear invasive *E. histolytica*. Invasion starts when trophozoites deplete the mucus layer and invade the colonic epithelium. In some cases this results in amoeba migration into the lamina propria and submucosa, where they can cause ulcerations and/or gain entry into the portal circulation to be carried to extraintestinal sites.

In response to invasion the host mounts a rapid inflammatory response. It appears that in most situations this sufficiently controls the parasite, as amebiasis usually does not progress beyond dysentery and diarrhea (though in terms of health and well being, these illnesses should not be deemed insignificant). In patients with amebic colitis and ALA the parasite employs multiple strategies that allow it to successfully subvert the immune response and establish a chronic infection. In such cases the host develops a defective adaptive response that cannot clear the parasite and there is evidence that host genetics play a role.

There are many parasite molecules that contribute to *E. histolytica* pathogenicity. Gal-lectin and the cysteine proteases, whose levels of expression and activity correlate positively with amoeba virulence, are crucial factors. In short, Gal-lectin enables amoeba to colonize via attachment to colonic mucus. During invasion, it mediates adherence to host cells, apoptosis and phagocytosis. The heavy subunit of this molecule triggers an inflammatory response and is involved in complement resistance by preventing assembly of the membrane attack complex on amoeba surfaces. The cysteine proteases dissolve colonic mucus, degrade the extracellular matrix, activate and inactivate components of complement, and limit the humoral response by cleaving anti-parasite antibodies. *E. histolytica* is also capable of disarming neutrophils and macrophages via a number of mechanisms. Namely, this involves parasite enzymes that neutralize ROS and parasite-host interactions that inhibit NO production.

Though our understanding of amebiasis has advanced far, there are a number of basic questions about the host-parasite relationship that remain unanswered. For example, how and why does *E. histolytica* transition from a harmless commensal to a destructive pathogen? Also, what host-parasite interactions are responsible for keeping the majority of amoeba at bay and why do most infections remain benign? Evidence indicates some individuals are genetically predisposed to developing invasive infections, while others are resistant. However, the mechanisms of human resistance to colonization or invasion are poorly understood.

Answers to these questions could help identify and target susceptible populations for vaccination. There are now several good vaccine candidates that have proved success in animal models. Clinical trials need to be carried out to determine their efficacy in humans. A successful amebiasis vaccine will elicit long-lasting memory that prevents the occurrence of both acute (diarrhea and dysentery) and chronic amebiasis (colitis and extraintestinal abscesses). In places where *E. histolytica* is endemic, people are faced with a multitude of problems, least of which concerns the prevention of amebiasis. Collaborations between investigators of basic science and the public and private health sectors could create viable solutions to prevent this disease.

ACKNOWLEDGEMENTS

Dr. Chadee is a Canada Research Chair (Tier 1) in Gastrointestinal Inflammation and his research is supported by grants from the Natural Sciences and Engineering Research Council of Canada, the Canadian Institute for Health Research, the Canadian Foundation for Innovation, the Crohn's and Colitis Foundation of Canada, and the Canadian Association of Gastroenterology-Astra Zeneca-CIHR Research and Fellowship Awards. L. Mortimer is supported by Achievers in Medicine Award, Dean's Entrance Scholarship (DES) and a FGS award from the University of Calgary.

REFERENCES

[1]   WHO/PAHO/UNESCO report: a consultation with experts on amoebiasis: Mexico City, Mexico 28-29 January, 1997. Epidemiol Bull 1997; 18:13-4.
[2]   Stanley SL. Amoebiasis. Lancet 2003; 361: 1025-34.
[3]   Abd-Alla MD, Ravdin JI. Diagnosis of amoebic colitis by antigen capture ELISA in patients presenting with acute diarrhoea in Cairo, Egypt.Trop Med Int Health 2002; 7: 365–70.
[4]   Haque R, Duggal P, Ali IM, Hossain MB, Mondal D, Sack RB, Farr BM, Petri WA. Innate and Acquired Resistance to Amebiasis in Bangladeshi Children. J Infect Dis 2002.; 186: 547-52.
[5]   Haque R, Mondal D, Duggal P, Kabirm M, Roy S, Farr BM, Sack RB, Petri W.A. *Entamoeba histolytica* Infection in Children and Protection from Subsequent Amebiasis. Infect Immun 2006; 74: 904-9.
[6]   Prathap K, Gilman R. The Histopathology of Acute Intestinal Amebiasis. Am J Pathol 1970; 60: 229-46.
[7]   Chadee K, Meerovitch E. *Entamoeba histolytica*: Early Progressive Pathology in the Cecum of the Gerbil (Meriones unguiculatus). Am J Trop Med Hyg 1985; 34: 283-291.
[8]   Espinosa-Cantellano M, Martinéz-Palomo A. Pathogenesis of Intestinal Amebiasis: From Molecules to Disease. Clin Microbiol Rev 2000; 13: 318-31.
[9]   Chadee K, Meerovitch E. The Pathogenesis of Experimentally Induced Amebic Liver Abscess in the Gerbil (Meriones unguiculatus). Am J Pathol 1984; 117: 71-80.
[10] Chadee K, Petri WA, Innes DJ, Ravdin JI. Rat and Human Colonic Mucins Bind to and Inhibit Adherence Lectin of Entamoeba histolytica. J Clin Invest 1987; 80: 1245-54.
[11] Dodson JM, Lenkowski PW, Eubanks AC, Jackson TF, Napodano J, Lyerly DM, Lockhart LA, Mann BJ, Petri WA. Infection and Immunity Mediated by the Carbohydrate Recognition Domain of the *Entamoeba histolytica* Gal/GalNAc Lectin. J Infect Dis 1999; 179: 460-6.
[12] Bracha R, Mirelman D. Adherence and Ingestion of *Escherichia coli* Serotype 055 by Trophozoites of *Entamoeba histolytica*. Infect Immun 1983; 40: 882-7.
[13] Ravdin J, Guerrant RL. Role of Adherence in Cytopathogenic Mechanisms of *Entamoeba Histolytica* Study with Mammalian Tissue Culture Cells and Human Erythrocytes. J Clin Invest 1981; 65: 1303-13.

[14] Petri WA, Smith RD, Schlesinger PH, Murphy CF, Ravdin JI. Isolation of the Galactose-binding Lectin That Mediates the In Vitro Adherence of *Entamoeba histolytica*. J Clin Invest 1987; 80: 1238-44.

[15] Tannich E, Ebert F, Horstmann RF. Primary structure of the 170-kDa surface lectin of pathogenic *Entamoeba histolytica*. P Natl Acad Sci USA 1991; 88: 1849-53.

[16] Bracha R, Mirelman D. Virulence of *Entamoeba histolytica* Trophozoites Effects of Bacteria, Microaerobic Conditions, and Metronidazole. J Exp Med 1984; 160: 353-58.

[17] Wittner M, Rosenbaum M. Role of Bacteria in Modifying Virulence of *Entamoeba histolytica* Studies of Amebae from Axenic Cultures. Am J Trop Med Hyg 1970; 19: 755-61.

[18] Padilla-Vaca F, Ankri S, Bracha R, *et al.* Down Regulation of *Entamoeba histolytica* Virulence by Monoxenic Cultivation with *Escherichia coli* O55 Is Related to a Decrease in Expression of the Light (35-Kilodalton) Subunit of the Gal/GalNAc Lectin. Infect Immun 1999; 67: 2096–102.

[19] Galván-Moroyoqui JM, Domínguez-Robles M, Franco E, Meza, I. The Interplay between *Entamoeba* and Enteropathogenic Bacteria Modulates Epithelial Cell Damage. PLOS Neglect Trop D 2008; 2: e266.

[20] Tse S, Chadee K. Biochemical Characterization of Rat Colonic Mucins Secreted in Response to *Entamoeba histolytica*. Infect Immun 1992; 60: 1603-12.

[21] Belley A, Chadee K. Prostaglandin E2 Stimulates Rat and Human Colonic Mucin Exocytosis Via the EP4 Receptor. Gastroenterology 1999; 117: 1352-62.

[22] Dey I, Keller K, Belley A, Chadee K. Identification and characterization of a cyclooxygenase-like enzyme from *Entamoeba histolytica*. P Natl Acad Sci USA 2003; 100: 13561-6.

[23] Moncada D, Keller K, Chadee K. *Entamoeba histolytica*-Secreted Products Degrade Colonic Mucin Oligosaccharides. Infect Immun 2005; 73: 3790-3.

[24] Lidell ME, Moncada D, Chadee K, *et al.* *Entamoeba histolytica* cysteine proteases cleave the MUC2 mucin in its C-terminal domain and dissolve the protective colonic mucus gel. P Natl Acad Sci USA 2006; 103: 9298-303.

[25] Eckmann L, Reed SL, Smith JR, Kagnoff MF. *Entamoeba histolytica* Trophozoites Induce an Inflammatory Cytokine Response by Cultured Human Cells through the Paracrine Action of Cytolytically Released Interleukin-Iα. J Clin Invest 1995; 96: 1269-79.

[26] Dey I, Chadee K. Prostaglandin E2 Produced by *Entamoeba histolytica* Binds to EP4 Receptors and Stimulates Interleukin-8 Production in Human Colonic Cells. Infect Immun 2008; 76: 5158-63.

[27] Seydel KB, Li E, Zhang Z, Stanley SL. Epithelial Cell–Initiated Inflammation Plays a Crucial Role in Early Tissue Damage in Amebic Infection of Human Intestine. Gastroenterology 1998; 115: 1446-53.

[28] Seydel KB, Li E, Swanson PE, *et al.* Human Intestinal Epithelial Cells Produce Proinflammatory Cytokines in Response to Infection in a SCID Mouse-Human Intestinal Xenograft Model of Amebiasis. Infect Immun 1997; 65: 1631-9.

[29] Kammanadiminti SJ, Dey I, Chadee K. Induction of Monocyte Chemotactic Protein 1 in Colonic Epithelial Cells by *Entamoeba histolytica* Is Mediated via the Phosphatidylinositol 3-Kinase/p65 Pathway. Infect Immun 2007; 75: 1765-70.

[30] Kammanadiminti SJ, Chadee K. Suppression of NF-κB Activation by *Entamoeba histolytica* in Intestinal Epithelial Cells Is Mediated by Heat Shock Protein 27. J Biol Chem 2006; 281: 26112-20.

[31] Leroy A, Lauwaet T, De Brunye G, *et al.* *Entamoeba histolytica* disturbs the tight junction complex in human enteric T84 cell layers. The FASEB J 2000; 14: 1139-46.

[32] Leroy A, De Bruyne G, Mareel M, *et al.* Contact-Dependent Transfer of the Galactose-Specific Lectin of *Entamoeba histolytica* to the Lateral Surface of Enterocytes in Culture. Infect Immun 1995; 63: 4253-60.

[33] Lauwaet T, José Oliveira M., De Bruyne G, *et al.* *Entamoeba histolytica* trophozoites transfer lipophosphopeptidoglycans to enteric cell layers. Int J Parasitol 2004; 34: 549-56.

[34] Maldonado C, Trejo W, Ramírez A, *et al.* Lipophosphopeptidoglycan of *Entamoeba histolytica* Induces an Antiinflammatory Innate Immune Response and Downregulation of Toll-Like Receptor 2 (TLR-2) Gene Expression in Human Monocytes. Arch Med Res 2000; 31: S71-73.

[35] Rawal S, Majumdar S, Vohra, H. Activation of MAPK kinase pathway by Gal/GalNAc adherence lectin of *Entamoeba histolytica*: gateway to host response. Mol Cell Biochem 2005; 268: 93-101.

[36] Ivory CP, Chadee, K. Activation of dendritic cells by the Gal-lectin of *Entamoeba histolytica* drives Th1 responses *in vitro* and *in vivo*. Eur J Immunol 2007; 37: 385-94.

[37] Séguin R., Mann BJ, Keller K, *et al.* Identification of the galactose-adherence lectin epitopes of *Entamoeba histolytica* that stimulate tumor necrosis factor-a production by macrophages. Proc Natl Acad Sci USA 1995; 92: 12175-9.

[38] Chadee K. J Innate Immun 2009; 1: 69- 174. Cover Image.

[39] Ravdin JI, Croft, BY, Geurrant RL. Cytopathogenic Mechanisms of *Entamoeba histolytica*. J Exp Med 1980; 152:3 77-90.

[40] HustonC.D, Boettner DR, Miller-Sims V, *et al.* Apoptotic Killing and Phagocytosis of Host Cells by the Parasite *Entamoeba histolytica*. Infect Immun 2003; 71: 964-72.

[41]   Ravdin JI, Moreau F, Sullivan JA, *et al.* Relationship of Free Intracellular Calcium to the Cytolytic Activity of *Entamoeba histolytica.* Infect Immun 1988; 56: 1505-12.

[42]   Saffer LD, Petri WA. Role of the Galactose Lectin of *Entamoeba histolytica* in Adherence-Dependent Killing of Mammalian Cells. Infect Immun 1991; 59: 4681-3.

[43]   Seydel KB, Stanley SL. *Entamoeba histolytica* Induces Host Cell Death in Amebic Liver Abscess by a Non-Fas-Dependent, Non-Tumor Necrosis Factor Alpha-Dependent Pathway of Apoptosis. Infect and Immun 1998; 66: 2980-3.

[44]   Huston CD, Houpt ER, Mann BJ, *et al.* Caspase 3-dependent killing of host cells by the parasite *Entamoeba histolytica.* Cell Microbiol 2000; 2: 617-25.

[45]   Teixeira JE, Huston CD. Participation of the Serine-Rich *Entamoeba histolytica* Protein in Amebic Phagocytosis of Apoptotic Host Cell. Infect Immun 2008; 76: 959-66.

[46]   Boettner DR, Huston CD, Linford AS, *et al. Entamoeba histolytica* Phagocytosis of Human Erythrocytes Involves PATMK, a Member of the Transmembrane Kinase Family. PLOS Pathog 2008; 4: e0122-33.

[47]   García-Rivera G, Rodríguez MA, Ocádiz R, *et al. Entamoeba histolytica*: a novel cysteine protease and an adhesin form the 112 kDa surface protein. Mol Microbiol 1999; 33: 556-68.

[48]   Okada M, Huston CD, Mann BJ, *et al.* Proteomic Analysis of Phagocytosis in the Enteric Protozoan Parasite *Entamoeba histolytica.* Eukaryot Cell 2005; 4: 827-31.

[49]   Rodríguez MA, García-Pérez RM, García-Rivera G, *et al.* An *Entamoeba histolytica* Rab-like encoding gene and protein: function and cellular location. Mol Biochem Parasitol 2000; 108: 199-206.

[50]   Saito-Nakano Y, Yasuda T, Shigeta Y, *et al.* Identification and Characterizaton of a Rab5 Homologue in *Entamoeba histolytica.* Arch Med Res 2000; 31: S155-6.

[51]   Welter BH, Laughlin RC, Temesvari LA. Characterization of a Rab7-like GTPase, EhRab7: a marker for the early stages of endocytosis in *Entamoeba histolytica.* Mol Biochem Parasitol 2002; 121: 254-64.

[52]   Ghosh SK, Samuelson J. Involvement of p21racA, Phosphoinositide 3-Kinase, and Vacuolar ATPase in Phagocytosis of Bacteria and Erythrocytes by *Entamoeba histolytica*: Suggestive Evidence for Coincidental Evolution of Amebic Invasiveness. Infect Immun 1997; 65: 4243-9.

[53]   Labruyère E, Zimmer C, Galy V, *et al.* EhPAK, a member of the p21-activated kinase family, is involved in the control of *Entamoeba histolytica* migration and phagocytosis. J Cell Sci 2003; 116: 61-71.

[54]   Leippe, M., Ebel, S., Schoenberger, O.L., *et al.* Pore-forming peptide of pathogenic *Entamoeba histolytica.* Proc Natl Acad Sci USA 1991; 88: 7659-63.

[55]   Leippe M, Andra J, Nickel R, *et al.* Amoebapores, a family of membranolytic peptides from cytoplasmic granules of *Entamoeba histolytica*: isolation, primary structure, and pore formation in bacterial cytoplasmic membranes. Mol Microbiol 1994; 14: 895-904.

[56]   Leippe M, Bruhn, H, Hecht O, *et al.* Ancient weapons: the three-dimensional structure of amoebapore A. Trends Parasitol 2005; 21: 5-7.

[57]   O'Neill LA. The interleukin-1 receptor/ Toll-like receptor superfamily: 10 years of progress. Immunol Rev 2008; 226: 10-18.

[58]   Bhakdi S, Muhly M, Korom S, *et al.* Effects of Escherichia coli Hemolysin on Human Monocytes- Cytocidal Action and Stimulation of Interleukin-1 Release. J Clin Invest 1990; 85: 1746-53.

[59]   Boise L, Collins C. Salmonella-induced cell death: apoptosis, necrosis or programmed cell death? Trends Microbiol 2001; 9: 64-7.

[60]   Chen C, Kono H, Golenbock D, *et al.* Identification of a key pathway required for the sterile inflammatory response triggered by dying cells. Nat Med 2007; 13: 851-6.

[61]   Zhang Z, Yan L, Wang L, *et al.* Entamoeba histolytica cysteine proteinases with interleukin-1 beta converting enzyme (ICE) activity cause intestinal inflammation and tissue damage in amoebiasis. Mol Microbiol 2000; 37: 542-8.

[62]   Meza I, Galvàn-Moroyoqui M, Dominguez-Robles MC, *et al. Entamoeba histolytica* and E. dispar interaction with enteropathogenic bacteria synergizes damage to epitheal cells amplifying the inflammatory response. Eur J Trop Med Inter Health 2007;12: S1,44.

[63]   Blázquez S, Zimmer C, Guigon G, *et al.* Human Tumor Necrosis Factor is a Chemoattractant for the Parasite *Entamoeba histolytica.* Infect Immun 2006; 74: 1407–11.

[64]   Hamano S, Asgharpour A, Stroup SE, *et al.* Resistance of C57BL/6 Mice to Amoebiasis Is Mediated by Nonhemopoietic Cells but Requires Hemopoietic IL-10 Production. J Immunol 2006; 177: 1208-13.

[65]   Houpt ER, Glembocki DJ, Obrig TG, *et al.* The Mouse Model of Amebic Colitis Reveals Mouse Strain Susceptibility to Infection and Exacerbation of Disease by CD4+ T Cells. J Immunol 2002; 169: 4496-503.

[66]   Asgharpour A, Gilchrist C, Baba D, *et al.* Resistance to Intestinal *Entamoeba histolytica* Infection Is Conferred by Innate Immunity and Gr-1+ Cells. Infect Immun 2005; 73: 4522-9.

[67]   Ruiz PA, Shkoda A, Kim SC, *et al.* IL-10 gene-deficient mice lack TGF-β/Smad signaling and fail to inhibit proinflammatory gene expression in intestinal epithelial cells after the colonization with colitogenic Enterococcus faecalis. J Immunol 2005; 174: 2990 – 9.

[68]   Schwerbrock NM, Makkink MK, van der Sluis M, *et al*. Interleukin 10-deficient mice exhibit defective colonic Muc2 synthesis before and after induction of colitis by commensal bacteria. Inflamm Bowel Dis 2004; 10: 811– 23.

[69]   Grazia Roncarolo M, Bacchetta R, Bordignon C, *et al*. Type 1 T regulatory cells. Immunol Rev 2001; 182: 68-79.

[70]   Zhou P, Streutker C, Borojevic R, *et al*. IL-10 modulates intestinal damage and epithelial cell apoptosis in T cell-mediated enteropathy. Am J Physiol 2004; 287: G599-604.

[71]   Denis M, Chadee, K. Human neutrophils activated by interferon-gamma and tumour necrosis factor-alpha kill *Entamoeba histolytica* trophozoites *in vitro*. J Leukoc Biol. 1989; 46: 270-4.

[72]   Guerrant RL, Brush J, Ravdin JI, *et al*. Interaction between *Entamoeba histolytica* and human polymorpho-nuclear neutrophils. J Infect Dis 1981; 143: 83-93.

[73]   Bruchhaus I, Tannich E. Induction of the iron-containing superoxide dismutase in *Entamoeba histolytica* by a superoxide anion-generating system or by iron chelation; Mol. Biochem. Parasitol. 1994; 67: 281-8.

[74]   Bruchhaus I, Tannich E. Identification of an *Entamoeba histolytica* gene encoding a protein homologous to prokaryotic disulphide oxidoreductases. Mol Biochem Parasitolo. 1995; 70: 187-91.

[75]   Bruchhaus I, Richter S, Tannich E, *et al*. Recombinant expression and biochemical characterization of an NADPH: flavin oxidoreductase from *Entamoeba histolytica*. Biochem. J. 1998; 330: 1217-21.

[76]   Choi M, Sajed D, Poole L, *et al*. An unusual surface peroxiredoxin protects invasive *Entamoeba histolytica* from oxidant attack. Mol Biochem Parasitol 2005; 143: 80-9.

[77]   Davis PH, Zhang X, Guo J, *et al*. Comparative proteomic analysis of two *Entamoeba histolytica* strains with different virulence phenotypes identifies peroxiredoxin as an important component of amoebic virulence. Mol Microbiol 2006; 61: 1523-32.

[78]   Murray HW, Aley SB, Scott WA. Susceptibility of *Entamoeba histolytica* to oxygen intermediates. Mol Biochem Parasitol 1981; 3: 381–91.

[79]   Ghadirian E, Somerfield SD, Kongshavn PA. Susceptibility of *Entamoeba histolytica* to Oxidants. Infect Immun 1986; 51: 263-7.

[80]   Riahi Y, Simon-Tov R, Ankri S. Molecular cloning, expression and characterization of a serine proteinase inhibitor gene from *Entamoeba histolytica*. Mol Biochem Parasitol 2004; 133: 153-62.

[81]   Sim S, Park S, Yong T, *et al*. Involvement of b2-integrin in ROS-mediated neutrophil apoptosis induced by *Entamoeba histolytica*. Microbes Infect 2007; 9: 1368-75.

[82]   Marion, S. and Guillén, N. Genomic and proteomic approaches highlight phagocytosis of living and apoptotic human cells by the parasite *Entamoeba histolytica*. Int J Parasitol 2006; 36: 131-9.

[83]   Velazquez C, Shibayama-Sala M, Aguirre-Garcia J, *et al*. Role of Neutrophils in Innate Resistance to *Entamoeba histolytica* liver infection in mice. Parasite Immunol 1998; 20: 255-62.

[84]   Seydel KB, Zhang T, Stanley SL. Neutrophils Play a Critical Role in Early Resistance to Amebic Liver Abscesses in Severe Combined Immunodeficient Mice. Infect Immun 2000; 65: 3951-3.

[85]   Siman-Tov R, Ankri, S. Nitric oxide inhibits cysteine proteinases and alcohol dehydrogenase 2 of *Entamoeba histolytica*. Parasitol Res 2003; 89: 146-9.

[86]   Lin JY, Chadee K. Macrophage Cytotoxicity Against *Entamoeba histolytica* Trophozoites is Mediated by Nitric Oxide from L-Arginine. J Immunol 1992; 148: 3999-4005.

[87]   Seydel KB, Smith SJ, Stanley SL. Innate Immunity to Amebic Liver Abscess Is Dependent on Gamma Interferon and Nitric Oxide in a Murine Model of Disease. Infect Immun 2000; 68: 400-2.

[88]   Salata RA, Martinez-Palomo A, Murray HW, *et al*. Patients Treated for Amebic Liver Abscess Develop Cell Mediated Responses Effective in vitro Against *Entamoeba histolytica*. J Immunol 1986; 136: 2633-9.

[89]   Campbell D, Gaucher D, Chadee K. Serum from *Entamoeba histolytica*–Infected Gerbils Selectively Suppresses T Cell Proliferation by Inhibiting Interleukin-2 Production. J Infect Dis 1999; 179: 1495-501.

[90]   Wang W, Keller K, Chadee K. Modulation of Tumor Necrosis Factor Production by Macrophages in *Entamoeba histolytica* Infection. Infect Immun 1992; 60: 3169-74.

[91]   Wang W, Keller K, Chadee K. *Entamoeba histolytica* modulates the nitric oxide synthase gene and nitric oxide production by macrophages for cytotoxicity against amoebae and tumour ceils. Immunology 1994; 83: 601-10.

[92]   Denis M, Chadee K. *In Vitro* and *In Vivo* Studies of Macrophage Functions in Amebiasis. Infect Immun 1988; 56: 3126-31.

[93]   Elnkave K, Siman-Tov R, Ankri S. Consumption of L-arginine mediated by *Entamoeba histolytica* L -arginase (EhArg) inhibits amoebicidal activity and nitric oxide production by activated macrophages. Parasite Immunol 2003; 25: 597-608.

[94]   Reed SL, Keene WE, McKerrow JH, Gigli I. Cleavage of C3 by a neutral cysteine proteinase of *Entamoeba histolytica*. J Immunol 1989; 143: 189-95.

[95]   Reed S, Gigli I. Lysis of Complement-sensitive *Entamoeba histolytica* by Activated Terminal Complement Components. J Clin Invest 1990; 86: 1815-22.

[96]   Gutiérrez-Kobeh L, Cabrera N, Pérez-Montfort R. A mechanism of acquired resistance to complement-mediated lysis by *Entamoeba histolytica*. J Parasitol 1997; 83: 234-41.

[97]   Hamelmann C, Foerster B, Burchard GD, Shetty N, Horstmann RD. Induction of complement resistance in cloned pathogenic *Entamoeba histolytica*. Parasite Immunol 1993; 15: 223-8.

[98]   Reed S, Curd JG, Gigli I, Gillin FD, Braude AI. Activation of complement by pathogenic and nonpathogenic *Entamoeba histolytica*. J Immunol 1986; 136: 2265-70.

[99]   Reed SL, Sargeaunt PG, Braude AI. Resistance to lysis by human serum of pathogenic *Entamoeba histolytica*. Trans R Soc Trop Med Hyg 1983; 77: 248-53.

[100]   Braga L, Ninomiya H, McCoy JJ, *et al.* Inhibition of the complement membrane attack complex by the galactose-specific adhesion of *Entamoeba histolytica*. J Clin Invest 1992; 90: 1131-7.

[101]   Ventura-Juárez J, Campos-Rodríguez R, Jarillo-Luna RA, *et al.* Trophozoites of *Entamoeba histolytica* express a CD59-like molecule in human colon. Parasitol Res 2009; 104: 821-6.

[102]   Spath GF, Garraway LA, Turco SJ, *et al.* The role(s) of lipophosphoglycan (LPG) in the establishment of *Leishmania major* infections in mammalian hosts. Proc Natl Acad Sci USA 2003; 100: 9536-41.

[103]   Weber C, Blazquez S, Marion S, *et al.* Bioinformatics and Functional Analysis of an *Entamoeba histolytica* Mannosyltransferase Necessary for Parasite Complement Resistance and Hepatical Infection. PLOS Neglect Trop D 2008; 2: e165.

[104]   Bhattacharya A, Arya R, Clark CG, *et al.* Absence of lipophosphoglycan-like glycoconjugates in *Entamoeba dispar*. Parasitology 2000; 120: 31–5r.

[105]   Reed SL, Ember J, Herdman D, *et al.* The Extracellular Neutral Cysteine Proteinaes of *Entamoeba histolytica* Degrade Anaphylatoxins C3a and C5a. J Immunol 1995; 155: 266-74.

[106]   Walport MJ. Complement Second of Two Parts. New Engl J Med 2001; 344: 1140-4.

[107]   Köhl J. Anaphylatoxins and infectious and non-infectious inflammatory diseases. Mol Immunol 2001; 38: 175-87.

[108]   Gasque P. Complement: a unique innate immune sensor for danger signals. Mol Immunol 2004; 41: 1089-98.

[109]   Snow M, Chen M, Guo J, *et al.* Short Report: Differences in Complement-mediated Killing of *Entamoeba histolytica* Between Men and Women—An Explanation for the Increased Susceptibility of Men to Invasive Amebiasis? Am J Trop Med Hyg 2008; 78: 922-3.

[110]   Stanley SL, Jackson TF, Reed SL, Calderon J, Kunz-Jenkins C, Gathiram V, Li E. Serodiagnosis of invasive amebiasis using a recombinant *Entamoeba histolytica* protein. JAMA 1991; 266: 1984-6.

[111]   Schain DC, Salata RA, Ravdin JI. Human T-Lymphocyte Proliferation, Lymphokine Production, and Amebicidal Activity Elicited by the Galactose-Inhibitable Adherence Protein of *Entamoeba histolytica*. Infect Immun 1992; 60: 2143-6.

[112]   Schain DC, Salata RA, Ravdin JI. Development of Amebicidal Cell-Mediated Immunity in Gerbils (Meriones unguiculatus) Immunized with the Galactose-Inhibitable Adherence Lectin of *Entamoeba histolytica*. Journal Parasitol 1995; 81: 563-8.

[113]   Ivory CP, Keller K, Chadee K. CpG-Oligodeoxynucleotide Is a Potent Adjuvant with an *Entamoeba histolytica* Gal-Inhibitable Lectin Vaccine against Amoebic Liver Abscess in Gerbils. Infect Immun 2006; 74: 528-36.

[114]   Ivory CP, Chadee K. Intranasal Immunization with Gal-Inhibitable Lectin plus an Adjuvant of CpG Oligodeoxynucleotides Protects against *Entamoeba histolytica* Challenge. Infect Immun 2007; 75: 4917-22.

[115]   Guo X, Stroup SE, Houpt E. Persistence of *Entamoeba histolytica* infection in CBA mice owes to intestinal IL-4 production and inhibition of protective IFN-γ. Mucosal Immunol 2008. 1: 139-46.

[116]   Houpt ER, Glembocki DJ, Obrig TG, *et al.* The Mouse Model of Amebic Colitis Reveals Mouse Strain Susceptibility to Infection and Exacerbation of Disease by CD4+ T Cells. J Immunol 2002; 169: 4496-503.

[117]   Lotter H, Jacobs T, Gaworski, I, *et al.* Sexual Dimorphism in the Control of Amebic Liver Abscess in a Mouse Model of Disease. Infect Immun 2006; 74: 118-24.

[118]   Haque R, Mondal D, Shu J, *et al.* Correlation of Interferon-γ Production by Peripheral Blood Mononuclear Cells with Childhood Malnutrition and Susceptibility to Amebiasis. Am J Trop Med Hyg 2007; 76: 340-4.

[119]   Petri WA, Joyce P, Broman J, Smith RD, Murphy CF, Ravdin JI. Recognition of the Galactose- or N-Acetylgalactosamine-Binding Lectin of *Entamoeba histolytica* by Human Immune Sera. Infect Immun 1987; 55: 2327-31.

[120]   Abd-Alla MD, Jackson TF, Soong GC, *et al.* Identification of the *Entamoeba histolytica* Galactose-Inhibitable Lectin Epitopes Recognized by Human Immunoglobulin A Antibodies following Cure of Amebic Liver Abscess. Infect Immun 2004; 72: 3974-80.

[121]   Abd-Alla MD, Jackson TF, Rogers T, *at al.* Mucosal Immunity to Asymptomatic *Entamoeba histolytica* and *Entamoeba dispar* Infection Is Associated with a Peak Intestinal Anti-Lectin Immunoglobulin A Antibody Response. Infect Immun 2006; 74: 3897-903.

[122]   Petri WA, Snodgrass TL, Jackson TF, *et al.* Monoclonal Antibodies Directed Against the Galactose-Binding Lectin of *Entamoeba histolytica* Enhance Adherence. J Immunol 1990; 144: 4803-9.

[123]   Haque R, Ali IM, Sack RB, *et al.* Amebiasis and Mucosal IgA Antibody against the *Entamoeba histolytica* Adherence Lectin in Bangladeshi Children. J Infect Dis 2001; 183: 1787-93.

[124]   Kelsall BL, Ravdin JI. Immunization of rats with the 260-kDa *Entamoeba histolytica* galactose-inhibitable lectin elicits an intestinal secretory immunoglobulin A response that has *in vitro* adherence inhibition activity. Infect Immun 1995; 63: 686-9.

[125] Lotter H, Zhang T, Seydel KB, *et al*. Identification of an Epitope on the *Entamoeba histolytica* 170-kD Lectin Conferring Antibody-mediated Protection against Invasive Amebiasis. J Exp Med 1997; 185: 1793-801

[126] Cieslak PR, Virgin HW, Stanley SL. A severe combined immunodeficient (SCID) mouse model for infection with *Entamoeba histolytica*. J Exp Med 1992. 176: 1605-9.

[127] Duggal P, Haque R, Roy S, *et al*. Influence of Human Leukocyte Antigen Class II Alleles on Susceptibility to *Entamoeba histolytica* Infection in Bangladeshi Children. J Infect Dis 2004; 189: 520-6.

[128] Macpherson AJ, McCoy KD, Johansen F, *et al*. The immune geography of IgA induction and function. Mucosal Immunol 2008; 1: 11-22.

[129] Carrero JC, Diaz MY, Viveros M, *et al*. Human Secretory Immunoglobulin A Anti-*Entamoeba histolytica* Antibodies Inhibit Adherence of Amebae to MDCK Cells. Infect Immun 1994; 62: 764-7.

[130] Kelsall BL, Ravdin JI. Degradation of human immunoglobulin A by *Entamoeba histolytica*. J Infect Dis 1993; 168: 1319-22.

[131] Garcia-Nieto, R.M., Rico-Mata, *et al*. Degradation of human secretory IgA1 and IgA2 by *Entamoeba histolytica* surface-associated proteolytic activity. Parasitol Int 2008; 57: 417-23.

[132] Tran VQ, Herdman S, Torian BE, *et al*. The Neutral Cysteine Proteinase of *Entamoeba histolytica* Degrades IgG and Prevents Its Binding. J Infect Dis 1998; 177: 508-11.

[133] Que X, Reed SL. Cysteine Proteinases and the Pathogenesis of Amebiasis. Clin Microbiol Rev 2000; 13: 196-206.

[134] Petri WA, Ravdin JI. Protection of Gerbils from Amebic Liver Abscess by Immunization with the Galactose-Specific Adherence Lectin of Entamoeba histolytica. Infect Immun 1991; 59: 97-101.

[135] Zhang T, Stanley SL. Protection of gerbils from amebic liver abscess by immunization with a recombinant protein derived from the 170-kilodalton surface adhesin of *Entamoeba histolytica*. Infect Immun 1994; 62: 2605-8.

[136] Soong CG, Kain KC, Abd-Alla M, *et al*. A recombinant cysteine-rich section of the *Entamoeba histolytica* galactose inhibitable lectin is efficacious as a subunit vaccine in the gerbil model of amebic liver abscess. J Infect Dis 1995; 171: 645-51.

[137] Campbell D, Mann BJ, Chadee K. A subunit vaccine candidate region of the *Entamoeba histolytica* galactose-adherence lectin promotes interleukin-12 gene transcription and protein production in human macrophages. Eur J Immunol 2000; 30: 423-30.

[138] Ivory CP, Chadee K. DNA vaccines: designing strategies against parasitic infections. Genet Vaccines Ther 2004; 2:17.

[139] Gaucher D, Chadee K. Construction and immunogenicity of a codon-optimized *Entamoeba histolytica* Gal-lectin-based DNA vaccine. Vaccine 2002; 20: 3244-53.

[140] Cooper CL, Davis HL, Morris ML, *et al*. Safety and immunogenicity of CPG 7909 injection as an adjuvant to Fluarix influenza vaccine. Vaccine 2004; 22: 3136–43.

[141] Ivory CP, Prystajecky M, and Chadee K. Toll-Like Receptor 9-Dependent Macrophage Activation by *Entamoeba histolytica* DNA. Infect Immun 2008; 76: 289-97.

[142] Suzuki J, Kobayashi S, Murata R, *et al*. Profiles of a Pathogenic *Entamoeba histolytica*-like Variant with Variations in the Nucleotide Binding Sequence of the Small Subunit Ribosomal RNA Isolated From a Primate (De Brazza's Guenon). J Zoo Wildlife Med 2007; 38: 471-4.

[143] Abd Alla MD, White GL, Roger TB, *et al*. Adherence-Inhibitory Intestinal Immunoglobulin A Antibody Response in Baboons Elicited by Use of a Synthetic Intranasal Lectin-Based Amebiasis Subunit Vaccine. Infect Immun 2007; 75: 3812-22.

[144] Utrera-Barillas D, Velaquez JR, Enciso A, *et al*. An anti-inflammatory oligopeptide produced by *Entamoeba histolytica* down-regulates the expression of pro-inflammatory chemokines. Parasite Immunol 2003; 25: 475-82.

[145] Giménez-Scherer A, Cárdenas G, Lopéz-Osuna M, *et al*. Immunization with a tetramer derivative of an anti-inflammatory pentapeptide produced by *Entamoeba histolytica* protects gerbils (Meriones unguiculatus) against experimental amoebic abscess of the liver. Parasite Immunol 2004; 26: 343-9.

[146] Zhang T, Cieslak PR, Foster L, *et al*. Antibodies to the serine rich *Entamoeba histolytica* protein (SREHP) prevent amoebic liver abscess in severe combined immunodeficient (SCID) mice. Parasite Immunol 1994; 16: 225-30.

[147] Zhang T, Cieslak PR, Stanley SL. Protection of Gerbils from Amebic Liver Abscess by Immunization with a Recombinant *Entamoeba histolytica* Antigen. Infect Immun 1994; 62: 1166-70.

[148] Zhang T, Stanley SL. DNA Vaccination with the serine Rich *Entamoeba histolytica* Protein (SREHP) Prevents Amebic Liver Abscess in Rodent models of Disease. Vaccine 2000; 18: 868-74.

[149] Zhang T, Stanley SL. Oral Immunization with an Attenuated Vaccine Strain of Salmonella typhimurium Expressing the Serine-Rich *Entamoeba histolytica* Protein Induces an Antiamebic Immune Response and Protects Gerbils from Amebic Liver Abscess. Infect Immun 1996; 65: 1526-31.

[150] Ryan ET, Butterton JR, Zhang T, *et al*. Oral Immunization with Attenuated Vaccine Strains of Vibrio cholerae Expressing a Dodecapeptide Repeat of the Serine-Rich *Entamoeba histolytica* Protein Fused to the Cholera Toxin B Subunit Induces Systemic and Mucosal Antiamebic and Anti-V. cholerae Antibody Responses in Mice. Infect Immun 1997; 65: 3118-25.

CHAPTER 6

Immunity to Giardiasis

Aleksander Keselman and Steven M. Singer*

Department of Biology, Georgetown University, Washington, DC, USA

Abstract: *Giardia duodenalis* is the most common protozoan cause of diarrhea in the world. A hallmark of this infection is the variation in clinical responses which are observed, ranging from asymptomatic, self-limited infections to chronic infections with persistent severe diarrhea, cramps, nausea and weight loss. Some of this variation likely derives from differences in the parasites themselves, while the remainder is likely due to differences in host immune responses. This chapter will focus on the role of immune responses in determining the outcome of infections with *Giardia*, both in eradicating parasites from the intestinal lumen and in contributing to the symptoms of infection.

OVERVIEW

Impact

Intestinal infections with *Giardia duodenalis* are the most commonly occurring protozoan diarrheal disorder in the world. *Giardia* is a flagellated, waterborne parasite and its infectious cysts can be detected in almost all surface waters. *Giardia* has two morphologically distinct life stages; the infectious cyst form is ingested by a host and, in response to signals from within the host's stomach and small intestine, releases vegetative trophozoite forms which then replicate in the small intestine. *Giardia* was first observed in (his own) human feces by Anton van Leeuwenhoek in 1681 [1]. Interestingly, *Giardia* is so common that for many years after its discovery it was thought to be commensal rather than parasitic. The link between *Giardia* and disease was not considered until the 1920s, when Dobell and Miller implicated it in causing malabsorption syndromes. This lack of recognition was partly due to its appearance in many healthy people at the time. With breakthroughs in water purification and overall improved hygiene, the distinction between giardiasis and commensal bacterial colonization became more clear. The capacity of *Giardia* to infect humans and cause disease was formally demonstrated in 1954 when Rendtorff orally inoculated human subjects with cysts [2].

The developing world has suffered the bulk of the economic and health burden resulting from chronic exposure to *Giardia*. Outbreaks of giardiasis are a common and chronic problem wherever proper water purification is not available. *Giardia* cysts are detectable in most surface waters including drinking wells where the degree of fecal contamination from wild animals and livestock correlates directly to the concentration of cysts [3, 4]. Abundant animal reservoirs tend to exacerbate outbreaks, especially in agricultural communities and hygienically compromised environments. Outbreaks in livestock present an additional health risk to farmers and potentially limit profits in already economically disparaged regions of the world. People living in close proximity to livestock or wildlife are also more susceptible to chronic or recurring infection as most animal infections are asymptomatic and many treatments available for humans do not provide long lasting protection against *Giardia*. Several groups have estimated that between 3% and 7% of the developing world is infected with *Giardia* [5-7]. An estimated 200 million cases of symptomatic giardiasis exist in developing regions of Africa, Asia, and Latin America [8]. Each year, roughly 500,000 new patients present with symptoms of infection with *Giardia* and this accounts for roughly 20% of all diarrheal disease in the developing world [8, 9]. Many of these cases are in children who are more susceptible to infection than adults [10]. The prevalence of giardiasis among children varies throughout the developing world; examples include 15.9% in Nicaragua [11], 16% in Yemen [12], 27.4 % in Brazil [13] and 36.6% in Australian aboriginal populations [14].

In developed nations, *Giardia* is considered the most common cause of waterborne diarrheal disease [15]. Increased incidence among children in day care centers and campers/hikers has resulted in the designation of *Giardia* as a re-emerging infectious disease in the developed world [16-18]. In the United States, the frequency of giardiasis ranges from 0.1 to 23.5 per 100,000 people and differs state to state and seasonally. There are two age groups at greatest risk for giardiasis: 1-9 years of age and 30 – 39 years of age. Most cases are reported between the months of June and October when warm climatic conditions, heightened exposure to river water, and increased human-human contact promote infection. Although the developed world is privileged in terms of the availability of purified water, local outbreaks have been reported where water

*Corresponding Author: Steven M. Singer, Department of Biology, Georgetown University, Washington, DC, USA; Email: sms3@georgetown.edu

Emilio Jirillo (Ed)
All rights reserved - © 2010 Bentham Science Publishers Ltd.

treatment systems have been breached. For example, in 2001 there was an outbreak of giardiasis in Colorado after the failure of a bag filtration system. Preceding that was a New York outbreak in which contaminated drinking water was not filtered, leaving infectious *Giardia* cysts in the water for consumption [19]. Overall, there have been over 100 reported waterborne outbreaks in the United States alone resulting from the consumption of sewer contaminated drinking water [20]. Other developed countries have also reported waterborne outbreaks, including New Zealand, Sweden, the UK, Australia and Canada [8].

Giardiasis and its impact on societies have recently begun to receive global attention. Giardiasis was included by the World Health Organization (WHO) in 2004 in the Neglected Pathogen Initiative [21]. This initiative was established to allocate research funding to diseases that are endemic to the underdeveloped world, including infections with *Giardia* and *Cryptosporidium*. Recognizing the economic and health impacts of these pathogens led the WHO to invest in the development of more sensitive detection methods as well as inquiries into new treatments, vaccines, and improved sanitation [22]. Furthermore, the National Institute of Allergies and Infectious Diseases (NIAID) has classified *Giardia* as a category B biodefense pathogen due to its route of transmission, low infectious dose and stability of cysts in the environment.

Life Cycle

Giardia has a relatively simple life cycle involving two main stages, the environmentally resistant cyst form and the infective trophozoite form. Cysts are oval-shaped, thin-walled, and measure between 10 and 14 μm in length. *Giardia* cysts have been shown to be temperature resistant, surviving in water at 4 °C for up to three months. The cyst form persists mainly outside of the host and is dormant until it is ingested by a host and releases trophozoites that colonize the small intestine. *Giardia* cysts are ubiquitous to most running water, especially where fecal matter from animal reservoirs contaminates drinking reserves. Excystation of ingested *Giardia* begins in the small intestine where two trophozoites emerge from each cyst. While these trophozoites reside in the small intestine they undergo numerous rounds of binary fission. Pathology is caused by trophozoites that remain attached to the mucosa of the lumen of the proximal small bowel. The colonization of the small intestine can last for up to several weeks, depending on the conditions of the infection. Each trophozoite is roughly 12 to 20 μm in length and 5 to 10 μm in width. Trophozoites have a convex dorsal surface, are binucleated and have four symmetrically-oriented flagella, and attach to the intestinal epithelium through the action of their ventral disk. The ventral disk is composed of microtubules, microribbons, and cross-bridges composed of giardins [23]. As trophozoites descend through the small intestine and into the colon they transform into cysts and are then shed in feces.

Epidemiology

Giardia parasites are found in a wide variety of animal species and there has been much debate over the relationship among different parasite isolates. In 1952, Felice originally recognized three species of *Giardia*; *G. muris* infecting mainly rodents, birds and reptiles, *G. agilis* infecting amphibians, and *G. duodenalis* infecting humans and most other mammals [24]. Since then, several additional species have been isolated and classified; *G. ardeae* from herons, *G. psittaci* from psittacine birds, and *G. microti* from muskrats. Each of these species designations was based on parasite morphology and/or host range. More recent genetic analyses of isolates that were collected from livestock as well as canine hosts suggested that *G. duodenalis* exhibited wide genetic variation and led to application of the term genetic assemblage [25]. There are currently seven recognized genotypes (Assemblages A through G) of *G. duodenalis*, although they all share similar morphology. Of the seven assemblages of *G. duodenalis,* only assemblages A and B appear to be capable of infecting humans, and both of these assemblages can also be found infecting other species including dogs, cats, rodents and livestock. Assemblages C-G also infect these other species, but have not yet been reported to infect humans [16].

Recent technological advances have allowed researchers to apply molecular and genetic based approaches to characterize *G. duodenalis*. Assemblage A has been divided into A-1 and A-2 isolates. Strains WB and Portand, belong to group A-1 are used widely for laboratory studies; WB was used as the template for the *Giardia* genome project [26]. The JH strain belongs in group A-2 and has also been used in several genomic studies. Assemblage B isolates (sometimes called Group 3) were described by Nash and Keister in 1985 [27]. This group includes GS, which has been central to the study of immune responses to infection with *G. duodenalis* since it infects adult laboratory mice. Recently, genome sequencing of one assemblage A strain (WB) and one assemblage B strain (GS) has been reported [26, 28]. These strains differ by over 20% in coding sequences, suggesting that they might best be considered as different species. Readers are referred to Franzen et al. for a more in-depth discussion of this proposal [28].

Proper identification of the infecting organisms is crucial in trying to better understand the epidemiology of *Giardia* infection. The distribution of the assemblages in humans, as determined by clinical surveys conducted in several communities, generally deviates only slightly from a ~7:3 ratio of assemblage B to assemblage A infections [29]. In a recent examination of 35 human clinical samples in the UK, 64% had infections with assemblage B parasites, 27% with assemblage A parasites, and 9% were infected with both [30]. An outbreak in a UK nursery demonstrated that 21 out of 24 patients (88% of infected individuals) were infected with assemblage B members [30]. Examination of a group of 18 patients in India revealed that 61% of these patients were infected with Assemblage B parasites [31]. Assemblage B infections may be less likely to be identified however, as one study in a day care center in Western Australia concluded that Assemblage A infections were 26 times more likely to induce diarrhea in children [29]. Thus, infections with Assemblage B parasites may go unreported and are likely more prevalent than they are assumed to be.

Several reports have tried to link the specific genotype of infecting parasite with the development of symptomatic or asymptomatic infections. However, the literature pertaining to strain dependent virulence is quite variable within different regions of the world. One study found a 100% correlation between the severity of diarrheal disease and infecting strains in a Dutch population [32]. This study found that assemblage A isolates were responsible for intermittent diarrhea, while assemblage B infections resulted in persistent diarrheal disease. This group correlated the severity of symptomatic disease to infection with assemblage A parasites. Other studies have provided similar reports, where assemblage A strains cause symptomatic disease [33]. A more molecular diagnostic approach was undertaken in a recent study, revealing contradictory correlations between genotype and clinical manifestations in a Malaysian population. Of the individuals testing positive for *Giardia* (55% of the sample population) in their stool samples, 98% were infected with assemblage B parasites, whereas the remaining 2% were infected by parasites from assemblage A [34]. This study found a correlation precisely opposite to that of the previously mentioned work, where infections with assemblage B parasites were more likely to result in diarrhea, abdominal discomfort, vomiting, and nausea than infections with Assemblage A parasites. Studies in the Netherlands [32] as well as Ethiopia [35] have similarly reported increased persistence of symptomatic disease with assemblage B parasites. Thus, correlations between genotype and virulence appear to vary by study and may reflect further differences in parasites or differences among hosts. Moreover, infections with multiple strains of *Giardia* are not uncommon and reliable diagnosis and detection is essential for better understanding these differences.

Giardia can be transmitted in several different ways. The consumption of contaminated drinking water poses the greatest risk for ingesting *Giardia*. There is an abundance of reported outbreaks due to the contamination of unfiltered drinking water with run-off or sewage discharges [36]. Zoonotic and human-human transmission provide alternative avenues for contracting giardiasis. Because both assemblage A and B strains can infect species other than humans, zoonotic transmission through cattle and domestic animal reservoirs poses a risk for humans. However, one study examining *Giardia* isolated from humans and dogs living in close proximity found that humans were primarily infected with assemblage A or B parasites, whereas dogs were infected with C or D assemblage members [37]. This suggests that either zoonotic transmission is not as prominent as waterborne transmission, since people and pets seem to be susceptible to distinct genotypic populations of *Giardia*. In contrast, one report from Ecuador suggested that the abundance of domestic animals was a predictor of pediatric giardiasis [38]. More common than zoonotic transmission, human to human transmission occurs with outbreaks being relatively frequent among children and staff in day care centers [39]. Sexual transmission has also been reported in some instances.

Control Strategies

Controlling giardiasis on a global scale is an arduous but necessary task. Solutions to this problem are multifactorial and will require an in-depth understanding of its epidemiological properties, the molecular factors that promote infection and the best ways in which socioeconomic efforts can improve sanitation in the developing world. Improvement in diagnostics is also an important factor in controlling giardiasis and the need for more sensitive molecular-based techniques is evident as most of the world currently relies on the detection of cysts using microscopy in both contaminated water and fecal samples. Indicator bacteria have also been used in determining contamination with *Giardia*.

Current drug treatments for human patients and veterinary cases remain largely ineffective as they do not provide long-lasting protection against infection, especially in areas where *Giardia* is highly endemic and reinfection occurs rapidly. Currently available drug treatments, including anti-protozoal agents such as Quinacrine, Furazolidone, Metronidazole, Albendazole, Tinidazole, and Nitazoxanide, can be expensive but provide effective short-term protection. Strong side effects associated with these drugs and resistance to metronidazole has been reported [40]. Furthermore, rigorous treatment regimens prove difficult to follow and often lead to treatment failure.

As with all endemic infections, vaccination is a promising method of disease control. A vaccine, GiardiaVax™, is available for veterinary use but no human vaccine is commercially available. This vaccine could still help reduce human disease by targeting zoonotic transmission of *Giardia*. This is important because domestic animals such as cats and dogs tend to be prone to asymptomatic infection. Unfortunately, the effectiveness of this vaccine is questionable [41]. One study found that vaccination reduced cyst shedding, cyst viability, and diarrheal disease in kittens but the low infective dose associated with giardiasis suggests that these vaccines may render domestic animals asymptomatic while retaining the capacity for transmission [42]. Likewise, a study in dogs found vaccination to be effective after treatment failure with anti-*Giardial* drugs in which the subjects appeared to have resolved infection at the time of a second booster shot and remained asymptomatic and cyst free for roughly a year after vaccination [43]. While vaccine studies appear promising based on the resulting *Giardia*-specific antibody production in animals, immunity studies suggest that the antibody role may be limited in eliminating *Giardia* infection and that minimizing cyst transmission may be a more effective control method. Immune tolerance from constant exposure to *Giardia* antigens in the gut may further limit the impact of antibody responses and vaccines that elicit them in controlling giardiasis. The process of antigenic variation (discussed later) further complicates the development of vaccines.

The trophozoite form of *Giardia* has classically been considered as a target for vaccine development, but in the last few years, the cyst form has received increased attention. Studies have shown that a significant proportion of the adaptive immune response is geared toward clearing the cyst forms of the parasite, as well as the infective trophozoite form [44]. Inhibiting transmission through vaccination has started to gain interest following studies that have implicated adaptive immunity against cysts in reducing disease. In fact, one study showed that treatment of *Giardia* with monoclonal antibodies against cyst wall proteins resulted in non-viable cysts, which could impart protection to humans both by helping to clear infection and by preventing transmission through cyst shedding [45]. Other groups have commented on the antigenic differences between the trophozoite and cyst stages revealing several exclusive as well as common antigenic targets for adaptive immunity. There remains the potential for successful vaccination against giardiasis but more attention to targets and immune mechanisms is necessary.

The most effective angle from which to contain human exposure to *Giardia* is water treatment; through disinfection and filtration. This undoubtedly requires substantial funding and research for global application but has proven effective in the developed world as it targets the linking factor between zoonotic and human infection, and therefore can diminish the risk of contracting giardiasis. Water filtration has been shown to remove 99% of *Giardia* cysts [46]. Adequate processing of sewage waste helps minimize environmental contamination and has proven effective [46, 47]. Maintenance of filtration plants is also important as backwashed filter water contains concentrated levels of cysts and poses a threat of outbreak.

Pathology

The stages of *Giardia* infection can be categorized into three distinct phases: the latent phase, the acute phase, and the elimination phase. The latent phase begins with the ingestion of the cysts and their emergence as trophozoites that colonize the small intestine. Usually between 7 and 10 days later, the acute phase marks the peak of trophozoite burden in the small intestine and is met with the start of cyst shedding by the host. As the host mounts an immune response and begins clearing the small intestine of trophozoites, cyst shedding diminishes and the elimination phase begins. Rapid elimination in immunocompetent hosts suggests that the disease is self limiting, however roughly 30 to 50% of acute infections extend into chronic giardiasis with intermittent diarrheal disease presenting with weight loss and malabsorption syndrome in many patients [48]. It is difficult in practice to distinguish relapsing infections from secondary infections due to re-exposure to the parasite, particularly in areas with high carriage rates. Better molecular diagnostic tools would help resolve this issue.

Infections in humans with *G. duodenalis* result in clinical manifestations in 50% or less of individuals, even when infections are with identical parasite genotypes [49]. Interestingly, isolates obtained from highly symptomatic patients generated similar rates of clinical disease (~50%) when used to experimentally inoculate volunteers [49]. Several underlying host factors have been suggested to contribute to pathological variability; host immunity [50-59], age and stage of development [60-63], sex [34, 64], nutrition [65-66] and the composition of intestinal bacterial flora [67] have been suggested to influence both the susceptibility to infection and the overall medical consequences of giardiasis.

In humans, giardiasis presents as a continuum ranging from asymptomatic cases to severe malabsorption syndrome [48]. The most commonly reported symptoms range from mild to persistent diarrhea, steatorrhea, flatulence, epigastric pain and weight loss [68]. Less common manifestations are nausea, vomiting and fever [8]. In most clinical cases, symptoms develop within one to two weeks after ingesting cysts and vanish as soon as 4 days after emerging [68]. Deviation from this window has been observed to range from 1 to 75 days after exposure to cysts [2, 69]. In symptomatic hosts, acute infection is accompanied by duodenal and jejunal injury, the extent of which does not always correlate to symptomatic manifestations [70]. Intestinal pathology in giardiasis is thought to arise from retracting villi, damaged microvilli (i.e. the brush border), impaired barrier function, and reduced absorptive capacity.

Malabsorption of nutrients is a major pathological manifestation arising from infection with *Giardia*. Several intestinal pathological factors contribute to malabsorption; increased epithelial permeability [71], secretion of sodium and chloride ions [72], reduced epithelial surface area, and structurally compromised brush border [73]. Classical malabsorption of fat, D-xylose, Vitamin A and Vitamin B_{12} has been described in patients [74]. Zinc and iron deficiencies have also been noted in giardiasis [75]. The role of parasite toxins and host immune responses in leading to these pathological changes is unclear.

Malnutrition, caused by diminished intestinal nutrient absorption, challenges proper development in children, especially those that reside in already nutritionally compromised settings [76]. Pediatric giardiasis poses a significant health risk, especially during developmentally critical stages of life between ages 1 and 4 [77]. A study in Guatemala has reported that infections with *G. duodenalis* in the first two years of life affect growth and development [77]. This is not surprising as nutrient absorption is essential for proper neural development and establishment of synapses during the first two years of life [78]. Indeed, children between the ages of 2 and 6 have been reported to be at greatest risk of giardiasis in certain parts of the world [76]. Pediatric cases have shown signs of developmental defects, cognitive disabilities, and failure to thrive as a result of parasite-mediated malabsorption syndrome [48, 79, 80]. Children exhibit vitamin A and B12 deficiencies as well as defects in lipid metabolism as a result of *Giardia*. A recent clinical study in Turkey found that out of 160 children up to age 5, 80 had enteric infections, of which *G. duodenalis* was the most common parasite. This survey found that *Giardia* infected children were at greater risk of growth stunting as well as poor psychomotor development [62].

Several clinical studies have demonstrated impaired development in children with chronic intestinal infection by *Giardia* [79, 80, 81]. Roughly 64% of weight and height deficits in Gambian children were attributed to chronic giardiasis [82]. Treatment of pediatric giardiasis in Bangladesh diminished the incidence of developmental stunting [83, 84]. In these studies, anti-*Giardia* antibodies were detectable in children as young as 2 months and persistent serum IgG and IgM were extremely common, indicating chronic and recurring infections. Rates of intestinal injury have been reported to be as high as 75% in children with chronic infection, coinciding with increased wasting, increased growth stunting and being underweight in the first two years of life [85]. A study in Malaysian children indicated incidences of growth stunting (61.3%) and being underweight (56.5%) that were comparable to previous studies [65]. A *G. duodenalis* study in Israeli children found decreased weight/height to age ratios in chronically infected children relative to *Giardia* free controls [61]. Thus, even in the absence of symptoms such as diarrhea and cramps, *Giardia* infection can be an insidious cause of impaired physical and cognitive development in children. These figures are however potentially misleading as the diagnostic criteria vary between studies. While some surveys focus on cases of symptomatic giardiasis, using diarrhea episodes as a diagnostic measure, others rely on detection of cysts in the stool or antibodies in sera. Larger, more uniform studies of the links between specific infections and child development are clearly needed.

Secondary *Giardia* infections have been generally described as less severe in nature; characterized by the merging of the three phases (latent, acute, and elimination). With chronic infections, cyst shedding peaks at only 10% of the amount of shedding observed with acute, primary infection [51]. These recurring infections are considered to be less dramatic because of adaptive responses mounted by the host, which further supports the potential for vaccine effectiveness. However, more studies are needed to fully understand the role of immunity in clearing infection.

IMMUNITY TO GIARDIA

Acquired immunity

Abundant data indicate that *Giardia* triggers a strong adaptive immune response. Anti-*Giardia* immunoglobulin A (IgA) antibodies are detected in humans and animals following infection [44, 86]. Furthermore, IgA was shown to be instrumental in clearing *G. muris* infection in mice and is likely important in human infection with *G. duodenalis* as human immunoglobulin deficiencies lead to prolonged infection [87, 88]. IgG specific for *Giardia* antigens can also be detected three weeks post infection in the majority of human giardiasis cases [49, 89]. There are many antigenic components of *Giardia* that have been proven to stimulate immune responses. For example, several of the antigens recognized by human antibodies include surface proteins (82 kDa and 65 kDa polypeptides), the cytoskeletal giardins, heat shock proteins, lectins, and tubulin in the disk and flagella [90-95].

Epidemiological analysis of human outbreaks provides substantial evidence for acquired immunity in giardiasis. Acquired immunity has been demonstrated in epidemic scenarios whereby local residents exhibit significantly reduced rates of infections and symptomatic disease compared to visiting foreigners. Outbreaks at popular tourist locations provide excellent platforms for such clinical studies. One 1948 outbreak in an apartment building in Tokyo resulted in a 46% infection rate among Japanese natives and a 76% infection rate among American residents [96]. Pre-epidemic infections among Japanese staff members in this building were detected at rates between 5 and 8%. A 1965 outbreak among skiers in Aspen, Colorado yielded an 11.3% rate of diarrheal disease caused by *Giardia* compared to only 5% in local residents [97]. A 1985 outbreak of *Giardia* in the Aspen Highlands community further demonstrated acquired immunity among locals [98]. Finally, Isaac-Renton and colleagues found clear evidence for prior infection leading to protection against *Giardia* infection in a second outbreak in British Columbia [99]. The mechanism of protection was not well defined in these studies, and it is possible that prior infection may provide resistance to symptomatic disease rather than re-infection, similar to acquired immunity in malaria.

Studies in hypogammaglobulinemic human patients have demonstrated susceptibility to chronic *Giardia* infections, implicating antibodies as a major mechanism for controlling this infection. There is increased cyst shedding coupled to decreased anti-*Giardia* serum IgA and IgG with prolonged infection [100]. Patients suffering from common variable immunodeficiency (CVID) and X-linked agammaglobulinemia (XLA) were at increased risk of symptomatic giardiasis [101]. CVID is characterized by B-cell and T-cell deficiency and agammaglobulinemia where the intestine is especially deprived of B-cells predisposing individuals to enteric infections [102]. However, the defects in CVID and XLA can affect cell types other than B cells, making it difficult to conclude that the lack of antibodies alone is responsible for the inability to control *Giardia* infections.

As opposed to B cells, studies in patients with T cell deficiencies indicate that other mechanisms can control *Giardia* infection. A common finding in HIV patients is an inverse correlation between the persistence of diarrheal disease and CD4+ T cell counts [103]. A study in Indonesia found that 74% of HIV patients with chronic diarrheal disease had severe T-cell depletion [104]. While the occurrence of diarrheal disease due to polyparasitism was significantly more common in this population, *Giardia* was not more prevalent in the patients with low T cell counts than in immunocompetent populations [105]. Also, HIV positive individuals with giardiasis have marginally lower anti-*Giardia* immunoglobulin levels along with severe CD4+ deficiencies, but are still able to resolve infections despite these immunological setbacks [105]. These data suggest that *Giardia* itself is not opportunistic and does not burden individuals with HIV; infection rates of as low as 6.2% have been reported in HIV positive individuals [106, 107]. Interestingly, there are conflicting reports of CD4+ T lymphocyte mediated immunity in human giardiasis. Similarly, immunodeficient patients with thymic dysplasia (DiGeorge syndrome) also do not commonly suffer severe diarrheal manifestations from giardiasis [108]. These data taken together suggest that compensatory mechanisms may be in place for dealing with giardiasis that enable immunocompromised hosts to clear infection and avoid the development of symptomatic disease.

Mechanistic studies of immunity are typically performed more easily in animal models than in humans. Analysis of immunity to *Giardia* in animal models has helped to clarify the observations made in humans. Several models have been used including infections in neonatal and adult mice with *G. duodenalis*, infections in adult mice with *G. muris* and infections in gerbils with *G. duodenalis*. These different models have occasionally produced discordant results, but understanding reasons for these discrepancies has sometimes highlighted important facets of this disease.

The Antibody Response

Antibodies and antibody producing B cells play key roles in immunity against *G. muris* but these roles may be more limited during *G. duodenalis* infections. The involvement of the antibody response in clearing *Giardia* was illustrated by Snider and Underwood in 1985 when they treated mice with anti-IgM antibodies and found that infection with *G. muris* was prolonged [109]. This does not imply, however, that IgM is central in *Giardia* immunity because this treatment effectively targets all classes of immunoglobulins by depleting naïve B cells. XID mice carrying a mutation in the same gene that is altered in human XLA (btk), also develop prolonged infections with *G. muris*, implicating both B cells and antibodies in clearing infection [51]. However, XID mice acquired resistance to secondary infections as well as their wild-type controls, suggesting that control of primary and secondary infections could involve different immune mechanisms. Infection with *G.*

duodenalis in mice seems to be less B cell dependent than *G. muris*. Mice which lack B cells due to deletion of the μ exons of the Ig heavy chain (μMT mice) controlled *G. duodenalis* infections as quickly as wild-type controls [54]. In contrast, control of infection required CD4+ T cells [54].

Because it is secreted into the intestinal lumen, IgA is believed to be the most effective in clearing infections with *Giardia*. IgA dimers are transported across the epithelium by the poly-Ig receptor (pIgR) into the intestinal lumen. IgA deficient mice infected with *G. muris* exhibit defects in clearing infection, similar to B cell deficient mice [87]. Neither IgA deficient nor B cell deficient mice are protected from secondary infection with *G. muris*, suggesting that the antibody response and IgA in particular are essential in acquired immunity in the mouse model [87]. However, cyst shedding was diminished considerably in the IgA knockout mice during secondary infection, suggesting other immune mechanisms can contribute to resistance to this parasite. These results contrast those previously mentioned, in which B cell deficient mice do clear infection with *G. duodenalis* [54]. IgA may be more important for eradication of *G. muris*, but less essential in the murine adaptive response against *G. duodenalis*. Indeed, human patients with selective IgA deficiencies have only slightly increased incidence of *Giardia* infection, consistent with a limited role of IgA in protective immunity against *G. duodenalis* [110]. Direct confirmation of differences in the role of IgA in controlling *G. muris* and *G. duodenalis* was obtained using mice lacking the poly-Ig receptor (pIgR). These mice developed chronic infections with *G. muris*, but not with *G. duodenalis* [56]. This implies that *G. duodenalis* may be sensitive to non-antibody immune factors in mice to which *G. muris* is resistant, or that *G. muris* is more sensitive to antibody-mediated cytotoxicity.

Giardia targeting antibodies can be cytotoxic to the parasite *in vitro*. Serum from *G. muris* infected mice has been shown to agglutinate trophozoites and induce lysis with complement [111]. Complement-independent cytotoxicity of monoclonal antibodies targeting *Giardia* has also been described [112]. Furthermore, when sera containing high levels of anti-*Giardia* IgA were systemically administered to mice, they provided transient protection for the host against *G. muris* [56]. Antibodies can also provide protection against *G. duodenalis* in mice, although this protection requires longer periods of time. In mice lacking IL-6, *G. duodenalis* infections were not rapidly controlled like in wild-type mice [113]. Interestingly, the IL-6 deficient mice did eliminate the infection after 60 days, at the same time they produced antibodies reacting with a diverse population of parasites [113]. These results suggest that antigenic variation by *G. duodenalis* (see below) prevents antibodies from effectively controlling infections until such time as the antibodies recognize either invariant epitopes or all potential variant antigens.

Immunoreactive sera have been used to identify antigens conserved between *Giardia* strains [56]. In these mouse studies, there were several 25 to 50 kDa antigens conserved between the GS(M) and WB/C6 strains, but most of the 22 to >200 kDa antigens belonged exclusively to WB/C6. A total of 12 proteins were identified by mass spectrometry: OCT, ADI, α-enolase, α-1, α-2, α-7.1, and α-11- giardins, as well as β-giardin, α2-tubulin, *Giardia* trophozoite antigen-2, uridine phosphorylase-like protein 1 and fructose-1,-6-bisphosphate aldolase. Antibodies to several of these antigens were detected in the breast milk of infected humans, suggesting similar immune responses across the host species [114]. Other antigens having been described include a 57 kDa antigen [90], a 49 kDa glycosylphosphatidylinositol (GPI) anchored protein [115] and an 8 kDa fatty acid binding protein [116]. Another promising study identified sixteen immunodominant antigens among strains Portland I, GS, and HP-88 when examining sera from human patients affected by an outbreak of *Giardia* in Sweden [117]. Although these antigens were discovered in trophozoites, they were also detected in cyst protein extracts. These proteins were identified with mass spectrometry and six of them were determined to be novel: SALP-1, GTA-1, GTA-2, UPL-1, α-7.1-giardin, and α-7.3-giardin. A common antigen among all strains would be extremely helpful in diagnosing the parasite and in vaccine design, but has yet to be identified.

The efforts to understand the antigens targeted by adaptive immunity in giardiasis have mainly focused on the trophozoites. However, Abdul-Wahid and Faubert demonstrated that the cyst form of the parasite is, to a degree, antigenically distinct and may therefore provide new targets for diagnosis and vaccine development. This group used proteomic analysis to demonstrate distinct expression profiles of trophozoite, encysting, and cyst populations of *G. muris* [118]. This study determined that there were roughly 40% differences in protein expression between these phases of the *Giardia* life cycle. Further antigenic diversity arises from varying antigens being expressed by genetically different strains. This has important implications for vaccine development, as it suggests that there are multiple sets of antigens which may be targeted by the immune system.

In addition to the changes in protein expression that occur as the parasite differentiates, *Giardia* trophozoites undergo extensive antigenic variation of their surface proteins. As noted above, this limits the ability of antibody responses to control infections and our ability to develop diagnostics or vaccines that target these surface proteins. *Giardia* trophozoites are completely covered with one of a family of structurally-related proteins, the variant-specific proteins, or VSPs [119]. Transition between VSPs is enhanced by anti-*Giardia* IgA targeting of these proteins [120]. Only one of 150- 200 VSPs is expressed on the surface of an individual trophozoite at a particular time [121]. VSPs vary in size from 30 kDa to 200 kDa and possess a variable cysteine-rich amino-terminal region and a conserved carboxy-terminal region that includes a hydrophobic transmembrane domain. VSP switching in *Giardia* trophozoites was shown to occur spontaneously *in vitro* every 6-13 generations by shedding of the major surface VSP [121]. In addition, the encystation and excystation processes have been shown to induce VSP switching [122].

The mechanisms that control antigenic variation in *Giardia* are poorly understood. Neither a gene-rearrangement process nor promoter-dependent switch-on/switch-off were demonstrated to be involved in *Giardia* antigenic switching. Kulakova et al. (2006) showed that transcription of *vsp* genes involves histone lysine acetylation in upstream chromatin, suggesting that epigenetic mechanisms were essential for antigenic variation in *Giardia* [123]. Another study by Prucca et al. showed that regulation of VSP switching involved a post-transcriptional gene silencing system involving RNA-dependent RNA polymerase and Dicer enzymes, known components of the RNA interference machinery [124]. Antisense RNA sequences were detected, but corresponded only to the silenced VSP genes. No antisense RNA was detected for the expressed VSP gene. In addition, silencing of Dicer and RNA-dependent RNA polymerase led to expression of multiple VSP in individual parasites. These findings suggested that antigenic variation in *Giardia* was controlled by post-transcriptional silencing.

The Cellular Immune Response

A large portion of the adaptive immune response against *Giardia* is T cell mediated. The involvement of the T_H response in controlling giardiasis was apparent from studies of *G. muris* and *G. duodenalis* infections in T cell deficient mice that showed prolonged infection with both *Giardia* species that were readily eliminated with the adoptive transfer of T cells [54, 125, 126]. CD4 depletion prolonged infection in B-cell deficient mice confirming the notion of an antibody independent role for T-cells [54]. Likewise, mice treated with anti-CD4 antibodies or depleted of TCRβ developed chronic infection with *G. duodenalis* and *G. muris*. Flow cytometry studies conducted on Peyer's patch cells in *G. muris* infected BALB/c mice demonstrated progressive intraepithelial infiltration by CD4+ T-cells, but not CD8+ T cells, during the transition from the acute phase (11% to 17% of intraepithelial cells) to the elimination phase (18% of intraepithelial cells) of infection [118]. Peyer's patch-derived B cell increases were observed to coincide with the presence of CD4+ T cells, increasing from 55% to 66% during acute infection and remaining high throughout the elimination phase. Infections in class I MHC deficient, β_2 microglobulin knockout, mice ruled out a role for CD8+ T cells in protective immunity since they did not result in prolonged infection with *G. duodenalis* [54]. Finally, αβ-TCR deficient mice were unable to control *G. duodenalis* infection, whereas γδ-TCR deficient mice cleared infections similarly to wild type [54].

T lymphocyte responses in giardiasis likely contribute to both protection and pathogenesis. One role of T cells in clearing this infection is carried out by both recruiting and activating innate and adaptive immune cells within the musoca and sub-mucosa. For example, one study noted that *G. muris* infections enhanced intraepithelial lymphocyte infiltration in histological cross sections of the murine small intestine [126]. This recruitment of lymphocytes to the intestinal epithelium was partially T cell dependent and correlated to the elimination of *Giardia* [126]. A second T cell function is mediating morphological and structural alterations within the epithelium that are thought to contribute to pathological manifestations. Athymic nude mice fail to develop intestinal pathologies that are observed in immunocompetent mice infected with *G. muris* [126]. These athymic nude mice not only had normal brush border and intestinal ultrastructure, they also did not exhibit maltase and sucrase deficiencies. Therefore, the role of T cells in giardiasis is multi-dimensional; they are involved in both clearing infection and pathology.

CD4+ T cells likely act by stimulating other immune responses through the release of cytokines. Clinical studies have demonstrated increased serum IL-6 and IFN-γ in *G. duodenalis* infections suggesting the systemic stimulation of T cell T_H1 and T_H2 responses [127]. Ebert provided *in vitro* evidence of *G. duodenalis* stimulating lymphocyte proliferation and IFN-γ production, but failed to show any cytotoxic effects on the parasite [128]. Exposure of IL-2 activated, naïve human intraepithelial lymphocytes (IEL), lamina propria lymphocytes (LPL) and peripheral blood lymphocytes (PBL) to *G. duodenalis* did not lead to overt lysis of the parasite at a 50:1 effector to target ratio. As well, *in vitro* chemotactic assays did not reveal enhanced migration on the part of these lymphocytes. Another group, however, did demonstrate cytotoxicity *in vitro* when using mature IEL, LPL, and splenic lymphocytes from *G. duodenalis* infected mice [129]. In humans, heavy CD4+ duodenal infiltration has been shown to couple with high levels of anti-*Giardia* IgA secretion, suggesting that T-cell activation may lead to an antibody response [130]. However, neither IL-4 elicited T_H2 responses nor IFN-γ elicited T_H1

responses are required for control of *G. duodenalis* infections [54]. Mucosal T_H-cells from *G. muris* infected mice were shown to release significant levels of IFN-γ and IL-4 when stimulated with Con A [131]. This suggests that both T_H1 and T_H2 cells are activated with giardiasis and that they readily secrete cytokines upon stimulation. Which types of T cell responses are required for protective immunity remains unclear and whether any single T_H subset is needed is unknown.

Cytokines in Giardiasis

There is a growing body of evidence suggesting IL-6 is an important cytokine in immunity against *Giardia* [113, 132]. IL-6 is a prominent cytokine of the T_H2 response and stimulates B cell differentiation and antibody production, T cell proliferation, and modulates the IgA response. It is produced by several cell types including enterocytes, monocytes, and a number of other T_H2 response cells. Increased levels of intestinal IL-6 have been reported in human cases of *G. duodenalis* infection [127]. Considering the contribution of the B cell and antibody responses to immunity it is surprising that reduced levels of IL-6 have been found the intestinal epithelium of immunocompetent mice with acute *G. muris* infection [126]. This is especially interesting as increased IL-6 has been linked to decreased sucrase-isomaltase activity in Crohn's disease, which results in brush border pathology similar to that observed in giardiasis [133]. However, one study revealed that infection with *G. muris* actually lowered duodenal IL-6 in immunocompetent mice but not in athymic mice, suggesting that T cells may serve a suppressive function in intestinal epithelial responses [126]. Reduced IL-6 correlated with intestinal injury as evident by reduced disaccharidase activity, breakdown of the brush border and microvilli shortening observed in immunocompetent mice. However, the uninfected athymic mice have IL-6 levels comparable to those of infected immunocompetent mice, suggesting that non-T cell sources of IL-6 may be quite important in the intestine. These findings suggest that while IL-6 is important for generating immunity to *Giardia*, it likely plays an indirect role in this response [126].

TNFα has recently been suggested to serve a protective role in giardiasis. Zhou et al. recently demonstrated that infection with *G. duodenalis* did not alter TNFα mRNA levels in C57BL/6 mice [134]. TNFα knockout and anti-TNFα treated mice eliminated *G. duodenalis* infection after 28 days, but had a much higher parasite load than control mice in the first two weeks of infection [134]. Interestingly, intestinal TNFα mRNA levels were significantly reduced during infection in IL-6 deficient mice, while TNFα deficiency did not in turn alter IL-6 production [134]. Furthermore, IL-6 deficient mice could not clear infection for up to 60 days despite having similar parasite counts to TNFα deficient mice. This suggests that IL-6 may function upstream of TNFα in giardiasis and that TNFα may have a more direct role in clearing infection. This is consistent with the finding that immunocompetent mice and humans have elevated TNFα in the intestinal epithelium with *G. duodenalis* infection [134, 135]. Also, the difference in clearing infection between IL-6 and TNFα deficient mice suggests that IL-6 deficiency affects more than TNFα signaling. TNFα is involved in the production of nitric oxide by inducing the expression of iNOS, which is repressed by IL-4. While increases in IL-4 mRNA have been measured in mice infected with *G. duodenalis*, IL-6 deficiency has been shown to augment IL-4 levels compared to wild-type mice. Thus, in the absence of IL-6, the production of anti-parasite effector mechanisms such as nitric oxide may be repressed by downregulating TNFα and upregulating IL-4.

Anti-parasite Effector Mechanisms

While *Giardia* infection generates adaptive immune responses, many of the factors actually responsible for eliminating the parasite from the intestine are part of innate defense mechanisms. For example, human milk and duodenal fluids have been shown to be lethal for *Giardia* trophozoites, demonstrating that they have anti-*Giardia* activities that contribute to the elimination of infection [136]. Antimicrobial peptides in the small intestine have been shown to play a role in the targeting and elimination of enteric pathogens [137]. Defensins are cationic antimicrobial peptides and show considerable sequence variation, suggesting promiscuity in pathogenic detection. Humans express two isoforms of α defensins in the gut (HD5 and HD6) whereas mice express 20, which are referred to as cryptdins [137]. The α and β defensins are distinguished based on their spacing of conserved cysteine residues. Human neutrophils express defensins, whereas mouse neutrophils do not [138]. In mice, stimulated paneth cells secrete proteolytically processed cryptdins into the small intestine. This proteolysis is carried out by the matrix metalloproteinase-7 (MMP-7) [139]. The β-defensins are constitutively expressed at low levels, but are inducible with bacterial infection [140]. The β-defensins are expressed ubiquitously throughout the mucosal surfaces lining the small intestine and colon in both mice and humans. Both α and β defensins have been implicated in pathogen elimination with infections of *Salmonella typhimurium* [141] and *Haemophilus influenzae* [142], respectively.

In 1994, Aley et al. demonstrated that a number of mouse defensins, were cytotoxic to *Giardia* trophozoites [143]. This group found that cryptdins 2 and 3 were toxic toward trophozoites, but not cryptdins 1 and 6. This is interesting as it suggests that despite broadly conserved sequences within the cryptdins or defensins, they demonstrate different specificity for a given pathogen. Also, this study showed that the neutrophil defensins NP-2 and indolicidin were extremely cytotoxic. In contrast, HNP-1 required much higher doses to achieve comparable cytotoxic effects.

There is a significant lack in data regarding the *in vivo* processes involving defensins in host defenses against *Giardia*. Some preliminary data suggests that defensins play a limited role in clearing *Giardia* infection; *G. muris* levels in the small intestine of MMP-7 deficient mice were not statistically greater than in wild-type mice at 1, 3 and 7 weeks post-infection [17]. Indeed, they actually had a lower parasite load at one week post infection [17]. It is speculated that inducible β−defensins like HBD-2 and cathelicidin LL-37/hCAP18 do not contribute to *Giardia* immunity as they are either induced by inflammation or simply not expressed in the small intestine [17]. There is, however, reason to believe that defensins may function indirectly in giardiasis by regulating the microbiota of the small intestine, which are known to effect the ability of *Giardia* to colonize in mice [67]. Still research is needed to better understand the physiological role of defensins in the mucosal immune response to *Giardia*.

Nitric oxide is an important secondary messenger for mammals and other animals and it facilitates a variety of physiological and in some cases pathological processes. In addition to mediating microbial toxicity, nitric oxide performs several other physiological functions, such as neurotransmission and maintenance of the mucosal barrier as well as inducing vascular smooth muscle relaxation. There are three known isotypes of the enzyme that catalytically synthesizes nitric oxide from arginine: these are neuronal nitric oxide synthase (nNOS/NOS1), inducible NOS (iNOS/NOS2) and endothelial NOS (eNOS/NOS3). Expression of iNOS is enhanced *in vivo* by inflammatory and parasitic factors and *in vitro* by cytokines like IFN-γ [17].

Nitric oxide was shown to be cytostatic for *Giardia in vitro* and to prevent transition between stages of the parasites life cycle [144]. Incubation of *G. duodenalis* with the NO donor GSNO resulted in complete inhibition of trophozoite growth without inducing apoptosis, suggesting that NO is cytostatic for *Giardia* [144]. Exposure to GSNO also prevented the formation of encystation-specific secretory vesicles (ESVs) as well as the expression of the cyst wall protein (CWP2) in parasites cultured in encysting conditions. This suggests that NO may prevent encystation and thus contribute to limiting transmission.

Along with having cytostatic effects on *Giardia*, NO also has cytotoxic potential but *in vitro* reports are confounding. It is speculated that macrophages may contribute to immunity in giardiasis by producing large amounts of NO. Fernendes *et al*. demonstrated that incubation of cytokine stimulated murine peritoneal macrophages with *G. duodenalis* Portland I strain for two hours resulted in NO mediated reduction in parasite viability [145]. The NOS inhibitor N-iminoethyl-L-ornithine (L-NIO) diminished the anti-*Giardial* potential of activated macrophages suggesting that this observed cytotoxicity is a consequence of NO production. The cytotoxic effects of NO were also confirmed in a macrophage free system, whereby incubating the parasite with the different NO donors S-Nitroso-acetyl-penicillamine (SNAP) and sodium nitroprusside (SNP) and 3-Morpholinosydnonimine hydrochloride (SIN-1) induced cell death. Importantly, this cytotoxicity was lost when the peroxide scavenger catalase was used in concert to the NO donors, suggesting that peroxynitrite may be the cell death causing agent rather than NO itself. This was consistent with the observation that superoxide dismutase (SOD) greatly enhanced the cytotoxicity of SIN-1 and that this enhancement was catalase sensitive. However, a different study exposed *G. duodenalis* WB strain trophozoites to the NO donor GSNO at concentrations as high as 5 mM and did not see significant cell death [144]. These different responses to NO may reflect genetic variation between strains WB and Portland I as well as the use of different NO donors and culturing conditions.

Giardia has been shown to competitively inhibit NO production by human intestinal epithelial cells *in vitro* [144]. Cultured monolayers of the human intestinal epithelial cell line HT-29 demonstrated reduced NO production when incubated with *G. duodenalis* after stimulation with the cytokines IL-1α, IFN-γ, and TNF-α. Uninfected cells demonstrated progressive increases in NO production after stimulation with cytokines for 10 hours. NO production was extremely sensitive to *Giardia*. This inhibition was demonstrated in other human epithelial cell lines Caco2 and HT-8 as well. Furthermore, the addition of exogenous arginine was shown to effectively replenish NO levels, supporting the hypothesis that *Giardia* consumes arginine and thereby limits the substrate for NOS rather than targeting NO or NOS directly.

Interestingly, there is evidence that nNOS, not iNOS plays a protective role in immunity against *Giardia in vivo*. The observation that iNOS deficient mice cleared infection with *G. duodenalis* similarly to wild-type mice, while treatment with the nonspecific NOS inhibitor L-NAME prolonged infection prompted the investigation of the role of nNOS in immunity

[146]. Indeed, it was shown that selective inhibition of nNOS with 7-nitroindasole and gene targeting of nNOS had delaying effects on parasite clearance, resembling L-NAME treatment. The contraction of smooth muscle within the intestinal epithelium results from cholinergic stimulation, while relaxation is accomplished through NO mediated inhibitory signals. Coordination of contraction and relaxation yields motility and propulsion. Inhibition of nNOS was found to reduce intestinal motility by inhibiting NO mediated muscle relaxation. Selective inhibition of nNOS resulted in prolonged infection with *G. duodenalis* infections in mice [146, 147]. *In vivo* studies such as these are, however, largely lacking and more emphasis is needed on such approaches to delineate the involvement of antimicrobial molecules in immunity to *Giardia*.

It has been known since 1983 that *Giardia* infections are not cleared in mice deficient in mast cells due to mutations in the gene c-kit [148]. More recently, Li et al. demonstrated that blockade of mast cell recruitment and activation using antibodies to c-kit also prolonged infections with *G. duodenalis* [149]. Interestingly, these c-kit mutants did not have any detectable anti-*Giardia* IgA two weeks after infection and also had lower levels of IL-6 mRNA in the intestine. Thus, mast cells could function as initiators, regulators and effectors of the immune response in this infection by releasing cytokines, proteases and neurotransmitters.

Innate Immunity

Innate immunity is an important component of the host defense against *Giardia*. Receptors in the innate response target common microbial macromolecules that are recognized as foreign. Upon recognition of foreign molecular patterns, the innate response releases cytokines and chemokines that recruit additional cells, helping to slow down pathogen replication and triggering an adaptive response. Infection with *Giardia* takes place at the intestinal epithelium, and this is considered the first line of immune defense against invasion by intestinal parasites. Release of chemokines by the intestinal epithelium may function to recruit both innate and adaptive immune cells upon infection with *Giardia*. Caco2 cells, a colon derived epithelial cell line, secrete CCL2, CCL20, and CXCL1-3 in response to *Giardia* [150]. These chemokines are responsible for the recruitment of immune cells, including dendritic cells, T cells and macrophages. CCL2 causes the degranulation of basophils and mast cells, while CCL20 plays a chemoattractive role in recruiting phagocytes and dendritic cells (DCs) to the site of infection. The chemokines CXCL1-3 function in recruiting neutrophils, polymorphonucleocytes, and monocytes, respectively. *In vivo* roles for these chemokines in giardiasis have not been examined.

The capacity of *Giardia* to inhibit the innate immune response has been described in dendritic cells (DCs). Our lab recently demonstrated that *G. duodenalis* had the capacity to suppress murine bone marrow derived dendritic cell proinflammatory cytokine production in response to LPS and other classical stimulators of innate immunity [151]. In this study, *G. duodenalis* was a poor inducer of proinflammatory cytokines, releasing no IL-10 or IL-12 and small amounts of IL-6 and TNFα. Although, the costimulatory molecules CD80, CD86 and CD40 were slightly upregulated by *Giardia*. LPS alone strongly induced both the secretion of proinflammatory cytokines IL-6, IL-12, IL-10, and TNFα as well as the costimulatory molecules CD80, CD86 and CD40. Co-incubation of DCs with LPS and parasite extracts suggested that *G. duodenalis* has the capacity to inhibit dendritic cell antigen presentation by blocking induction of MHC II proteins and co-stimulatory molecules. Furthermore, LPS induced IL-12 secretion was significantly diminished by coincubation with *Giardia* extract, compared to LPS alone. In contrast, an ERK1/2 dependent IL-10 upregulation was observed when incubating DCs with *Giardia* and LPS, compared to LPS alone. IL-12 production was shown to be significantly enhanced by treatment with an anti-IL-10R antibody, suggesting that IL-12 is under partial repression by IL-10. Addition of wortmannin, an inhibitor of phosphoinositide-3 kinase (PI-3K), greatly enhanced IL-12 production in DCs incubated with LPS and parasite extracts. These data suggest that *Giardia* may activate PI-3K in dendritic cells, resulting in reduced production of proinflammatory signals. The inhibition of DC IL-12 production by *Giardia*, suggests that an inflammatory environment could contribute to immune-mediated parasite elimination or even prevention of colonization. Although inflammation is not a consistent component of *Giardia* infection, evidence described above suggests that inflammatory factors like TNFα are involved in this response. How DCs that have been exposed to *Giardia* direct T cell development remains to be examined.

IMMUNITY & PATHOLOGY

There is significant variability in the symptoms exhibited by patients infected with *Giardia*. Some of this variability may be due to differences among the parasites present, but differences in host immune responses likely also contribute to this variability. Several mechanisms have been described that contribute to pathogenesis in giardiasis [152]. These include changes in intestinal motility, permeability of the intestinal mucosa, function of the brush border and ion secretion into the intestinal lumen. The role of immune responses in each of these is described below.

Intestinal Motility

There is ample evidence that *Giardia* infection increases intestinal motility and that this contributes to epigastric pain and diarrheal disease. The finding that infection with *G. duodenalis* increased intestinal transit rates in gerbils prompted research into the regulatory mechanisms involved in this process [153]. Increased contractility of intestinal smooth muscle and intestinal transit rates have both been observed following infection with *G. duodenalis* [146, 154]. Moreover, increased rates of intestinal transit were demonstrated in immunocompetent mice but not SCID mice infected with *G. duodenalis and G. muris,* suggesting that this is in part immune regulated [146, 147]. In all cases, increased intestinal motility correlated to clearing infection. These changes were diminished when mice infected with *G. duodenalis* or *G. muris* were treated with the NOS inhibitor L-NAME or with the μ-opiate receptor agonist loperamide [146, 147]. Thus, adaptive immune responses contribute to symptoms of disease associated with intestinal motility changes.

While nitric oxide is likely important for affecting intestinal motility through mediating muscle relaxation, the neurotransmitter cholecystokinin (CCK) was recently shown to be important for mediating enhanced muscle contractility following *Giardia* infection. [154]. Intestinal muscle preparations from mice infected with *Giardia* responded to acetylcholine, 5-HT and PAR-1 agonists similar to uninfected mice [154]. In contrast, exposure to CCK was shown to have a much greater stimulatory effect on intestinal muscle contraction from infected mice than uninfected mice. This CCK response was subsequently shown to be mast cell dependent as pre-treatment with compound 48/80 to deplete mast cell granules abolished the response. Blockage of mast cell degranulation with ketotifen also blocked the muscular response to CCK. These findings suggest that CCK alters muscle function by activating mast cells and that mast cells have a regulatory role in *Giardia* mediated alterations in intestinal motility. Interestingly, elevated CCK levels were observed with giardiasis in humans [155]. Moreover, CCK is central in stimulating the intestinal release of bile by the gallbladder and bile is also essential for trophozoite replication. Thus, CCK may both promote parasite replication and contribute to symptomatic disease in human infections.

Malabsorption

Many of the severe pathological manifestations that follow infection with *Giardia*, such as diarrhea, cramps and nausea, are quite variable among patients. Changes in the intestinal epithelium contributing to nutrient malabsorption, however, appear to occur even in the absence of overt symptoms. The epithelial dysfunction resulting from giardiasis resembles that of various non-parasitic enteric disorders such as bacterial enteritis, chronic food anaphylaxis, Crohn's disease and coeliac disease [152, 156]. This suggests that *Giardia* may utilize overlapping pathways with these non-parasitic diseases to trigger pathology in the intestine and that these common pathologies may be partially immune mediated. Epithelial dysfunction with giardiasis is a multicomponent set of pathologies that manifest physiologically through nutrient malabsorption. Malabsorption from infection with *Giardia* is considered to consist of three components; increased epithelial permeability, reduced brush border function and a secretory component. These factors are not exclusive, but are overlapping; malabsorption of glucose and other nutrients is thought to result from reduced absorptive surface area of the epithelium due to shortening of the microvilli as well as reduced chemical gradients due both to hypersecretion of ions and paracellular flux. Other defects have been also reported with giardiasis, such as impaired pancreatic enzyme secretion and bile salt abnormalities [152].

Epithelial Permeability

Compromised molecular ultrastructural integrity in the intestinal epithelium is a pathological consequence of *Giardia* infection that contributes to malabsorption by causing increased epithelial permeability. This is considered to result from cytoskeletal abnormalities within the intestinal epithelium and defects in the tight junctions between the individual cells that comprise the intestinal barrier. Abnormal epithelial permeability has been considered a key contributor to many pathological gastrointestinal diseases [156-159]. Several molecular factors that may contribute to the breakdown of the epithelial barrier in humans have been studied in *Giardia* infected human cell lines. Addition of parasites to monolayers of Caco2 and SCBN epithelial cell cultures has been shown to induce changes in F-actin, α-actinin, and ZO-1, and to induce apoptosis [73, 160-162]. Caspase 3 dependent apoptosis was demonstrated in HCT-8 epithelial cells infected with *G. duodenalis* [163]. Apoptosis of intestinal epithelial cells was shown to be strain dependent [162]. Recently, changes in permeability, tight junction proteins and apoptosis of epithelial cells were documented in biopsies of human giardiasis patients [164]. Better understanding of the parasite factors that induce these changes is needed.

Studies conducted in mice have been helpful in our understanding of the molecular events that mediate increased intestinal permeability with giardiasis. Several *in vivo* mouse studies have demonstrated increased permeability and breakdown of barrier function of the small intestine in response to infection with *Giardia* [134, 161]. Persistently increased permeability in the small intestine was shown in both euthymic and athymic mice, although to a greater extent in euthymic mice [161]. This suggests that malabsorption is to some extent T cell independent. Cellular relocation of ZO-1 was observed in infected mice as well [161]. A recent *in vitro* study demonstrated that increased intestinal permeability due to the activation of sodium/glucose cotransporters via by SGLT-1 may have preventative effects on cell death [165]. Activation of glucose uptake through this pathway was disrupted by myosin light chain kinase (MLCK) [165]. The extent of immune system involvement in effecting changes in epithelial permeability remains unclear. Studies with cell lines indicate that some changes occur in the complete absence of immune cells, while others in vivo suggest that the situation may be more complex.

Brush Border

Acquired immunity in giardiasis triggers the shortening of the microvilli structures lining the intestinal epithelium and thereby reducing the absorptive capacity of the gut. The reduced surface area of the intestine is one of the main causes of malabsorption and contributes to diarrheal disease in giardiasis [45]. Impaired disaccharidase activity correlates with reduced microvilli surface area [126, 166]. Lactase deficiencies were also reported in humans, although these patients did not demonstrate maltase and sucrase deficiencies [167]. The exact role of adaptive immunity in brush border breakdown is not fully understood but several insights have been gained from clinical examinations and experimental studies using animal models of giardiasis.

While *in vivo* human studies are extremely difficult to carry out, clinical cases of symptomatic giardiasis have provided valuable isolates of *G. duodenalis* for *in vitro* investigations into the mechanisms governing intestinal pathology. Histological reports in humans failed to detect significantly increased infiltration of intraepithelial CD8+ T lymphocytes in sections where retracted villi and altered enterocyte morphology were observed [168]. One study used isolates obtained from children suffering from diarrheal disease in Mexico City and used them to *in vitro* study the effects of giardiasis on the morphology of the intestinal epithelium [169]. This group found that exposing canine MDCK epithelial cells to these *G. duodenalis* isolates obtained from humans resulted in the depletion of microvilli. Furthermore, a clinical study observed villus retraction in 41% of giardiasis patient biopsies [70]. Although, interestingly the biopsies obtained from uninfected control subjects also presented with villus flattening based on morphology. Thus, while role of villus shortening in giardiasis is controversial, microvillus retraction appears to be a common occurrence in this disease.

Experimental studies in mice have revealed that the breakdown of the intestinal brush border in giardiasis is a main cause of nutrient malabsorption and is at least in part T cell induced. Wild-type mice infected with *G. muris* developed microvillus shortening, while athymic mice infected in parallel did not [126]. A recent report demonstrated that adoptive transfer of CD8+, but not CD4+, T cells from *G. muris* infected mice to naïve recipients resulted in intestinal injury, similar to that seen in infected mice [166]. This study demonstrated that *G. muris* infection led to CD8+ T cell mediated brush border defects, retracted microvilli, and an increased crypt/villus ratio. However, both CD4+ and CD8+ mesenteric lymph node T cells contributed to the infiltration of lymphocytes into the epithelium [166]. It remains unclear how this extracellular pathogen stimulates a CD8+ T cell response. Nevertheless, since parasite control has been shown to be independent of CD8+ T cell responses [54], these results suggest that blocking CD8+ T cell responses to the parasite could ameliorate some pathology without compromising the ability to eradicate infections.

Secretory Products

It has been shown that *Giardia* produces excretory-secretory products that have enterotoxic properties and induce secretion of sodium and chloride in murine intestinal segments [72]. Electrolyte imbalances of chloride have been observed in humans with chronic giardiasis [164]. In 2001, Kaur et al, identified a 58 kDa biologically active glycoprotein extracted from *Giardia* which seemed to have enterotoxic properties eliciting the intestinal secretion of sodium and chloride [169]. Subsequently, antibodies against this toxin were shown to cross react with the cholera toxin (CT) suggesting potential toxin conservation [170]. Other evidence suggests that *Giardia* imposes alterations on electrolyte homeostasis within the intestinal epithelium in a direct manner.

Excretory/secretory products (ESP) from *Giardia* have been demonstrated to have apoptotic capacity within the epithelium. GP49, a GPI anchored antigen of *G. duodenalis* was shown to alter electrolyte fluxes in the human intestinal epithelial cell line, T84 [115]. *Giardia* ESPs have been shown to be immunoreactive and coincubation with antibodies prevents intestinal apoptosis *in vitro* [170]. Culture filtrates have been shown to damage fibroblasts *in vitro* and to reduce salt and water absorption in rats *in vivo* [171, 172]. There is evidence for an immune response to ESPs *in vivo* as the immunization of mice with these proteins significantly shortened the duration of disease after challenge with *Giardia* [173]. Unfortunately, the excretory/secretory toxins in *Giardia* have not been identified at the molecular level. Better understanding of these toxins would greatly facilitate molecular epidemiology investigations, vaccine development and new therapeutics for giardiasis.

CONCLUSIONS

Giardia is a highly adaptive, molecularly and morphologically diverse, intestinal parasite. The diversity of this protozoon is illustrated by the wide range of hosts that it infects. Its colonization of the small intestine elicits an immune response (both innate and adaptive) which plays an essential role in clearing infection. The generation of immunity in (at least some) individuals previously infected with the parasite suggests that vaccination may be a promising and practical route of disease control. There are, however, many challenges associated with the development of effective vaccines.

The genetic and environmental factors that may predispose a host to infection with a certain species of *Giardia* remain to be elucidated and fully understood. However, in both mouse models and human infections, it has been demonstrated that biological host factors, such as age, nutritional status, and immune status may render one more susceptible to infection with particular species or strains of the parasite. For example suckling mice have been readily infected with *G. duodenalis* whereas adult mice were more resistant [60]. Moreover, the range of clinical presentations seen in human infections and the potential role for immune responses in contributing to the development of symptoms further complicates immunological intervention in this disease. The variation in the severity and nature of pathological manifestations in hosts alludes to the multiple levels of diversity in parasite and host that may complicate the development of therapeutics. Host specificity has been demonstrated in giardiasis but distinctions between host specific strains are constantly drawn and identification of all possible isolates that may be infectious to a particular host is lacking. Life cycle specific antigens have been demonstrated in *Giardia* as well as antigenic variation within single organisms of the parasite and these factors also complicate vaccine development. Nevertheless, the rapid pace of advancement in our understanding of these issues should hopefully lead to new clinical interventions.

REFERENCES

[1]   Meyer E A. *Giardia* as an organism. In: Thompson RCA, Reynoldson JA, and Lymbery AJ Ed. Giardia: from molecules to disease. University Press, Cambridge, UK 1994; p.3

[2]   Rendtorff RC. The experimental transmission of human intestinal protozoan parasites. II. *Giardia lamblia* cysts given in capsules. Am J Hyg 1954; 59: 209-20.

[3]   Hansen JS, Ongerth JE. Effects of time and watershed characteristics on the concentration of *Cryptosporidium* oocysts in river water. Appl Environ Microbiol 1991; 57: 2790-5.

[4]   LeChevallier MW, Norton WD, Lee RG. *Giardia* and *Cryptosporidium* spp. in filtered drinking water supplies. Appl Environ Microbiol 1991; 57: 2617-21.

[5]   Hoogenboom-Verdegaal AM, de Jong JC, During M, Hoogenveen R, Hoekstra JA. Community-based study of the incidence of gastrointestinal diseases in The Netherlands. Epidemiol Infect 1994; 112: 481-7.

[6]   Adam RD. The biology of *Giardia* spp. Microbiol Rev: 1991; 55: 706-32.

[7]   Quinn KJ. The river in a rural community. J Ir Med Assoc 1971; 64: 602-4.

[8]   Fricker, C.R., Medema, G.D. and Smith, H.V. Protozoan parasites (*Cryptosporidium, Giardia, Cyclospora*). In Guidelines for Drinking-Water Quality. Geneva: World Health Organization 2002; pp. 70–118. http://www.who.int/water_sanitation_health/-dwq/en/admicrob5.pdf

[9]   Islam, A. *Giardiasis* in developing countries. Giardiasis. Meyer E A, Ed.1990; pp. 235-266. Amsterdam: Elsevier

[10]   Mahmud MA, Chappell C, Hossain MM, Habib M, Dupont HL. Risk factors for development of first symptomatic *Giardia* infection among infants of a birth cohort in rural Egypt. Am J Trop Med Hyg 1995; 53: 84-8.

[11]   Téllez A, Morales W, Rivera T, Meyer E, Leiva B, Linder E. Prevalence of intestinal parasites in the human population of León, Nicaragua. Acta Trop 1997; 66: 119-25.

[12]   Azazy AA, Raja'a YA. Malaria and intestinal parasitosis among children presenting to the paediatric centre in Sana'a, Yemen. East Mediterr Health J 2003; 9: 1048-53.

[13]   Roberts A, Kemp C. Infectious diseases of refugees and immigrants: giardiasis (*Giardia lamblia*). J Am Acad Nurse Pract 2001; 13: 532-3.

[14]   Reynoldson JA, Behnke JM, Gracey M, *et al*. Efficacy of albendazole against *Giardia* and hookworm in a remote Aboriginal

community in the north of Western Australia. Acta Trop 1998; 71: 27-44.

[15]   Slifko TR, Smith HV, Rose JB. Emerging parasite zoonoses associated with water and food. Int J Parasitol 2000; 30: 1379-93.

[16]   Thompson RC. The zoonotic significance and molecular epidemiology of *Giardia* and giardiasis. Vet Parasitol 2004; 126:15-35.

[17]   Eckmann L. Mucosal defences against *Giardia*. Parasite Immunol 2003; 25: 259-70.

[18]   Thompson RC, Monis PT. Variation in *Giardia*: implications for taxonomy and epidemiology. Adv Parasitol 2004; 58: 69-137.

[19]   Barwick RS, Levy DA, Craun GF, Beach MJ, Calderon RL. Surveillance for waterborne-disease outbreaks--United States, 1997-1998. Surveill Summ 2000; 49: 1-21.

[20]   Craun GF. Waterborne disease outbreaks in the United States of America: causes and prevention. World Health Stat Q 1992; 45: 192-9.

[21]   Savioli L, Smith H, Thompson A. *Giardia* and *Cryptosporidium* join the 'Neglected Diseases Initiative'. Trends Parasitol 2006; 225: 203-8.

[22]   Cacciò SM, Thompson RC, McLauchlin J, Smith HV. Unravelling *Cryptosporidium* and *Giardia* epidemiology. Trends Parasitol 2005; 21: 430-7.

[23]   Elmendorf HG, Dawson SC, McCaffery JM. The cytoskeleton of *Giardia lamblia*. Int J Parasitol 2003; 33: 3-28.

[24]   Felice, F. P. Studies on the cytology and life history of a *Giardia* from the laboratory rat. Univ Calif Publ Zool 1952; 57: 53-143.

[25]   Monis PT, Andrews RH, Mayrhofer G, *et al.* Novel lineages of *Giardia intestinalis* identified by genetic analysis of organisms isolated from dogs in Australia. Parasitology 1998; 116: 7-19.

[26]   Morrison, H.L., et al., Genomic Minimalism in the Ealry Diverging Intestinl Parasite *Giardia lamblia*. Science 2007; 317: 1921-1926.

[27]   Nash TE, Keister DB. Differences in excretory-secretory products and surface antigens among 19 isolates of *Giardia*. J Infect Dis. 1985; 152: 1166-71.

[28]   Franzen O, et al. Draft Genome Sequencing of *Giardia intestinalis* Assemblage B Isolate GS: Is Human Giardiasis Caused by Two Different Species? PLoS Pathogens 2009; 5: e1000560.

[29]   C. Read, J. Walters, I. D. Robertson and R. C. A. Thompson. Correlation between genotype of *Giardia duodenalis* and diarrhoea. Letter to the Editor. Society for Parasitology 2002

[30]   F. L. Amar, P. H. Dear, S. Pedraza-Díaz, N. Looker, E. Linnane, and J. McLauchlin. Sensitive PCR-Restriction Fragment Length Polymorphism Assay for Detection and Genotyping of *Giardia duodenalis* in Human Feces. J Clin Microbiol 2002; 40: 446-452

[31]   Traub RJ, Robertson ID, Irwin P, Mencke N, Monis P, Thompson RC. Humans, dogs and parasitic zoonoses--unravelling the relationships in a remote endemic community in northeast India using molecular tools. Parasitol Res 2003; 90 Suppl 3: S156-7.

[32]   Homan WL, and Mank TG, Human giardiasis: genotype linked differences in clinical symptomatology. Int J Parasitol 2001; 31: 822-6.

[33]   Sahagún J, Clavel A, Goñi P, Seral C, Llorente MT, Castillo FJ, Capilla S, Arias A, Gómez-Lus R,. Correlation between the presence of symptoms and the *Giardia duodenalis* genotype. Eur J Clin Microbiol Infect Dis 2008; 27: 81-83.

[34]   Mohammed Mahdy AK, Surin J, Wan KL, Mohd-Adnan A, Al-Mekhlafi MS, Lim YA. *Giardia intestinalis* genotypes: Risk factors and correlation with clinical symptoms. Acta Trop. 2009; 112: 67-70.

[35]   Gelanew T, Lalle M, Hailu A, Pozio E, Cacciò SM. Molecular characterization of human isolates of *Giardia duodenalis* from Ethiopia. Acta Trop 2007; 102: 92-9.

[36]   Jakubowski, W, Graun GF, Olson BE, Olson ME,Wallis PM. Update on the control of *Giardia* in water supplies. In: *Giardia*: the cosmopolitan parasite. Wallingford, UK, CAB International 2002; pp. 217-238.

[37]   Hopkins RM, Meloni BP, Groth DM, Wetherall JD, Reynoldson JA, Thompson RC. Ribosomal RNA sequencing reveals differences between the genotypes of *Giardia* isolates recovered from humans and dogs living in the same locality. J Parasitol 1997; 83: 44-51.

[38]   Sackey ME, Weigel MM, Armijos RX. Predictors and nutritional consequences of intestinal parasitic infections in rural Ecuadorian children. J Trop Pediatr 2003; 49: 17-23.

[39]   Walterspiel JN, Pickering LK. *Giardia* and giardiasis. Prog Clin Parasitol 1994; 4: 1-26.

[40]   Upcroft J, Upcroft P. My favorite cell: *Giardia*. Bioessays 1998; 3:256-63.

[41]   Olson ME, Ceri H, Morck DW. *Giardia* vaccination. Parasitol Today 2000; 16: 213-7.

[42]   Olson ME, Morck DW, Ceri H. The efficacy of a *Giardia lamblia* vaccine in kittens. Can J Vet Res. 1996; 4:249-56.

[43]   Olson ME, Hannigan CJ, Gaviller PF, Fulton LA. The use of a *Giardia* vaccine as an immunotherapeutic agent in dogs. Can Vet J 2001; 11: 865-8.

[44]   Faubert G. Immune response to *Giardia duodenalis*. Clin Microbiol Rev 2000; 13: 35-54

[45]   Campbell JD, Faubert GM. Recognition of *Giardia lamblia* cyst-specific antigens by monoclonal antibodies. Parasite Immunol 1994; 16: 211-9.

[46]   Sykora. J. L., Sorber, C. A., Jakubowski W., *et al.* Distribution of *Giardia* cysts in wastewater. Water Sci Technol 1991; 24: 187-192

[47]   Grimason AM, Smith HV, Parker JF, Jackson MH, Smith PG, Girdwood RW. Occurrence of *Giardia* sp. cysts and *Cryptosporidium* sp. oocysts in faeces from public parks in the west of Scotland. Epidemiol Infect 1993; 110: 641-5.

[48]   Farthing MJ. Diarrhoeal disease: current concepts and future challenges. Pathogenesis of giardiasis. Trans R Soc Trop Med Hyg 1993; 3: 17-21.

[49]   Nash TE, Herrington DA, Losonsky GA, Levine MM. Experimental human infections with *Giardia lamblia*. J Infect Dis 1987; 156: 974-84.

[50]   Hermans PE, Diaz-Buxo JA, Stobo JD. Idiopathic late-onset immunoglobulin deficiency. Clinical observations in 50 patients. Am J Med 1976; 61: 221-7.

[51]   Skea DL, Underdown BJ. Acquired resistance to *Giardia muris* in X-linked immunodeficient mice. Infect Immun 1991; 59: 1733-8.

[52]   Petro TM, Watson RR, Feely DE, Darban H. Suppression of resistance to *Giardia muris* and cytokine production in a murine model of acquired immune deficiency syndrome. Reg Immunol 1992; 4: 409-14.

[53]   Moolasart P. Giardia lamblia in AIDS patients with diarrhea. J Med Assoc Thai 1999; 82: 654-9.

[54]   Singer SM, Nash TE. T-cell-dependent control of acute *Giardia lamblia* infections in mice. Infect Immun 2000; 68: 170-5.

[55]   Scott E. Food safety and foodborne disease in 21st century homes. Can J Infect Dis 2003; 14: 277-80.

[56]   Davids BJ, Palm JE, Housley MP, *et al.* Polymeric immunoglobulin receptor in intestinal immune defense against the lumen-dwelling protozoan parasite *Giardia*. J Immunol 2006; 177: 6281-90.

[57]   Pengsaa K, Sirivichayakul C, Vithayasai N, Senawong S, Luangwedchakarn V. Chronic diarrhea and abnormal serum immunoglobulin levels: a case report. Southeast Asian J Trop Med Public Health 2007; 38: 424-6.

[58]   Sawatzki M, Peter S, Hess C. Therapy-resistant diarrhea due to *Giardia lamblia* in a patient with common variable immunodeficiency disease. Digestion 2007; 75: 101-2.

[59]   Dib HH, Lu SQ, Wen SF. Prevalence of *Giardia lamblia* with or without diarrhea in South East, South East Asia and the Far East. Parasitol Res 2008; 103: 239-51.

[60]   Hill DR, Guerrant RL, Pearson RD, Hewlett EL. *Giardia lamblia* infection of suckling mice. J Infect Dis 1983; 147: 217-21.

[61]   Fraser D, Bilenko N, Deckelbaum R J, Dagan R, El-On J, and Naggan L. *Giardia lamblia* carriage in Israeli Bedouin infants: risk factors and consequences. Clin Infect Dis 2000; 30: 419-24

[62]   Simsek Z, Zeyrek FY Kurcer MA. Effect of *Giardia* infection on growth and psychomotor development of children aged 0-5 years. J Trop Pediatr 2004; 50: 90-3.

[63]   Goto R, Mascie-Taylor CG, Lunn PG. Impact of anti-*Giardia* and anthelminthic treatment on infant growth and intestinal permeability in rural Bangladesh: a randomised double-blind controlled study. Trans R Soc Trop Med Hyg 2009; 103: 520-9.

[64]   Daniels CW, Belosevic M. Serum antibody responses by male and female C57Bl/6 mice infected with *Giardia muris*. Clin Exp Immunol 1994; 97: 424-9.

[65]   Al-Mekhlafi HM, Azlin M, Aini UN, *et al.* Protein-energy malnutrition and soil-transmitted helminthiases among Orang Asli children in Selangor, Malaysia. Asia Pac J Clin Nutr 2005; 14: 188-94.

[66]   Carvalho-Costa FA, Gonçalves AQ, Lassance SL, Silva Neto LM, Salmazo CA, Bóia MN. *Giardia lamblia* and other intestinal parasitic infections and their relationships with nutritional status in children in Brazilian Amazon. Rev Inst Med Trop Sao Paulo 2007; 49: 147-53.

[67]   Singer SM, Nash TE. The role of normal flora in *Giardia lamblia* infections in mice. J Infect Dis 2000; 181: 1510-2.

[68]   Raizman RE. Giardiasis: an overview for the clinician. Am J Dig Dis 1976; 21: 1070-4.

[69]   Brodsky RE, Spencer HC Jr, Schultz MG. Giardiasis in American travelers to the Soviet Union. J Infect Dis 1974; 130: 319-23.

[70]   Oberhuber G, Stolte M. Giardiasis: analysis of histological changes in biopsy specimens of 80 patients. J Clin Pathol 1990; 43: 641-3.

[71]   Buret A, Hardin JA, Olson ME, Gall DG. Pathophysiology of small intestinal malabsorption in gerbils infected with *Giardia lamblia*. Gastroenterology 1992;103: 506-13.

[72]   Samra HK, Ganguly NK, Garg UC, Goyal J, Mahajan RC. Effect of excretory-secretory products of *Giardia lamblia* on glucose and phenylalanine transport in the small intestine of Swiss albino mice. Biochem Int 1988; 17: 801-12.

[73]   Buret AG, Mitchell K, Muench DG, Scott KG. *Giardia lamblia* disrupts tight junctional ZO-1 and increases permeability in non-transformed human small intestinal epithelial monolayers: effects of epidermal growth factor. Parasitology 2002; 125: 11-9.

[74]   Hesham MS, Edariah AB, Norhayati M. Intestinal parasitic infections and micronutrient deficiency: a review. Med J Malaysia 2004; 59: 284-93.

[75]   Ertan P, Yereli K, Kurt O, Balcioğlu IC, Onağ A. Serological levels of zinc, copper and iron elements among *Giardia lamblia* infected children in Turkey. Pediatr Int 2002; 44: 286-8.

[76]   Flanagan PA. Giardia--diagnosis, clinical course and epidemiology. A review. Epidemiol Infect 1992;109: 1-22.

[77]   Farthing MJ, Mata L, Urrutia JJ, Kronmal RA. Natural history of *Giardia* infection of infants and children in rural Guatemala and its impact on physical growth. Am J Clin Nutr 1986; 43: 395-405.

[78]   Petri WA Jr, Miller M, Binder HJ, Levine MM, Dillingham R, Guerrant RL. Enteric infections, diarrhea, and their impact on function and development. J Clin Invest 2008;118: 1277-90.

[79]   Berkman DS, Lescano AG, Gilman RH, Lopez SL, and Black MM. Effects of stunting, diarrhoeal disease, and parasitic infection during infancy on cognition in late childhood: a follow-up study. Lancet 2002; 359: 564-71.

[80]   Lorntz B, Soares AM, Moore SR, *et al.* Early childhood diarrhea predicts impaired school performance. Pediatr Infect Dis J 2006; 25: 513-20.

[81]   Lunn PG. The impact of infection and nutrition on gut function and growth in childhood. Proc Nutr Soc 2000; 59: 147-54.

[82]   Campbell DI, Elia M, Lunn PG. Growth faltering in rural Gambian infants is associated with impaired small intestinal barrier function, leading to endotoxemia and systemic inflammation. J Nutr 2003; 133: 1332-8.

[83]   Rousham EK. An increase in *Giardia duodenalis* infection among children receiving periodic Anthelmintic treatment in Bangladesh. J Trop Pediatr 1994; 40: 329-33.

[84]   Northrop-Clewes CA, Rousham EK, Mascie-Taylor CN, Lunn PG. Anthelmintic treatment of rural Bangladeshi children: effect on host physiology, growth, and biochemical status. Am J Clin Nutr 200; 73: 53-60.

[85]   Goto R, Mascie-Taylor CG, Lunn PG. Impact of intestinal permeability, inflammation status and parasitic infections on infant growth faltering in rural Bangladesh. Br J Nutr 2009; 101: 1509-16.

[86]   Velazquez C, Beltran M, Ontiveros N, *et al. Giardia lamblia* infection induces different secretory and systemic antibody responses in mice. Parasite Immunol 2005; 27: 351-6.

[87]   Langford TD, Housley MP, Boes M, *et al.* Central importance of immunoglobulin A in host defense against *Giardia* spp. Infect Immun 2002; 70: 11-8.

[88]   Eren M, Saltik-Temizel IN, Yüce A, Cağlar M, Koçak N. Duodenal appearance of giardiasis in a child with selective immunoglobulin A deficiency. Pediatr Int 2007; 49: 409-11.

[89]   Ljungström I, Castor B. Immune response to *Giardia lamblia* in a water-borne outbreak of giardiasis in Sweden. J Med Microbiol 1992; 36: 347-52.

[90]   Einfeld DA, Stibbs HH. Identification and characterization of a major surface antigen of *Giardia lamblia*. Infect Immun 1984; 46: 377-83.

[91]   Moss DM, Mathews HM, Visvesvara GS, Dickerson JW, Walker EM. Antigenic variation of *Giardia lamblia* in the feces of Mongolian gerbils. J Clin Microbiol 1990; 28: 254-7.

[92]   Crossley R, Holberton D. Assembly of 2.5 nm filaments from giardin, a protein associated with cytoskeletal microtubules in *Giardia*. J Cell Sci 1985; 78: 205-31.

[93]   Char S, Cevallos AM, Farthing MJ. An immunodominant antigen of *Giardia lamblia* is a heat shock protein. Biotechnol Ther. 1992; 3(3-4): 151-7.

[94]   Farthing MJ, Pereira ME, Keusch GT. Description and characterization of a surface lectin from *Giardia lamblia*. Infect Immun. 1986; 51: 661-7.

[95]   Crossley R, Holberton DV. Characterization of proteins from the cytoskeleton of *Giardia lamblia*. J Cell Sci 1983; 59: 81-103.

[96]   Ritchie, L. S., and Davis, Cooper. Parasitological findings and epidemiological aspects of epidemic amebiasis occurring in occupants of the Mantetsu apartment building, Tokyo, Japan. Am. J Trop Med 1948 28: 803-816.

[97]   Gleason NN, Horwitz MS, Newton LH, Moore GT. A stool survey for enteric organisms in Aspen, Colorado. Am J Trop Med Hyg 1970; 3: 480-4.

[98]   Istre GR, Dunlop TS, Gaspard GB, Hopkins RS. Waterborne giardiasis at a mountain resort: evidence for acquired immunity. Am J Public Health 1984; 6: 602-4.

[99]   Isaac-Renton JL, Lewis LF, Ong CS, Nulsen MF. A second community outbreak of waterborne giardiasis in Canada and serological investigation of patients. Trans R Soc Trop Med Hyg. 1994; 88: 395-9.

[100] Webster AD. Giardiasis and immunodeficiency diseases. Trans R Soc Trop Med Hyg. 1980; 74: 440-3.

[101] Perlmutter DH, Leichtner AM, Goldman H, Winter HS. Chronic diarrhea associated with hypogammaglobulinemia and enteropathy in infants and children. Dig Dis Sci 1985; 12: 1149-55.

[102] Herbst EW, Armbruster M, Rump JA, Buscher HP, Peter HH. Intestinal B cell defects in common variable immunodeficiency. Clin Exp Immunol. 1994; 95: 215-21.

[103] Attili SV, Gulati AK, Singh VP, Varma DV, Rai M, Sundar S. Diarrhea, CD4 counts and enteric infections in a hospital - based cohort of HIV-infected patients around Varanasi, India. BMC Infect Dis 2006; 6: 39.

[104] Kurniawan A, Karyadi T, Dwintasari SW, Sari IP, Yunihastuti E, Djauzi S, Smith HV. Intestinal parasitic infections in HIV/AIDS patients presenting with diarrhoea in Jakarta, Indonesia. Trans R Soc Trop Med Hyg 2009; 103: 892-8.

[105] Janoff EN, Smith PD, Blaser MJ. Acute antibody responses to *Giardia lamblia* are depressed in patients with AIDS. J Infect Dis 1988; 157: 798-804.

[106] Barrett DM, Steel-Duncan J, Christie CD, Eldemire-Shearer D, Lindo JF. Absence of opportunistic parasitic infestations in children living with HIV/AIDS in children's homes in Jamaica: pilot investigations. West Indian Med J. 2008; 57: 253-6.

[107] Viriyavejakul P, Nintasen R, Punsawad C, Chaisri U, Punpoowong B, Riganti M. High prevalence of Microsporidium infection in HIV-infected patients. Southeast Asian J Trop Med Public Health 2009; 40: 223-8.

[108] Webster AD. Giardiasis and immunodeficiency diseases. Trans R Soc Trop Med Hyg. 1980; 74:440-3.

[109] Snider DP, Gordon J, McDermott MR, Underdown BJ. Chronic *Giardia muris* infection in anti-IgM-treated mice. I. Analysis of immunoglobulin and parasite-specific antibody in normal and immunoglobulin-deficient animals. J Immunol 1985; 134: 4153-62.

[110] Lai Ping So A, Mayer L. Gastrointestinal manifestations of primary immunodeficiency disorders. Semin Gastrointest Dis 1997; 1:22-32.

[111] Belosevic M, Faubert GM. Lysis and immobilization of *Giardia muris* trophozoites in vitro by immune serum from susceptible and resistant mice. Parasite Immunol. 1987; 1: 11-9.

[112] Nash TE, Aggarwal A. Cytotoxicity of monoclonal antibodies to a subset of *Giardia* isolates. J Immunol. 1986; 7: 2628-32.

[113] Zhou P, Li E, Zhu N, Robertson J, Nash T, Singer SM. Role of interleukin-6 in the control of acute and chronic *Giardia lamblia* infections in mice. Infect Immun 2003; 71: 1566-8.

[114] Téllez A, Palm D, Weiland M, *et al.* Secretory antibodies against *Giardia intestinalis* in lactating Nicaraguan women. Parasite Immunol 2005; 27: 163-9.

[115] Das S, Traynor-Kaplan A, Kachintorn U, Aley SB, Gillin FD. GP49, an invariant GPI-anchored antigen of *Giardia lamblia*. Braz J Med Biol Res 1994; 27: 463-9.

[116] Hasan SM, Maachee M, Córdova OM, Diaz de la Guardia R, Martins M, Osuna A. Human secretory immune response to fatty acid-binding protein fraction from *Giardia lamblia*. Infect Immun. 2002; 4: 2226-9.

[117] Palm JE, Weiland ME, Griffiths WJ, Ljungström I, Svärd SG. Identification of immunoreactive proteins during acute human giardiasis. J Infect Dis 2003; 12: 1849-59.

[118] Abdul-Wahid A, Faubert G. Int J Parasitol. Characterization of the local immune response to cyst antigens during the acute and elimination phases of primary murine giardiasis. Int J Parasitol 2008; 38: 691-703.

[119] Nash TE, Herrington DA, Levine MM, Conrad JT, Merritt JW Jr. Antigenic variation of *Giardia lamblia* in experimental human infections. J Immunol 1990; 144: 4362-9.

[120] Stager S, Muller N. Giardia lamblia infections in B-cell-deficient transgenic mice.Infect Immun. 1997; 9:3944-6.

[121] Nash TE, Mowatt MR. Characterization of a *Giardia lamblia* variant-specific surface protein (VSP) gene from isolate GS/M and estimation of the VSP gene repertoire size. Mol Biochem Parasitol 1992; 2: 219-27.

[122] Svärd SG, Meng TC, Hetsko ML, McCaffery JM, Gillin FD. Differentiation-associated surface antigen variation in the ancient eukaryote *Giardia lamblia*. Mol Microbiol. 1998; 30: 979-89.

[123] Kulakova L, *Singer SM, Conrad J, Nash TE. Epigenetic mechanisms are involved in the control of Giardia* lamblia antigenic variation. Mol Microbiol 2006; 61: 1533-42.

[124] Prucca CG, Slavin I, Quiroga R, *et al.* Antigenic variation in *Giardia lamblia* is regulated by RNA interference. Nature 2008; 456: 750-4.

[125] Stevens DP, Frank DM, Mahmoud AA. Thymus dependency of host resistance to *Giardia muris* infection: studies in nude mice. J Immunol 1978; 120: 680-2.

[126] Scott KG, Logan MR, Klammer GM, Teoh DA, Buret AG. Jejunal brush border microvillous alterations in *Giardia muris*-infected mice: role of T lymphocytes and interleukin-6. Infect Immun 2000; 68: 3412-8.

[127] Matowicka-Karna J, Dymicka-Piekarska V, Kemona H. IFN-gamma, IL-5, IL-6 and IgE in patients infected with *Giardia intestinalis*. Folia Histochem Cytobiol 2009; 47: 93-7.

[128] Ebert EC. Giardia induces proliferation and interferon gamma production by intestinal lymphocytes. Gut 1999; 44: 342-6.

[129] Kanwar SS, Ganguly NK, Walia BN, *Mahajan RC. Direct and antibody dependent cell mediated cytotoxicity against* Giardia lamblia by splenic and intestinal lymphoid cells in mice. Gut 1986; 1: 73-7.

[130] El-Shazly AM, El-Bendary M, Saker T, Rifaat MM, Saleh WA, El Nemr HI. Cellular immune response in giardiasis. J Egypt Soc Parasitol 2003; 33: 887-904.

[131] Djamiatun K, Faubert GM. Exogenous cytokines released by spleen and Peyer's patch cells removed from mice infected with *Giardia muris*. Parasite Immunol 1998; 20: 27-36.

[132] Bienz M, Dai WJ, Welle M, Gottstein B, Müller N.. Interleukin-6-deficient mice are highly susceptible to *Giardia lamblia* infection but exhibit normal intestinal immunoglobulin A responses against the parasite. Infect Immun. 2003; 71: 1569-73.

[133] Ziambaras T, Rubin DC, Perlmutter DH. Regulation of sucrase-isomaltase gene expression in human intestinal epithelial cells by inflammatory cytokines. J Biol Chem. 1996; 2: 1237-42.

[134] Zhou P, Li E, Shea-Donohue T, Singer SM. Tumour necrosis factor alpha contributes to protection against *Giardia lamblia* infection in mice. Parasite Immunol 2007; 29: 367-74.

[135] Bayraktar MR, Mehmet N, Durmaz R. Serum cytokine changes in Turkish children infected with *Giardia lamblia* with and without allergy: Effect of metronidazole treatment. Acta Trop. 2005; 95: 116-22.

[136] Reiner DS, Wang CS, Gillin FD. Human milk kills *Giardia lamblia* by generating toxic lipolytic products. J Infect Dis 1986; 154: 825-32.

[137] Zasloff M. Antimicrobial peptides in health and disease. N Engl J Med. 2002; 347: 1199-200.

[138] Eisenhauer PB, Lehrer RI. Mouse neutrophils lack defensins. Infect Immun 1992; 60: 3446-7.

[139] Ayabe T, Satchell DP, Pesendorfer P, *et al.* Activation of Paneth cell alpha-defensins in mouse small intestine. J Biol Chem 2002; 277: 5219-28.

[140] O'Neil DA, Porter EM, Elewaut D, *et al.* Expression and regulation of the human beta-defensins hBD-1 and hBD-2 in intestinal epithelium. J Immunol 1999; 163: 6718-24.

[141] Salzman NH, Chou MM, de Jong H, Liu L, Porter EM, Paterson Y. Enteric salmonella infection inhibits Paneth cell antimicrobial peptide expression. Infect Immun 2003; 71: 1109-15.

[142] Moser C, Weiner DJ, Lysenko E, Bals R, Weiser JN, Wilson JM. Beta-Defensin 1 contributes to pulmonary innate immunity in mice. Infect Immun 2002; 70: 3068-72.

[143] Aley SB, Zimmerman M, Hetsko M, Selsted ME, Gillin FD. Killing of *Giardia lamblia* by cryptdins and cationic neutrophil peptides. Infect Immun 1994; 62: 5397-403.

[144] Eckmann L, Laurent F, Langford TD, *et al.* Nitric oxide production by human intestinal epithelial cells and competition for arginine as potential determinants of host defense against the lumen-dwelling pathogen *Giardia lamblia*. J Immunol 2000; 164: 1478-87.

[145] Fernandes PD, Assreuy J. Role of nitric oxide and superoxide in *Giardia lamblia* killing. Braz J Med Biol Res 1997; 30: 93-9.

[146] Li E, Zhou P, Singer SM. Neuronal nitric oxide synthase is necessary for elimination of *Giardia lamblia* infections in mice. J Immunol 2006; 176:516-21.

[147] Andersen YS, Gillin FD, Eckmann L. Adaptive immunity-dependent intestinal hypermotility contributes to host defense against *Giardia* spp. Infect Immun 2006; 74: 2473-6.

[148] Erlich JH, Anders RF, Roberts-Thomson IC, Schrader JW, Mitchell GF. An examination of differences in serum antibody specificities and hypersensitivity reactions as contributing factors to chronic infection with the intestinal protozoan parasite, *Giardia muris*, in mice. Aust J Exp Biol Med Sci. 1983; 61: 599-615.

[149] Li E, Zhou P, Petrin Z, Singer SM. Mast cell-dependent control of *Giardia lamblia* infections in mice. Infect Immun 2004; 11: 6642-9.

[150] Roxström-Lindquist K, Ringqvist E, Palm D, Svärd S. *Giardia lamblia*-induced changes in gene expression in differentiated Caco-2 human intestinal epithelial cells. Infect Immun. 2005; 73: 8204-8.

[151] Kamda JD, Singer SM. Phosphoinositide 3-kinase-dependent inhibition of dendritic cell interleukin-12 production by *Giardia lamblia*. Infect Immun 2009; 77:685-93.

[152] Buret AG. Pathophysiology of enteric infections with *Giardia duodenalis*. Parasite 2008; 15:261-5.

[153] Deselliers LP, Tan DT, Scott RB, Olson ME. Effects of *Giardia lamblia* infection on gastrointestinal transit and contractility in Mongolian gerbils. Dig Dis Sci 1997; 42: 2411-9.

[154] Li E, Zhao A, Shea-Donohue T, Singer SM. Mast cell-mediated changes in smooth muscle contractility during mouse giardiasis. Infect Immun 2007; 75: 4514-8.

[155] Leslie FC, Thompson DG, McLaughlin JT, Varro A, Dockray GJ, Mandal BK. Plasma cholecystokinin concentrations are elevated in acute upper gastrointestinal infections QJM 2003; 96: 870-1.

[156] Rubin W, Ross LL, Sleisenger MH, Weser E. An electron microscopic study of adult celiac disease. Lab Invest 1966; 15: 1720-47.

[157] Madara JL, Barenberg D, Carlson S. Effects of cytochalasin D on occluding junctions of intestinal absorptive cells: further evidence that the cytoskeleton may influence paracellular permeability and junctional charge selectivity. J Cell Biol 1986; 102: 2125-36.

[158] Hecht G, Pothoulakis C, LaMont JT, Madara JL. *Clostridium difficile* toxin A perturbs cytoskeletal structure and tight junction permeability of cultured human intestinal epithelial monolayers. J Clin Invest 1988; 82: 1516-24.

[159] Tsukita S, Furuse M. Pores in the wall: claudins constitute tight junction strands containing aqueous pores. J Cell Biol 2000; 149: 13-6.

[160] Teoh DA, Kamieniecki D, Pang G, Buret AG. *Giardia lamblia* rearranges F-actin and alpha-actinin in human colonic and duodenal monolayers and reduces transepithelial electrical resistance. J Parasitol 2000; 86: 800-6.

[161] Scott KG, Meddings JB, Kirk DR, Lees-Miller SP, Buret AG. Intestinal infection with *Giardia* spp. reduces epithelial barrier function in a myosin light chain kinase-dependent fashion. Gastroenterology 2002; 123: 1179-90.

[162] Chin AC, Teoh DA, Scott KG, Meddings JB, Macnaughton WK, Buret AG. Strain-dependent induction of enterocyte apoptosis by *Giardia lamblia* disrupts epithelial barrier function in a caspase-3-dependent manner. Infect Immun 2002; 70: 3673-80.

[163] Panaro MA, Cianciulli A, Mitolo V, *et al.* Caspase-dependent apoptosis of the HCT-8 epithelial cell line induced by the parasite *Giardia intestinalis*. FEMS Immunol Med Microbiol 2007; 51: 302-9.

[164] Troeger H, Epple HJ, Schneider T, *et al.* Effect of chronic *Giardia lamblia* infection on epithelial transport and barrier function in human duodenum. Gut 2007; 56: 328-35.

[165] Yu LC, Huang CY, Kuo WT, Sayer H, Turner JR, Buret AG. SGLT-1-mediated glucose uptake protects human intestinal epithelial cells against *Giardia duodenalis*-induced apoptosis. Int J Parasitol 2008; 38: 923-34.

[166] Scott KG, Yu LC, Buret AG. Role of CD8+ and CD4+ T lymphocytes in jejunal mucosal injury during murine giardiasis. Infect Immun 2004; 72: 3536-42.

[167] Singh KD, Bhasin DK, Rana SV, *et al.* Effect of *Giardia lamblia* on duodenal disaccharidase levels in humans. Trop Gastroenterol 2000; 21: 174-6.

[168] Koot BG, Ten Kate FJ, Juffrie M, Rosalina I, Taminiau JJ, Benninga MA. Does *Giardia lamblia* cause villous atrophy in children?: a retrospective cohort study of the histological abnormalities in Giardiasis. J pediatr Gastroenterol Nutr 2009; 49: 304-8.

[169] Kaur H, Ghosh S, Samra H, Vinayak VK, Ganguly NK. Identification and characterization of an excretory-secretory product from *Giardia lamblia*. Parasitology. 2001; 123: 347-56.

[170] Shant J, Bhattacharyya S, Ghosh S, Ganguly NK, Majumdar S. A potentially important excretory-secretory product of *Giardia lamblia*. Exp Parasitol 2002; 102: 178-86.

[171] Katelaris P, Seow F, Ngu M. The effect of *Giardia lamblia* trophozoites on lipolysis *in vitro*. Parasitology 1991; 103: 35-9.

[172] Cevallos AM, James M, Farthing MJG. Small intestinal injury in a neonatal rat model is strain dependent. *Gastroenterology* 1995; 109: 766-73.

[173] Kaur H, Samra H, Ghosh S, Vinayak VK, Ganguly NK. Immune effector responses to an excretory-secretory product of *Giardia lamblia*. FEMS Immunol Med Microbiol 1999; 23: 93-105.

CHAPTER 7

Toll-Like Receptors and their Role in Host Resistance to *Toxoplasma gondii*

Felix Yarovinsky*

Department of Immunology, University of Texas Southwestern Medical Center, 5323 Harry Hines Blvd, Dallas, TX 75390-9093, USA

Abstract: *Toxoplasma gondii* and other apicomplexan parasites are widely distributed obligate intracellular protozoa. A critical host mediator produced in response to *T. gondii* infection is IL-12. This cytokine is synthesized by dendritic cells, macrophages and neutrophils and plays a pivotal role in the production of IFN-gamma, which in turn activates anti-microbial effector cells. In the past several years, many of the receptors and signaling pathways that link pathogen detection to induction of IL-12 have been identified and characterized. Among these receptors the Toll-like Receptor (TLR) family can recognize all classes of pathogens and induce different types of immune responses. In the following review, the evidence for specific TLR function in host resistance to *T. gondii* is summarized.

INTRODUCTION TO TOXOPLASMA GONDII

Toxoplasma gondii is an obligate intracellular protozoan pathogen of the phylum Apicomplexa [1]. Other members of this phylum include the human pathogens *Plasmodium* (the causative agent of malaria) and *Cryptosporidium* as well as the animal pathogens *Eimeria, Theileria,* and *Babesia* [2]. Apicomplexan parasites have a major effect on human health and cause more than two million deaths every year. All apicomplexans are intracellular parasites with polarized cell structures, and complex cytoskeletal and organellar arrangements at their apical end are essential for host cell invasion [3,4]. *T. gondii* is a remarkably successful member of this phylogenetic group. While many apicomplexans infect a narrow range of hosts, *T. gondii* can infect a broad range of mammals and birds. It is also unusual in the diversity of ways that it can be transmitted, which likely play a major role in its wide geographic distribution [1]. It is estimated that over one billion people are infected with this parasite, with essentially the entire human population at risk of infection.

Infection with *T. gondii* can be separated into two distinct stages: acute and chronic infections [1]. The acute stage is characterized by the rapidly growing form of the parasite called a tachyzoite ('tachos' means speed, and 'zoite' means animal being; both words originate from Greek). Tachyzoites can infect almost any nucleated cell, and once the host cell becomes infected, tachyzoites rapidly proliferate within an intracellular compartment called a 'parasitophorous vacuole.' Once the infected cell is ruptured, tachyzoites continue spreading and replicating throughout host tissues. In infected individuals, tachyzoites differentiate into bradyzoites ('bradys' meaning slow, from Greek), which form tissue cysts predominantly in the central nervous system. The development of tissue cysts defines the chronic stage of infection [1]. Encephalitis is one of the most common diseases caused by the parasite. This disease results from reactivation of the parasite in patients whose immune system was not fully functional (e.g., immunocompromised patients), typically due to the progression of acquired immunodeficiency syndrome or immunosuppressive therapy accompanying organ transplantation. *T. gondii* can also infect fetuses. Congenital toxoplasmosis frequently results in fetal hydrocephalus, seizures, mental retardation, blindness, and even death.

The population structure of *Toxoplasma* is dominated by three lineages, designated strain types I, II, and III [5,6]. While strains of type I are uniformly lethal in mice prior to establishment of cyst-associated persistence in the central nervous system (the LD100 is a single parasite), type II and III strains are less virulent (LD100>1000) and can establish chronic infections.

The immune response to *T. gondii* requires rapid sensing of the invading pathogen, production of proinflammatory

---

*Corresponding Author: Felix Yarovinsky, Department of Immunology, University of Texas Southwestern Medical Center, 5323 Harry Hines Blvd, Dallas, TX 75390-9093, USA. Email: Felix.Yarovinsky@UTSouthwestern.edu

Emilio Jirillo (Ed)
All rights reserved - © 2010 Bentham Science Publishers Ltd.

cytokines, and lymphocyte activation. The idea that parasitic molecules can activate innate effector functions was well appreciated in the context of macrophages, neutrophils, and dendritic cells (DCs) during infection [7]. It has been established that the interaction of macrophages with *T. gondii* or a *T. gondii* extract called STAg (soluble tachyzoite antigen, also called soluble toxoplasma antigen) results in activation of the mitogen-activated protein kinase (MAPK) signaling cascade and induction of proinflammatory cytokine production [8]. The major focus of these studies was identification of the cellular and molecular mechanisms leading to induction of the cytokine IL-12. This is because IL-12 plays a major role in orchestrating immunity to the parasite [9-11]. It has become understood that identification of the parasite molecules involved in IL-12 induction would reveal key elements of the innate immune system involved in detection of this parasite [7].

A separate line of studies demonstrated that another cytokine, IFN-γ, is essential for host resistance to the parasite [12-16]. Inactivation of IFN-γ by the administration of neutralizing antibodies [12, 14] or by deletion of the *ifnγ* gene [9] results in enhanced susceptibility to *T. gondii*. In addition, in vivo treatment with recombinant IFN-γ has a protective effect against *T. gondii* [17]. It was further established that IFN-γ production, primarily by T cells and NK cells, plays a major role in host resistance to the parasite [12-16]. Deficiency in IFN-γ during the acute or chronic phase of infection results in high susceptibility to the parasite. These observations explain the cellular mechanism responsible for *T. gondii* reactivation in individuals infected with human immunodeficiency virus. Because of the importance of IFN-γ in the development of host protection against the parasite, signaling cascades involved in the regulation of IFN-γ expression have been extensively characterized. It was established that IFN-γ production depends on IL-12 [10, 15, 16, 18-20]. At the same time, experiments involving macrophages showed that IFN-γ is required for the induction of IL-12 [21, 22]. Furthermore, it was observed that lack of a transcriptional factor called interferon consensus sequence binding protein, ICSBP (known in standard nomenclature as interferon regulatory factor 8, IRF-8), results in complete loss of IL-12 production and high susceptibility to *T. gondii* infection [23]. The question of whether IL-12 induces IFN-γ or IFN-γ primes innate immune cells for IL-12 induction was further clouded by mapping the IRF-8 binding site in the promoter region of IL-12p40 and IL-12p35, two subunits of biologically active IL-12 (IL-12p70) [24,25]. Because IFN-γ triggers IRF-8 production, and IRF-8 regulates transcription of IL-12p40 and IL-12p35, the chain of initial events involved in sensing *T. gondii* was not initially clear. The central paradox of the reciprocal regulation of IL-12 and IFN-γ was solved by the identification of a cell type involved in the initial sensing of the parasite and induction of IL-12 independently of IFN-γ, T cells, and costimulatory molecules [26]. Time kinetic analysis of the cells responsible for the immediate production of IL-12 in response to *T. gondii* or STAg established that splenic DCs but not macrophages play a major role in production of this cytokine [26]. Furthermore, a study by Caetano Reis e Sousa, Alan Sher, Chris Hunter, and other colleagues established that a particular population of DCs expressing the surface marker CD8 is responsible for the immediate response to *T. gondii* and the bulk of IL-12 production [27-29]. Results from Eric Denkers' laboratory identified that, in addition to DCs, neutrophils can rapidly produce IL-12 in the absence of IFN-γ [7]. In striking contrast, the ability of macrophages to produce IL-12 in response to *T. gondii* required prior exposure to IFN-γ (i.e., priming). Thus, it was concluded that to understand the initial steps involved in sensing *T. gondii*, it would be essential to identify the molecular mechanisms triggering IL-12 production by DCs and neutrophils.

A Brief Introduction to Toll-Like Receptors (TLRS)

Innate immune receptors are involved in the sensing of all types of pathogens and consist of several distinct types of receptors, including TLRs, NOD-like receptors, and RIG-I-like molecules [30]. By far, the best characterized innate immune receptors are the TLRs. Members of this receptor family recognize viral and microbial pathogens via sensing of so-called 'pathogen-associated molecular patterns' or PAMPs [31-34]. Examples of these PAMPs are lipopolysaccharide (LPS) from Gram-negative bacteria, bacterial flagellin, and viral single- and double-stranded RNA (Fig. **1**).

Activation of TLRs by these microbial products results in rapid initiation of innate immune responses and production of proinflammatory cytokines, including IL-12, followed by maturation of DCs and regulation of adaptive immune responses [35,36]. TLRs were named after the Toll protein of *Drosophila melanogaster*, which confers protection against fungi [37,38]. Since the discovery of the first human ortholog, TLR4, 10 human and 12 mouse TLRs have been identified, and for the majority of them, their ligands have been identified [30,39].

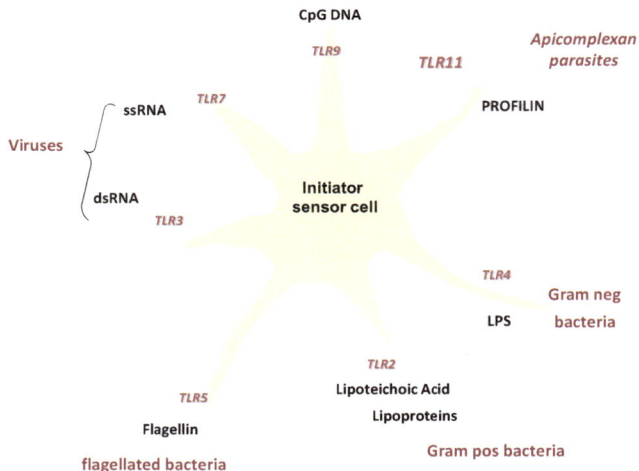

Figure 1: TLR and their ligands

All TLRs have similar structures. They contain extracellular leucine-rich repeats responsible for pathogen recognition and transmembrane (TM) and cytoplasmic Toll/interleukin-1 receptor (TIR) domains essential for intracellular signaling [40,41]. The extracellular leucine-rich repeat (LRR) domain consists of 19-27 repeats of the 24-amino acid conserved consensus sequence xLxxLxLxxNxΦxxΦxxxFxxLx, in which x is any amino acid. L and F can be substituted by other hydrophobic amino acids. Φ indicates any hydrophobic amino acid. The LRR is capped on both sides by characteristic N- and C-terminal structures that are likely involved in stabilizing the extracellular portion of the protein [40]. A single transmembrane domain not only connects the LRR to the signaling TIR motif but also plays an important role in TLR localization [42]. The intracellular TIR domain consists of approximately 150 amino acids and is highly conserved in its sequence across all known TLRs [43]. The TIR domain is essential for the recruitment of adaptor proteins that facilitate signaling after TLR activation [41]. The TIR domains can form homo- or heterodimers with other TLR TIR domains, leading to the recruitment of adaptor proteins. The key adaptor protein in this process is called MyD88 [44], but in addition, four other TLR adaptor proteins have been identified: TRIF, TIRAP/Mal, TRAM, and SRAM [41]. All of these adaptor proteins contain TIR domains and can be recruited by TLRs to transduce signals upon TLR ligand engagement [41].

The MyD88 adaptor protein plays a special role because all TLRs except TLR3 depend on this molecule [45-47] (Fig. 2). The recruitment of MyD88 leads to activation of IRAK kinases and recruitment of TRAF6. The activated complex associates with TAK1 and the TAK1-interacting proteins TAB1 and TAB2, which results in the activation of TAK1. Activated TAK1 phosphorylates the IKK complex and allows the activation of the transcriptional factor NF-kB (Fig. 2). The importance of MyD88, IRAK4, and TRAF6 has been confirmed by genetic inactivation of these molecules [45].

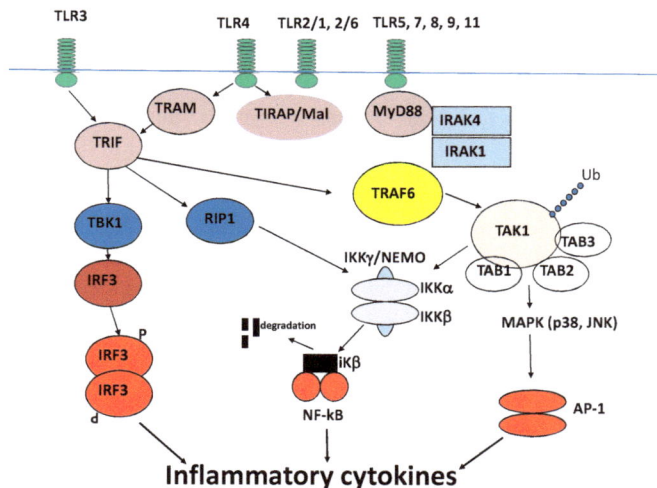

Figure 2: TLR signaling

Recent crystallization studies of LRR and TIR domains confirmed both theoretical and mutagenesis-based data proposing structure-signaling interactions among TLRs, their ligands, and signal transduction elements involved in the TLR signaling cascade [48-51].

MYD88 and *Toxoplasma Gondii*: On the Track to TLR Recognition

The discovery that TLR4 can initiate the NF-kB inflammatory program in the presence of LPS [31, 32, 45] led to the hypothesis that a dedicated TLR is also involved in sensing *T. gondii*. This idea was indirectly confirmed by an observation from Vogel and Sher's group, who demonstrated that signaling cascades initiated in response to LPS and the *T. gondii* extract STAg share many common elements, especially the ability to induce MAPK activation [52, 53]. However, it was noticed that while LPS recognition depends on TLR4, this innate immune receptor was not required for the induction of IL-12 in response to STAg [53].

The first direct evidence of TLR involvement in *T. gondii* recognition came from studies performed by Scanga and colleagues [54]. They infected MyD88-/- mice with the ME49 parasite strain (type II) and monitored survival of the animals. MyD88-/- mice failed to control acute *T. gondii* infection, and the mortality kinetics closely resembled the phenotype of IL-12p40-/- mice infected with the parasite [54]. A dramatic increase in parasite load seen in MyD88-/- animals was also independently reported by Yano and colleagues [55]. Most importantly, Scanga *et al.* examined whether MyD88 controlled the IL-12 response of DCs and neutrophils to *T. gondii*. They found that the IL-12 response was greatly impaired in neutrophils stimulated with either live tachyzoites or STAg extract [54]. Later studies with live parasites revealed a more complex picture. Surprisingly, when live RH tachyzoites (type I strain) were used to stimulate macrophages, IL-12 release did not require MyD88. At the same time, IL-12 production in response to ME49 tachyzoites (type II strain) was largely dependent on the MyD88 adaptor [56]. An even more complex scenario was observed with DCs. It was postulated that DC IL-12 production is controlled by two independent signaling pathways relying on the chemokine receptor CCR5 and MyD88 [57]. This hypothesis was formulated based on the observation that the DC IL-12 response to the parasite extract STAg was only partially dependent on the MyD88 pathway [58]. Moreover, it was shown that a *T. gondii*-derived 18-kDa cyclophilin called C-18 was capable of initiating CCR5-dependent (but MyD88-independent) IL-12 production from splenic DCs [58]. The mechanism of CCR5-dependent regulation of IL-12 is still not completely understood. While it is not surprising that different host signaling pathways contribute to innate recognition of *T. gondii*, MyD88 activation is clearly a critical step in the initiation of the IL-12-dependent response to *T. gondii* [54, 59].

TLR11 Plays a Central Role in Recognition of *T. gondii*

Despite the importance of MyD88 in the regulation of IL-12, it was not clear which innate immune receptor(s) may be involved in triggering MyD88 activation in response to *T. gondii*. An initial screen with two obvious candidates, TLR2 and TLR4, was unsuccessful. Dendritic cells isolated from mice deficient in either of these receptors showed unimpaired IL-12 response to the parasite, arguing against a major role for these receptors in the regulation of the MyD88-dependent IL-12 response to the parasite [54]. An additional screen carried out with a panel of animals deficient in TLR3, TLR5, TLR7, and TLR9 failed to identify a single receptor involved in *T. gondii* recognition (our unpublished observations). Moreover, the nature of the *T. gondii* molecule(s) responsible for the induction of IL-12 secretion by DCs is not clear. Since the ability of *T. gondii* to trigger DC IL-12 production can be completely eliminated by proteinase K treatment [60], it was logical to assume that the IL-12-inducing factor is likely to be a protein. By means of a combination of traditional biochemical techniques, a low molecular weight molecule that potently stimulated IL-12 production by DCs in a MyD88-dependent manner was isolated from STAg [61]. Mass spectrometry analysis identified this protein as a *T. gondii* profilin [61]. Most importantly, in a dose-response analysis, cloned recombinant *T. gondii* profilin was more active than unfractionated STAg over a range of several orders of magnitude. Taken together, these experiments suggest that *T. gondii* profilin is a major IL-12-inducing molecule present in the parasite [61]. The receptor for this molecule was identified using two different approaches. By the use of transfected cell lines, it was observed that profilin interacted with TLR11 but not with other tested TLRs. Moreover, when splenic DCs from TLR11-/- mice were stimulated with profilin, STAg, or live parasites they failed to produce IL-12, TNF, or IL-6 [61]. Taken together, these results identify TLR11 as an innate immune receptor for *T. gondii* profilin, one that is required for DC IL-12 production *in vitro* and *in vivo*.

TLRs recognize conserved molecules that perform essential functions in microorganisms. TLR ligands thus function as 'molecular signatures' for a class of pathogens [62,63]. Identification of *T. gondii* profilin as a TLR11 ligand raised several important questions. First, does TLR11 function as a general pattern-recognition receptor for apicomplexan parasites? Second, what is the biological function of profilin in the life cycle of *T. gondii*? Profilins are small, actin-binding proteins that regulate actin polymerization in other eukaryotic cells [64]. There are several essential actin-dependent steps that *T. gondii* tachyzoites must complete to survive: gliding and spreading on the surface of the host cell layer, host cell invasion, intracellular growth, and egress [65]. Until recently, the function of profilin in *T. gondii* was not clear [66].

In our follow-up studies, we established that *T. gondii* is not unique in triggering TLR11, but rather is one member of a family of apicomplexan parasites that express profilins capable of activating this TLR and inducing IL-12 production. We observed that profilins isolated from *Cryptosporidium parvum*, *Eimeria tenella*, and *Theileria parva* induce TLR11 activation in a manner similar to the *T. gondii* protein. An independent study with *Eimeria* profilin confirmed that this protein can activate DCs and initiate potent IL-12 production [67]. These results establish TLR11 as a pattern-recognition receptor for apicomplexan protozoa through its recognition of a conserved family of profilin molecules present in these intracellular pathogens (Fig. 1).

By conditional disruption of the profilin gene, Dominique Soldati and colleagues formally established a biological function for profilin in *T. gondii* [66]. It was shown that while *T. gondii* profilin is not required for parasite growth and replication, it is necessary for gliding, invasion, and egress of the parasite. Moreover, *T. gondii* profilin is essential for the parasite's virulence *in vivo* [66]. It is intriguing that, in addition to TLR11, the other major TLR that interacts with proteins, TLR5, recognizes highly conserved structural motifs in flagellin, a protein required for bacterial movement [68, 69]. Taken together, the results suggest that microbial motility-related functions are important targets for TLR recognition.

Another crucial issue concerns the in vivo function of TLR11 during infection with *T. gondii*. Much of what we currently know about the interaction of DCs with the parasite is limited to studies with the injected parasite extract STAg, which contains a complex mixture of *T. gondii* antigens but lacks the ability to mimic all steps of infection. Interestingly, when wild-type mice were immunized with STAg, profilin was found to be a dominant antigen in the CD4+ T-cell response to *T. gondii* [70]. Moreover, this response was completely abolished in mice deficient in TLR11 or MyD88. It was further established that CD4+ T-cell priming in response to *T. gondii* was initiated by the CD8+ DC subset [70]. These results are intriguing, since this DC subset is known to be the major initial source of IL-12 in response to *T. gondii* [26, 61, 71]. On the molecular level, it was shown that responsiveness to this parasite protein was regulated at the level of antigen presentation by DC and required both TLR11 signaling and major histocompatibility complex (MHC) class II recognition acting in the same cell [70]. While these findings support a major influence of TLR11 activation on antigen presentation by DCs in vivo, once infected with *T. gondii*, DCs may behave differently, and further studies are required to understand more completely the fate of DCs and T cells in TLR11-/- mice infected with the parasite. Indeed, it was shown that while *T. gondii*-infected TLR11-deficient mice displayed dramatically reduced serum IL-12 levels and developed more brain cysts in the chronic phase of infection, TLR11-/- (in contrast to MyD88-/- animals) survived the acute phase of the infection better [61]. These observations indicate that while TLR11 plays a major role in IL-12-dependent control of *T. gondii* infection, other MyD88-dependent TLR/IL-1 family members also contribute to the generation of host resistance to this protozoan pathogen.

In addition, TLR11 is not expressed in humans because its gene is encoded in the human genome as a pseudogene [39]. These results strongly suggest that in addition to TLR11, other TLRs are involved in the regulation of IL-12-dependent host protection against the parasite.

The Role of TLR2 in the Host Response to *Toxoplasma gondii*

TLR2 can be activated by a wide variety of microbial components. These include lipoproteins from various pathogens, peptidoglycan and lipoteichoic acid from Gram-positive bacteria, and zymosan from fungi [33]. The realization that TLR2 plays a fundamental role in the initiation of immune responses to various groups of pathogens led to the hypothesis that a similar recognition system may function during the sensing of parasites. The role for this TLR was initially established for the protozoan parasites *Leishmania* [72, 73] and *Trypanosoma cruzi* [74, 75]. In the case of *T. gondii*, several independent groups have investigated the role of TLR2 in parasite recognition and demonstrated that while TLR2-deficient mice display normal IL-12 production and host resistance to *T. gondii* infection at conventional doses, TLR2 signaling plays a non-redundant role when animals are challenged with higher infectious doses [54, 76]. It was shown that all TLR2-deficient mice died within 10 days after infection with 300 cysts, whereas a lower dose of the parasite resulted in 100% survival of TLR2-/- animals [76]. While the non-essential role of TLR2 in the regulation of IL-12 is likely explained by a dominant role for TLR11 in the induction of the DC IL-12 response and the central role for these cells in controlling the initial cytokine response to the parasite [61], the susceptibility of TLR2-/- mice to *T. gondii* revealed the complex nature of TLR signaling in different innate immune cells. While TLR2-deficient DCs and neutrophils are indistinguishable from wild-type cells in terms of IL-12 production [54], macrophage activation strictly depends on TLR2 activation by the parasite [77]. Yano and colleagues observed that TLR2 regulates *T. gondii*-induced nitric oxide (NO) production [76]. A central role for NO as the primary toxoplasmacidal mediator of activated macrophages has been established from studies employing NO synthase inhibitors and iNOS-/- animals [78-81]. Nevertheless, iNOS-/- mice are able to control acute infection [81], and additional effector mechanisms are likely controlled by TLR2. For example, this receptor was recently shown to regulate the *T. gondii*-induced production of the neutrophil attracting chemokine CCL2 [77]. This observation is relevant because of the known involvement of neutrophils in host resistance to the parasite [82-84]. On a broader level, it is intriguing that despite similarities in MyD88-dependent TLR signaling pathways, the major outcomes of TLR ligation are distinct. While TLR11 primarily controls an IL-12-dependent arm of host defenses, TLR2 is involved in regulation of CCL2 and TNF production in response to the parasite [61,77]. These data are consistent with the pioneering observation by Vogel and Sher that *T. gondii* contains distinct factors responsible for the induction of TNF and IL-12 [53, 60]. The definitive ligands for TLR2 appear to be core glycans and diacylglycerols isolated from purified *T. gondii* GPI [85]. These data are in agreement with findings from the related apicomplexan parasite *Plasmodium falciparum,* since malaria GPI recognition is mediated mainly through TLR2 [86, 87].

Other TLRs: Understanding the Complex Role of Toll-Like Receptor Signaling in Host Resistance to *T. gondii* Infection

In a non-biased study utilizing in vivo bioluminescence imaging, Barragan and colleagues investigated the dynamics of *T. gondii* infection in a panel of mice deficient in TLR signaling in comparison with MyD88-/- mice. Their data confirmed that MyD88 is essential for the control of parasite growth. However, they observed that mice deficient in TLR1, TLR2, or TLR6 are indistinguishable from wild-type animals in the ability to control the parasite *in vivo* [88]. These results stimulated additional searches for innate immune receptors involved in the cooperative regulation of the innate immune response against *T. gondii.*

Two additional TLRs have been implicated in host resistance to the parasite. First, purified *T. gondii* GPI triggers TLR4 signaling pathways [85]. Moreover, mice deficient in both TLR2 and TLR4, but not in TLR2 alone, showed complete abrogation of TNF production in response to GPI. These results suggest that TLR4 may cooperate with TLR2 during *T. gondii* infection [85]. Using a different approach, it has been shown that *T. gondii*-derived heat shock protein 70 stimulates maturation of murine bone marrow-derived DCs via TLR4 [89]. Since mice deficient in TLR4 showed only minimal enhancement in susceptibility to the parasite infection, this receptor is unlikely to play a significant role in *T. gondii* recognition [54, 76]. Nevertheless, an important but indirect effect of this TLR on small intestinal inflammation following peroral *T. gondii* infection was revealed [90]. It was noticed that oral infection with the parasite is accompanied by a substantial overgrowth of commensals in the ileum, leading to severe immunopathology. Lack of TLR4 prevented *T. gondii*-induced ileitis [90]. Similar results were reported in TLR9-/- animals [91]. It was shown that TLR9-deficient mice are relatively resistant to ileitis following oral infection with the parasite. Importantly, a reduced Th1 response to the parasite in the small intestine was observed [91]. These results may suggest that TLR9 is directly involved in the recognition of *T. gondii.* Indeed, several apicomplexan parasites can activate this innate immune receptor. The defined apicomplexan parasite ligands for TLR9 include genomic DNA from *Babesia* and hemozoin from *P. falciparum* [92, 93]. In contrast to these pathogens, our results utilizing either TLR9 transfectants or TLR9-deficient cells revealed that *T. gondii* genomic DNA does not trigger TLR9 activation (unpublished observations).

One explanation for the definitive role of TLR4 and TLR9 in the regulation of the Th1 response to the parasite was revealed during experiments using an oral (natural) route of infection with *T. gondii.* As mentioned above, oral infection with *T. gondii* leads to severe intestinal epithelial damage, associated with translocation of gut commensal bacteria. Because TLR4 and TLR9 (as well as TLR2) are most commonly involved in sensing bacteria, we investigated whether these 'bacterial' TLRs are activated by gut commensals rather than by the parasite itself [94]. We observed that when infected orally, mice lacking TLR2, TLR4, or TLR9 demonstrated profound deficiencies in their abilities to mount IFN-γ responses to the parasite. Remarkably, when these animals were infected intraperitoneally (a 'sterile' route of infection that bypasses involvement of gut commensal bacteria in the regulation of the Th1 response to the parasite), no detectable effects of these TLRs on the regulation of Th1 responses to the protozoan were seen [94]. Furthermore, it was found that depletion of gut commensal bacteria by antibiotic treatment during *T. gondii* infection had a major impact on the induction of the Th1 response to the parasite. When TLR11-/- animals were treated with broad-spectrum antibiotics, mice depleted of commensals were not able to mount IL-12 responses against the parasite. In addition, the IL-12 response was reduced but not abolished in antibiotic-treated wild-type animals, suggesting a model where intestinal cell damage triggered by parasitic infection allows commensal bacteria to initiate TLR2-, TLR4-, and TLR9-dependent host responses to the parasite, cooperating with TLR11-dependent activation signals in DCs initiated by *T. gondii* itself [94]. Importantly because all of these TLRs (TLR2, TLR4, TLR9, and TLR11) signal via MyD88, inactivation of this adaptor protein had a major impact on the IL-12 response to *T. gondii* irrespective of the route of infection with the parasite.

FUTURE PERSPECTIVES

There is common agreement that TLRs play a major role in the recognition of *T. gondii* and initiation of the parasite-specific immune response. However, it is not clear how TLR activation in dendritic cells, macrophages, and other innate immune cell types regulates inflammatory reactions during microbial infections. Furthermore, while it was initially assumed that TLR functions are restricted to innate immune cells, recent studies with *T. gondii* and other pathogens have revealed that MyD88 activation in T cells plays an important role in mounting a protective Th1 response against pathogens [95-98]. Studies addressing the cell-specific mechanisms of TLR functions will establish the molecular mechanisms involved in the initial sensing of the parasite and the complex cell-cell communications events essential for mounting a protective host response to the parasite.

In addition, while TLR signaling plays a central role in regulation of the protective response against *T. gondii*, other pattern-recognition receptors are likely involved in host resistance to the parasite. Identification of these receptors and their mechanisms of cooperation with TLRs is an important direction for future research. This is especially important for understanding the host resistance to *T. gondii* in humans because while TLR11 is a major regulator of the IL-12 response in mice, this receptor in not functional in humans. Furthermore, while extremely rare, nine children with MyD88 deficiencies were recently identified [99]. These patients suffer from infections with pyogenic bacteria, but not parasites, and at least one child mounted a resistance to *T. gondii* [99]. The existence of TLR- and MyD88-independent host resistance to the parasite has also been recently reported in a murine model of toxoplasmosis [100, 101]. Studies addressing these issues would certainly increase our knowledge in the area of innate immunity. Furthermore, it is important to remember that *T. gondii* is a master regulator of immunity. The parasite has profound effects on the activation of NF-κB and MAPK signaling cascades, which are essential for signal transduction by TLRs and other innate immune receptors. Thus, while interaction of *T. gondii* with innate immune cells leads to potent, largely TLR-dependent induction of IL-12, it is likely that manipulation of the signaling cascade by the parasite may mask the recognition systems involved in the recognition of *T. gondii*. This may be especially relevant for intracellular recognition systems such as Nod-like proteins, which have been implicated in the recognition of different groups of pathogens and tissue damage signals. For example, it is well documented that the NF-κB activation cascade is impaired in *T. gondii*-infected macrophages [102-106]. Macrophages infected with the parasite have impaired ability to secrete IL-12 and TNF after activation with a model TLR4 agonist, LPS [102, 106]. A similar observation has been made with DCs, where infection with the parasite led to impaired antigen presentation capacity as a result of the inability to upregulate MHC class II molecules [107]. Furthermore, it was reported that *T. gondii* interferes with IFN-γ signaling pathways [108]. Thus, it is logical to assume that identification of IFN-γ induced recognition systems will be compromised in *T. gondii*-infected cells. At the same time, progress in understanding the key events leading to *T. gondii* recognition depends on identification of parasite molecules that are recognized by the innate immune system. It is also equally important to reveal the *T. gondii*-specific proteins that are involved in altering host cell responses through NF-kB and other transcriptional factors. These studies will, without any doubt, be fruitful in understanding the molecular mechanisms involved in TLR-dependent and independent host resistance to the parasite.

ACKNOWLEDGEMENTS

This work was supported by grants from the National Institutes of Health (NIH) R21 AI079371 and 1R01AI085263.

REFERENCES

[1]   Black MW, Boothroyd JC. Lytic cycle of *Toxoplasma gondii*. Microbiol Mol Biol Rev 2000; 64: 607-23.

[2]   Kim K, Weiss LM . *Toxoplasma gondii*: the model apicomplexan. Int J Parasitol 2004; 34: 423-32.

[3]   Carruthers V, Boothroyd JC. Pulling together: an integrated model of Toxoplasma cell invasion. Curr Opin Microbiol 2007; 10: 83-89.

[4]   Keeley A, Soldati D . The glideosome: a molecular machine powering motility and host-cell invasion by *Apicomplexa*. Trends Cell Biol 2004; 14: 528-32.

[5]   Howe DK, Sibley LD. *Toxoplasma gondii* comprises three clonal lineages: Correlation of parasite genotype with human disease. J Infect Dis 1995; 172: 1561-66.

[6]   Grigg ME, Bonnefoy S, Hehl AB, *et al.* Success and virulence in *Toxoplasma* as the result of sexual recombination between two distinct ancestries. *Science* 2001; 294: 161-65.

[7]   Denkers EY, Butcher BA, Del Rio L, Kim L . Manipulation of mitogen-activated protein kinase/nuclear factor-kappaB-signaling cascades during intracellular *Toxoplasma gondii* infection. Immunol Rev 2004; 201: 191-205.

[8]   Li ZY, Manthey CL, Perera PY, *et al. Toxoplasma gondii* soluble antigen induces a subset of lipopolysaccharide-inducible genes and tyrosine phosphoproteins in peritoneal macrophages. *Infect Immun* 1994 ; 62: 3434-40.

[9]   Scharton Kersten TM, Wynn TA, Denkers EY, *et al.* In the absence of endogenous IFN-gamma, mice develop unimpaired IL-12 responses to *Toxoplasma gondii* while failing to control acute infection. *J Immunol* 1996; 157: 4045-54.

[10]   Gazzinelli RT, Hieny S, Wynn TA, *et al.* Interleukin 12 is required for the T-lymphocyte-independent induction of interferon gamma by an intracellular parasite and induces resistance in T-cell-deficient hosts. Proc. Natl. Acad Sci U S A 1993; 90: 6115-19.

[11]   Lieberman LA, Cardillo F, Owyang AM, *et al.* IL-23 provides a limited mechanism of resistance to acute toxoplasmosis in the absence of IL-12. J. Immunol 2004; 173: 1887-93.

[12]   Suzuki Y, Orellana MA, Schreiber RD, Remington JS. Interferon-gamma: the major mediator of resistance against *Toxoplasma gondii.* Science 1988; 240: 516-518.

[13]   Sher A, Oswald IP, HienyS, Gazzinelli RT. *Toxoplasma gondii* induces a T-independent IFN-gamma response in natural killer cells that requires both adherent accessory cells and tumor necrosis factor-alpha. J Immunol 1993; 150: 3982-89.

[14]   Johnson LL, VanderVegt FP, Havell EA. Gamma interferon-dependent temporary resistance to acute *Toxoplasma gondii* infection independent of CD4+ or CD8+ lymphocytes. Infect Immun 1993; 61: 5174-80.

[15]   Hunter CA, Subauste CS, Van Cleave VH, Remington JS. Production of gamma interferon by natural killer cells from *Toxoplasma gondii*-infected SCID mice: Regulation by interleukin-10, interleukin-12, and tumor necrosis factor alpha. Infect Immun 1994; 62: 2818-24.

[16]   Johnson LL, Sayles PC. Strong cytolytic activity of natural killer cells is neither necessary nor sufficient for preimmune resistance to *Toxoplasma gondii* infection. Nat Immun 1995; 4: 209-15.

[17]   Suzuki Y, Joh K, Kobayashi A. Tumor necrosis factor-independent protective effect of recombinant IFN-gamma against acute toxoplasmosis in T cell-deficient mice. J Immunol 1991; 147: 2728-33.

[18]   Scharton-Kersten T, Denkers EY, Gazzinelli R, Sher A. Role of IL-12 in induction of cell-mediated immunity to *Toxoplasma gondii.* Res Immunol 1995; 146: 539-45.

[19]   Scharton Kersten T, Caspar P, Sher A, Denkers EY. *Toxoplasma gondii*: evidence for interleukin-12-dependent and-independent pathways of interferon-gamma production induced by an attenuated parasite strain. Exp Parasitol 1996; 84: 102-14.

[20]   Hunter CA, Chizzonite R, Remington JS. IL-1 beta is required for IL-12 to induce production of IFN-gamma by NK cells. A role for IL-1 beta in the T cell-independent mechanism of resistance against intracellular pathogens. J Immunol 1995; 155: 4347-54.

[21]   Gazzinelli RT, Wysocka M, Hayashi S, *et al.* Parasite-induced IL-12 stimulates early IFN-gamma synthesis and resistance during acute infection with *Toxoplasma gondii.* J Immunol 1994; 153: 2533-43.

[22]   Khan IA, Matsuura T, Kasper LH. Interleukin-12 enhances murine survival against acute toxoplasmosis. Infect Immunol 1994; 62: 1639-42.

[23]   Scharton Kersten T, Contursi C, Masumi A, *et al.* Interferon consensus sequence binding protein-deficient mice display impaired resistance to intracellular infection due to a primary defect in interleukin 12 p40 induction. J Exp Med 1997; 186: 1523-34.

[24]   Wang IM, Contursi C, Masumi A, *et al.* An IFN-gamma-inducible transcription factor, IFN consensus sequence binding protein (ICSBP), stimulates IL-12 p40 expression in macrophages. J Immunol 2000; 165: 271-79.

[25]   Liu J, Guan X, Tamura T, *et al.* Synergistic activation of interleukin-12 p35 gene transcription by interferon regulatory factor-1 and interferon consensus sequence-binding protein. J Biol Chem 2004; 279: 55609-617.

[26]   Reis Sousa, Hieny S, Scharton Kersten T, *et al. In vivo* microbial stimulation induces rapid CD40 ligand-independent production of interleukin 12 by dendritic cells and their redistribution to T cell areas. J Exp Med 1997; 186: 1819-1829.

[27]   Scott P, Hunter C A. Dendritic cells and immunity to leishmaniasis and toxoplasmosis. Curr Opin Immunol 2002; 14: 466-70.

[28]   Yap GS, Sher A. Cell-mediated immunity to *Toxoplasma gondii*: initiation, regulation and effector function. Immunobiology 1999; 201: 240-47.

[29]   Sher A, Hieny S, Charest H, *et al.* The role of dendritic cells in the initiation of host resistance to *Toxoplasma gondii.* Adv Exp Med Biol 1998; 452: 103-10.

[30]   Ishii KJ, Koyama S, Nakagawa A, *et al.* Host innate immune receptors and beyond: making sense of microbial infections. Cell Host Microbe 2008; 3: 352-63

[31]   Medzhitov R, Preston Hurlburt P, Janeway J. A human homologue of the *Drosophila* toll protein signals activation of adaptive immunity Nature 1997; 388: 394-97.

[32.] Poltorak A, He X, Smirnova I, *et al.* Defective LPS signaling in C3H/HeJ and C57BL/10ScCr mice: Mutations in Tlr4 gene. Science 1998; 282: 2085-88.

[33] Takeda K, Kaisho T, Akira S. Toll-like receptors. Ann Rev Immunol 2003; 21: 335-76.

[34] Akira S , Takeda K, Kaisho T. Toll-like receptors: Critical proteins linking innate and acquired immunity. Nat Immunol 2001; 2: 675-80.

[35] Kopp E, Medzhitov R. Recognition of microbial infection by Toll-like receptors. Curr Opin Immunol 2003; 15: 396-401.

[36] Iwasaki A, Medzhitov R. Toll-like receptor control of the adaptive immune responses. Nat Immunol 2004; 5: 987-95.

[37] Lemaitre B, Nicolas E, Michaut L, *et al.* The dorsoventral regulatory gene cassette spatzle/Toll/cactus controls the potent antifungal response in *Drosophila* adults. Cell 1996; 86: 973-983.

[38] Lemaitre B. The road to Toll. Nat Rev Immunol 2004; 4: 521-527.

[39] Roach JC, Glusman G, Rowen L, *et al.* The evolution of vertebrate Toll-like receptors. Proc Natl Acad Sci U S A 2005; 102: 9577-82.

[40] Bell JK, Mullen GE, Leifer CA, *et al.* Leucine-rich repeats and pathogen recognition in Toll-like receptors. Trends Immunol 2003; 24: 528-33.

[41] O'Neill LA, Bowie AG. The family of five: TIR-domain-containing adaptors in Toll-like receptor signalling. Nat Rev Immunol 2007; 7: 353-64.

[42] Barton GM, Kagan JCA. Cell biological view of Toll-like receptor function: regulation through compartmentalization. Nat Rev Immunol 2009; 9: 535-42.

[43] Xu Y, Tao X, Shen B, *et al.* Structural basis for signal transduction by the Toll/interleukin-1 receptor domains. Nature 2000; 408: 111-15.

[44] Kawai T, Adachi O, Ogawa T, *et al.* Unresponsiveness of MyD88-deficient mice to endotoxin. Immunity 1999; 11: 115-22.

[45] Kawai T, Akira S. TLR signaling. Semin Immunol 2007; 19: 24-32.

[46] Yamamoto M, Sato S, Mori K, *et al.* Cutting edge: a novel Toll/IL-1 receptor domain-containing adapter that preferentially activates the IFN-beta promoter in the Toll-like receptor signaling. J Immunol 2002; 169: 6668-72.

[47] Yamamoto M, Sato S, Hemmi H, *et al.* Role of adaptor TRIF in the MyD88-independent toll-like receptor signaling pathway. Science 2003; 301: 640-43.

[48] Park BS, Song DH, Kim HM, *et al.* The structural basis of lipopolysaccharide recognition by the TLR4-MD-2 complex. Nature 2009; 458: 1191-95.

[49] Jin MS, Kim SE, Heo JY, *et al* . Crystal structure of the TLR1-TLR2 heterodimer induced by binding of a tri-acylated lipopeptide. Cell 2007; 130: 1071-82.

[50] Liu L, Botos I, Wang Y, Structural basis of toll-like receptor 3 signaling with double-stranded RNA. Science 2008; 320: 379-81.

[51] Choe J, Kelker MS, Wilson IA. Crystal structure of human toll-like receptor 3 (TLR3) ectodomain. Science 2005; 309: 581-85.

[52] Grunvald E, Chiaramonte M, Hieny S, *et al.* Biochemical characterization and protein kinase C dependency of monokine-inducing activities of *Toxoplasma gondii.* Infect Immun 1996; 64: 2010-18.

[53] Li ZY, Manthey CL, Perera PY, *et al. Toxoplasma gondii* soluble antigen induces a subset of lipopolysaccharide- inducible genes and tyrosine phosphoproteins in peritoneal macrophages. Infect Immun 1994; 62: 3434-40

[54] Scanga CA, Aliberti J, Jankovic D, *et al.* Cutting edge: MyD88 is required for resistance to *Toxoplasma gondii* infection and regulates parasite-induced IL-12 production by dendritic cells. J. Immunol 2002; 168: 5997-01.

[55] Chen M, Aosai F, Norose K, *et al.* Involvement of MyD88 in host defense and the down-regulation of anti-heat shock protein 70 autoantibody formation by MyD88 in *Toxoplasma gondii*-infected mice. J. Parasitol 2002; 88: 1017-19.

[56] Kim L, Butcher BA, Lee CW, *et al. Toxoplasma gondii* genotype determines MyD88-dependent signaling in infected macrophages. J. Immunol 2006; 177: 2584-91.

[57] Aliberti J, Jankovic D, Sher A. Turning it on and off: Regulation of dendritic cell function in *Toxoplasma gondii* infection. Immunol Rev 2004; 201: 26-34.

[58] Aliberti J, Valenzuela JG, Carruthers VB, *et al.* Molecular mimicry of a CCR5 binding-domain in the microbial activation of dendritic cells. Nat Immun 2003; 4: 485-90.

[59] Yarovinsky F, Sher A. Toll-like receptor recognition of *Toxoplasma gondii.* Int J Parasitol 2006; 36: 255-59.

[60] Grunvald E, Chiaramonte M, Hieny S, *et al.* Biochemical characterization and protein kinase C dependency of monokine-inducing activities of *Toxoplasma gondii.* Infect Immun 1996; 64: 2010-18.

[61] Yarovinsky F, Zhang D, Andersen JF, *et al.* Immunology: TLR11 activation of dendritic cells by a protozoan profilin-like protein. Science 2005; 308: 1626-29.

[62] Akira S, Uematsu S, Takeuchi O. Pathogen recognition and innate immunity. Cell 2006; 124: 783-01.

[63] Medzhitov R. Recognition of microorganisms and activation of the immune response. Nature 2007; 449: 819-26.

[64] Witke W. The role of profilin complexes in cell motility and other cellular processes. Trends Cell Biol 2004; 14: 461-69.

[65] Soldati D, Meissner M. *Toxoplasma* as a novel system for motility. Curr Opin Cell Biol 2004; 16: 32-40.

[66]   Plattner F, Yarovinsky F, Romero S, *et al* .*Toxoplasma* Profilin Is Essential for Host Cell Invasion and TLR11-Dependent Induction of an Interleukin-12 Response. Cell Host Microbe 2008; 3: 77-87.

[67]   Hedhli D, Dimier-Poisson L, Judge JW, *et al*.. Protective immunity against *Toxoplasma* challenge in mice by coadministration of *T. gondii* antigens and *Eimeria* profilin-like protein as an adjuvant. Vaccine 2009; 27: 2274-81.

[68]   Hayashi F, Smith KD, Ozinsky A, *et al*. The innate immune response to bacterial flagellin is mediated by Toll-like receptor 5. Nature 2001; 410: 1099-03.

[69]   Smith KD, Andersen-Nissen E, Hayashi F, *et al*. Toll-like receptor 5 recognizes a conserved site on flagellin required for protofilament formation and bacterial motility. Nat Immunol 2003; 4: 1247-53.

[70]   Yarovinsky F, Kanzler H, Hieny S, *et al*. Toll-like Receptor Recognition Regulates Immunodominance in an Antimicrobial CD4+ T Cell Response. Immunity 2006; 25: 655-64.

[71]   Liu CH, Fan YT, Dias A, *et al*. Cutting edge: Dendritic cells are essential for in vivo IL-12 production and development of resistance against *Toxoplasma gondii* infection in mice. J Immunol 2006; 177: 31-35.

[72]   Hawn TR, Ozinsky A, Underhill DM, *et al*. *Leishmania major* activates IL-1 alpha expression in macrophages through a MyD88-dependent pathway. Microbes Infect 2002; 4: 763-71

[73]   De Veer MJ, Curtis JM, Baldwin TM, *et al*. MyD88 is essential for clearance of *Leishmania major*: Possible role for lipophosphoglycan and Toll-like receptor 2 signaling. Eur J Immunol 2003; 33: 2822-31.

[74]   Coelho PS, Klein A, Talvani A, *et al*. Glycosylphosphatidylinositol-anchored mucin-like glycoproteins isolated from *Trypanosoma cruzi trypomastigotes* induce *in vivo* leukocyte recruitment dependent on MCP-1 production by IFN-gamma-primed-macrophages. J Leukoc Biol 2002; 71: 837-44.

[75]   Campos MA, Closel M, Valente EP, *et al*. Impaired production of proinflammatory cytokines and host resistance to acute infection with *Trypanosoma cruzi* in mice lacking functional myeloid differentiation factor 88. J Immunol 2004; 172: 1711-18.

[76]   Mun HS, Aosai F, Norose K, *et al*. TLR2 as an essential molecule for protective immunity against *Toxoplasma gondii* infection. Int Immunol 2003; 15: 1081-87.

[77]   Del Rio L, Butcher BA, Bennouna S, *et al*. *Toxoplasma gondii* triggers myeloid differentiation factor 88-dependent IL-12 and chemokine ligand 2 (monocyte chemoattractant protein 1) responses using distinct parasite molecules and host receptors. J Immunol 2004; 172: 6954-60.

[78]   Adams LB, Hibbs J, Taintor RR, Krahenbuhl JL. Microbiostatic effect of murine-activated macrophages for *Toxoplasma gondii*. Role for synthesis of inorganic nitrogen oxides from L-arginine. J Immunol 1990; 144: 2725-29.

[79]   Chao CC, Anderson WR, Hu S, *et al*. Activated microglia inhibit multiplication of *Toxoplasma gondii* via a nitric oxide mechanism. Clin Immunol Immunopathol 1993; 67: 178-83.

[80]   Bohne W, Heesemann J, Gross U. Reduced replication of *Toxoplasma gondii* is necessary for induction of bradyzoite-specific antigens: A possible role for nitric oxide in triggering stage conversion. Infect Immun 1994; 62: 1761-67.

[81]   Scharton-Kersten TM, Yap G, Magram J, Sher A. Inducible nitric oxide is essential for host control of persistent but not acute infection with the intracellular pathogen *Toxoplasma gondii*. J Exp Med 1997; 185: 1261-73.

[82]   Bliss SK, Marshall AJ, Zhang Y, Denkers EY. Human polymorphonuclear leukocytes produce IL-12, TNF-alpha, and the chemokines macrophage-inflammatory protein-1 alpha and -1 beta in response to *Toxoplasma gondii* antigens. J Immunol 1999; 162: 7369- 75.

[83]   Bliss SK, Gavrilescu LC, Alcaraz A, Denkers EY. Neutrophil depletion during *Toxoplasma gondii* infection leads to impaired immunity and lethal systemic pathology. Infect Immun 2001; 69: 4898-05.

[84]   Mordue,D.G. & Sibley,L.D. A novel population of Gr-1+-activated macrophages induced during acute toxoplasmosis. J Leukoc Biol 2003; 74: 1015-25.

[85]   Debierre-Grockiego F, Campos MA, Azzouz N, *et al*. Activation of TLR2 and TLR4 by glycosylphosphatidylinositols derived from *Toxoplasma gondii*. J Immunol 2007; 179: 1129-37.

[86]   Zhu J, Krishnegowda G, Gowda DC. Induction of proinflammatory responses in macrophages by the glycosylphosphatidylinositols of *Plasmodium falciparum*: the requirement of extracellular signal-regulated kinase, p38, c-Jun N-terminal kinase and NF-kappaB pathways for the expression of proinflammatory cytokines and nitric oxide. J Biol Chem 2005; 280: 8617-27.

[87]   Krishnegowda G, Hajjar AM, Zhu J, *et al*. Induction of proinflammatory responses in macrophages by the glycosylphosphatidylinositols of *Plasmodium falciparum*: Cell signaling receptors, glycosylphosphatidylinositol (GPI) structural requirement, and regulation of GPI activity. J Biol Chem 2005; 280: 8606-16.

[88]   Hitziger N, Dellacasa I, Albiger B, Barragan A. Dissemination of *Toxoplasma gondii* to immunoprivileged organs and role of Toll/interleukin-1 receptor signalling for host resistance assessed by in vivo bioluminescence imaging. Cell Microbiol 2005; 7: 837-48.

[89]   Aosai F, Rodriguez Pena MS, Mun HS, *et al*. *Toxoplasma gondii*-derived heat shock protein 70 stimulates maturation of murine bone marrow-derived dendritic cells via Toll-like receptor 4. Cell Stress Chaperones 2006; 11: 13-22.

[90]   Heimesaat MM, Fischer A, Jahn HK, *et al*. Exacerbation of murine ileitis by Toll-like receptor 4 mediated sensing of lipopolysaccharide from commensal *Escherichia coli*. Gut 2007; 56: 941-48.

[91]   Minns LA, Menard LC, Foureau DM, *et al*. TLR9 is required for the gut-associated lymphoid tissue response following oral infection of *Toxoplasma gondii*. J Immunol 2006; 176: 7589-97.

[92]   Shoda LKM, Kegerreis KA, Suarez CE, *et al*. DNA from protozoan parasites *Babesia bovis*, *Trypanosoma cruzi,* and *T. brucei* is mitogenic for B lymphocytes and stimulates macrophage expression of interleukin-12, tumor necrosis factor alpha, and nitric oxide. Infect Immun 2001; 69: 2162-71.

[93]   Coban C, Ishii KJ, Kawai T, *et al* . Toll-like receptor 9 mediates innate immune activation by the malaria pigment hemozoin. J Exp Med 2005; 201: 19-25.

[94]   Benson A, Pifer R, Behrendt CL, *et al*.Gut commensal bacteria direct a protective immune response against *Toxoplasma gondii*. Cell Host Microbe 2009; 6: 187-96.

[95]   LaRosa DF, Stumhofer JS, Gelman AE, *et al*. T cell expression of MyD88 is required for resistance to *Toxoplasma gondii*. Proc Natl Acad Sci U S A 2008; 105: 3855-60.

[96]   Rahman AH, Taylor DK, Turka LA. The contribution of direct TLR signaling to T cell responses. Immunol Res 2009; 45: 25-36.

[97]   Quigley M, Martinez J, Huang X, Yang Y. A critical role for direct TLR2-MyD88 signaling in CD8 T-cell clonal expansion and memory formation following vaccinia viral infection. Blood 2009; 113: 2256-64.

[98]   Zhou S, Kurt-Jones EA, Cerny AM, *et al*. MyD88 intrinsically regulates CD4 T-cell responses. J Virol 2009; 83: 1625-34.

[99]   Von Bernuth H, Picard C, Jin Z, *et al*. Pyogenic bacterial infections in humans with MyD88 deficiency. Science 2008; 321: 691-96.

[100] Lee CW, Sukhumavasi W, Denkers EY. Phosphoinositide-3-kinase-dependent, MyD88-independent induction of CC-type chemokines characterizes the macrophage response to *Toxoplasma gondii* strains with high virulence. Infect Immun 2007; 75: 5788-97.

[101] Masek KS, Zhu P, Freedman BD, Hunter CA. *Toxoplasma gondii* induces changes in intracellular calcium in macrophages. Parasitology 2007; 134: 1973-79.

[102] Leng J, Butcher BA, Egan CE, *et al*. *Toxoplasma gondii* prevents chromatin remodeling initiated by TLR-triggered macrophage activation. J Immunol 2009; 182: 489-97.

[103] Carmen JC, Southard RC, Sinai AP. The complexity of signaling in host-pathogen interactions revealed by the *Toxoplasma gondii*-dependent modulation of JNK phosphorylation. Exp Cell Res 2008; 314: 3724-36.

[104] Molestina RE, Sinai AP. Host and parasite-derived IKK activities direct distinct temporal phases of NF-kappaB activation and target gene expression following *Toxoplasma gondii* infection. J Cell Sci 2005; 118: 5785-96.

[105] Shapira S, Harb OS, Margarit J, *et al*. Initiation and termination of NF-kappaB signaling by the intracellular protozoan parasite *Toxoplasma gondii*. J Cell Sci 2005; 118: 3501-08.

[106] Denkers EY, Butcher BA, Del Rio L, Kim L. Manipulation of mitogen-activated protein kinase/nuclear factor-kappaB-signaling cascades during intracellular *Toxoplasma gondii* infection. Immunol Rev 2004; 201: 191-05.

[107] McKee AS, Dzierszinski F, Boes M, *et al*. Functional inactivation of immature dendritic cells by the intracellular parasite *Toxoplasma gondii*. J Immunol 2004; 173: 2632-40.

[108] Pollard AM, Knoll LJ, Mordue DG. The role of specific *Toxoplasma gondii* molecules in manipulation of innate immunity. Trends Parasitol 2009; 25: 491-94.

CHAPTER 8

Manipulation of Host-Cell Apoptosis during Infection with *Toxoplasma gondii*

Yoshifumi Nishikawa*

National Research Center for Protozoan Diseases, Obihiro University of Agriculture and Veterinary Medicine, Inada-cho, Obihiro, Hokkaido 080-8555, Japan

Abstract: Apoptosis play a crucial role in the interaction between hosts and parasites. Apoptotic response includes innate and adaptive immunities to restrict intracellular parasite replication and regulatory functions to modulate host immune responses. The obligate intracellular protozoan *Toxoplasma gondii* extensively modifies apoptosis of its own host cell or of uninfected bystander cells. Upon infection with *T. gondii*, apoptosis is triggered in T lymphocytes, macrophages and other leukocytes, thereby suppressing immune responses against the parasite. On the other hand, *T. gondii* inhibits host-cell apoptosis by direct or indirect mechanisms in the infected cells to facilitate parasite survival. The dual activity of *T. gondii* to both promote and inhibit apoptosis requires tight regulation to stabilize host and parasite interaction and establish toxoplasmosis. Here, molecular mechanisms behind the inhibition or induction of apoptosis by *T. gondii* infection and their pathogenesis are focused on.

INTRODUCTION

Toxoplasma gondii is an intracellular coccidian belonging to the phylum Apicomplexa. The parasite is distributed globally and can be found within many different species of mammals and birds. Although *T. gondii* is usually non-pathogenic to humans, it becomes an opportunistic pathogen, causing severe toxoplasmosis in immunocompromised hosts, such as AIDS patients [1]. In the host, after infection of intestinal epithelial cells, the infective stages (oocysts or bradyzoites) transform into tachyzoites, which display rapid multiplication by endodyogeny within an intracellular parasitophorous vacuole (PV). When the cells become packed with tachyzoites, the host cell plasma membrane ruptures, and free parasites are released into the extracellular milieu [2]. Induction of immune responses and resistance at the tachyzoite stage is a key step in the *T. gondii* life cycle, and will determine the survival of the host and the parasite itself [3]. After development of immunity, the tachyzoite stage is cleared from host tissues, and bradyzoites, the slowly-multiplying, essentially dormant and harmless form of the parasite, persist [4]. The bradyzoites survive within cysts, and are effectively isolated from the host immune system by the cyst wall [5]. Bradyzoites are found in proportionately larger numbers in the central nervous system (CNS). Indeed, cyst reactivation occurs most often in the brain. During infection, host-cell apoptosis plays a crucial role in the interaction between *T. gondii* and its hosts. Interestingly, *T. gondii* both promotes and inhibits host-cell apoptosis. Inhibition of host cell apoptosis might allow undistributed intracellular development, thus facilitating parasite survival. On the other hand, increased apoptosis of immune cells after infection is thought to partially downregulate effective immune responses against *T. gondii*. Host-cell apoptosis and its modulation by the parasite are also required to restrict tissue destruction by inflammatory responses (i.e. immunopathology).

Apoptosis

Apoptosis, a morphologically and biochemically distinct form of programmed cell death, plays a major role in the removal of damaged or unwanted cells during development, tissue homeostasis, aging of multicellular organisms and selection of the lymphocyte repertoire [6]. In addition, apoptosis has been recognized as an important defense mechanism against viral, bacterial and parasitic pathogens during innate and adaptive immunity [7]. Apoptosis, induced in infected cells by cytotoxic immune effector cells or other stress from hosts, is a critical defense against intracellular pathogens [8]. If the production of viable microorganisms is diminished, the sacrifice of infected host cells might facilitate the survival of the host organism. Apoptosis in distinct cell populations may contribute to the regulation of pathogen-induced immune responses [9]. Despite this cell-mediated immunity, many viral [10], bacterial [11] and protozoan pathogens [12-14] have developed mechanisms to invade and multiply within host cells without inducing apoptosis. As shown in Figure 1, direct effects of parasites and their products, as well as indirect mechanisms via the induction of antigen-specific T cells, participate in the modulation of host cell death. Apoptosis can be either initiated or downregulated by the parasite, thereby contributing to dissemination within the host, inhibiting or modulating host immune responses, or facilitating the intracellular survival of the pathogen.

*Corresponding Author: Yoshifumi Nishikawa, National Research Center for Protozoan Diseases, Obihiro University of Agriculture and Veterinary Medicine, Inada-cho, Obihiro, Hokkaido 080-8555, Japan; Tel.: +81-155-49-5886; Fax: +81-155-49-5643; Eamil: : nisikawa@obihiro.ac.jp

Emilio Jirillo (Ed)
All rights reserved - © 2010 Bentham Science Publishers Ltd.

Apoptotic death follows a regulated and prescribed dismantling of the cell. Morphological features include condensation of chromatin and disruption of the nuclear architecture, vacuolation of the cytoplasm, membrane blebbing, detachment from the substrate, and cell shrinkage; once apoptosis has been initiated, it cannot be reversed. In contrast, necrotic death results in cell lysis in a manner that is not particularly ordered. Apoptosis can be initiated by the binding of death ligands to their specific cell-surface receptors, such as Fas/APO-1 (CD95) or tumor necrosis factor receptor (TNFR), or by other stimuli, such as chemotherapeutic agents, irradiation, cellular stress and serum or growth factor deprivation [6, 15] (Fig. **2**). In addition, the release of perforin and granzymes by natural killer (NK) cells or antigen-specific cytotoxic T lymphocytes (CTLs) can induce apoptosis of target cells [16] (Fig. **1**). Transduction of these pro-apoptotic stimuli via different signaling pathways results in the activation of a family of cysteine proteases with specificity for aspartic acid residues, referred to as caspases, which represent the central component of the apoptotic machinery [17] (Fig. **2**).

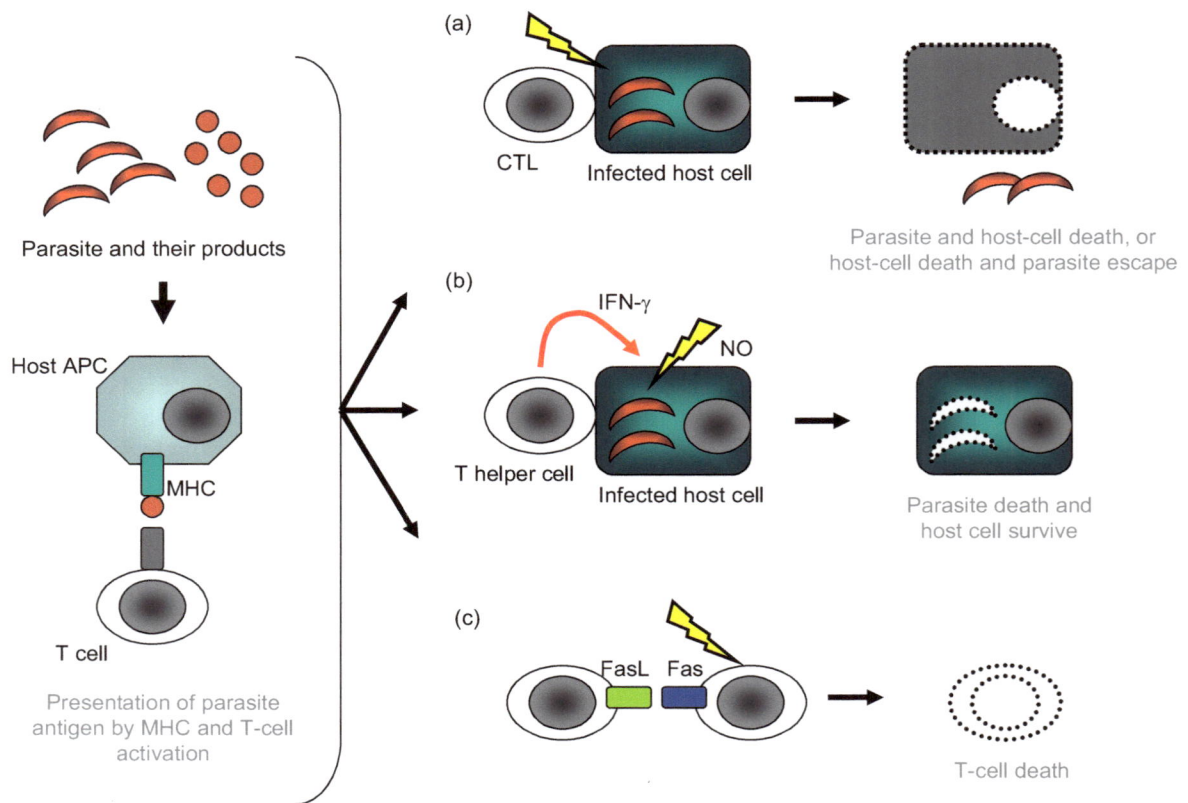

Fig. 1

Figure 1: Cell death by apoptosis during infection with *T. gondii*. In the course of infection with the parasites, their antigens are processed by host antigen-presenting cells (APC) and presented to T cells in the context of the major histocompatibility complex (MHC). (**a**) Activated cytotoxic T cells (CTL) attack the parasite-infected cells. (**b**) IFN-γ produced by T helper cells stimulates synthesis of nitric oxide (NO) to kill intracellular parasites. (**c**) Activated T cells express Fas and Fas ligand (FasL), and become susceptible to death by apoptosis induced by Fas signaling.

Given their potential to kill the cell upon activation, metazoan cells have elaborate regulatory safeguards to prevent accidental apoptotic activation. These safeguards act at the level of triggering (induction of the signal), signaling (transmission of the apoptotic signal) and execution (directed at caspase activity) of the apoptotic cascade (Fig. **2**). Several 'intrinsic' factors, such as the inhibitor of apoptosis proteins (IAPs), contribute to the control of caspase activity [18, 19]. Inhibitors of apoptosis proteins interfere with both pro-caspases and activated enzymes to effectively block their activity [18, 19]. A balance between the action of the pro-apoptotic and anti-apoptotic activities ultimately controls the life and death of cells.

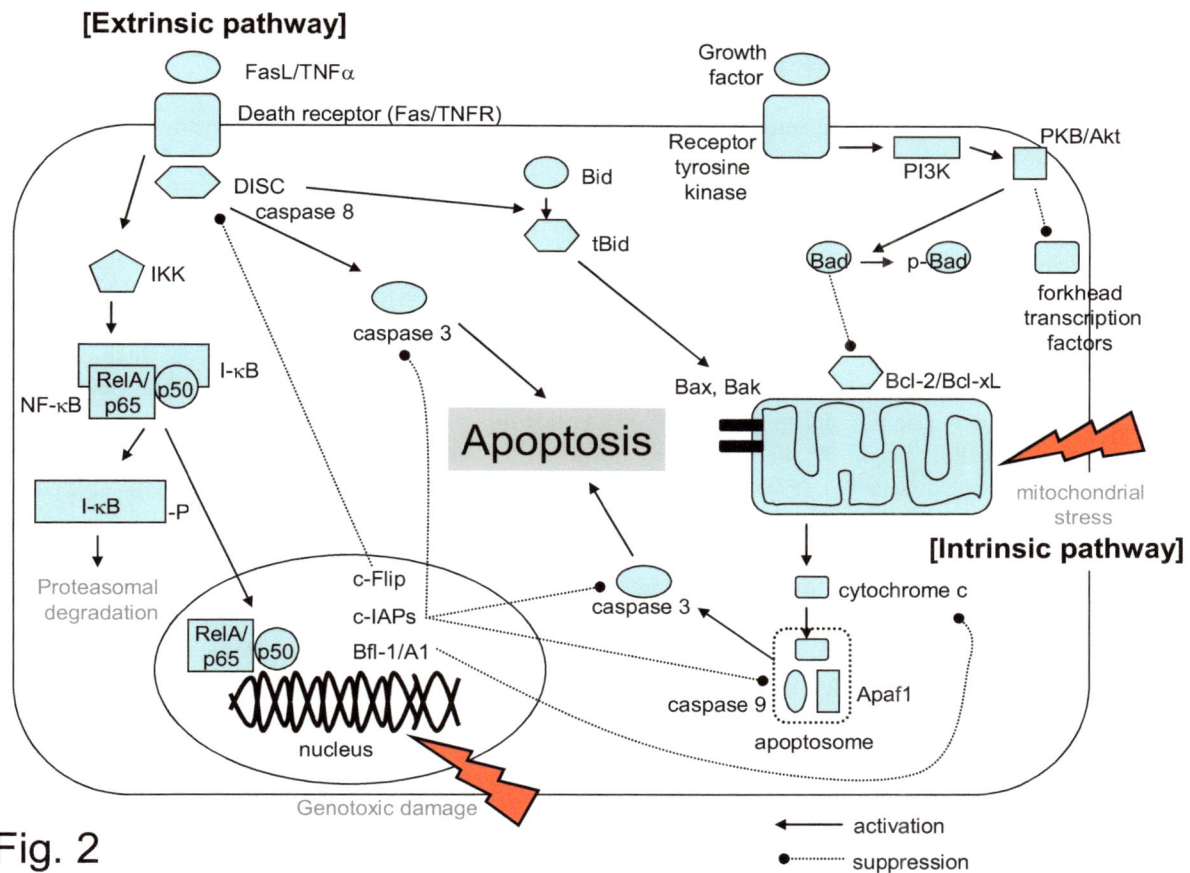

Figure 2: Simplified model of transduction pathways that induce or inhibit apoptosis. Apoptosis may be triggered by extrinsic stimuli such as FasL or TNF-α, which induce the recruitment and activation of caspase 8 upon binding to Fas or TNFR (death receptors), respectively. Caspase 8 activates an executioner caspase, caspase 3, which cleaves multiple proteins resulting in the removal of the cell. Similarly, intrinsic stimuli such as DNA damage lead to the activation of caspase 3. However, instead of caspase 8, intrinsic stimuli trigger the release of cytochrome c from mitochondria and the subsequent activation of caspase 9. Caspase 9 activates caspase 3 leading to apoptosis. The release of cytochrome c is regulated by the Bcl-2 family of proteins which consists of three groups: the anti-apoptotic proteins (e.g. Bcl-2, Bcl-xL), the multidomain pro-apoptotic proteins (e.g. Bax and Bak), and the BH3-domain only pro-apoptotic proteins (e.g. Bid and Bad). Caspase 8 activation also leads to the release of cytochrome c following the cleavage of Bid to tBid. The two pro-survival responses are due to the activation of NF-κB and PI3K. The transcription factor, NF-κB, is maintained in the cytosol due to the binding of IκB. Activation of NF-κB occurs when the Iκ kinase (IKK) is activated and phosphorylates IκB, targeting it for degradation. Following the degradation of IκB, NF-κB translocates to the nucleus and induces the transcription of multiple genes including anti-apoptotic genes like c-Flip (inhibits caspase 8 activation), c-IAP1 and c-IAP2 (inhibits caspases), and Bfl-1/A1 (prevents the release of cytochrome c). Cell surface receptors (growth factor receptors) recruit and activate PI3K upon binding their ligand. Once active, PI3K phosphorylates PKB/Akt which then inactivates the pro-apoptotic Bcl-2 protein Bad and the forkhead transcription factors blocking the transcription of pro-apoptotic genes. PKB/Akt also activates IKK resulting in the activation of the NF-κB response (Modified from ref. [12]).

As shown in Figure 2, the extrinsic pathway is activated following the binding of a ligand to a death receptor on the cell surface such as FasL/Fas and TNF-α/TNFR [20-22]. Activation of the receptor results in the formation of the death-inducing signaling complex (DISC) [20, 21], which recruits and activates the initiator caspase, caspase 8 [21, 22]. Active caspase 8 then cleaves and activates an executioner caspase, caspase 3, which is responsible for cleaving multiple proteins and the subsequent death of the cell [22]. The intrinsic pathway, initiated by intracellular signals (e.g. DNA damage), relies on the release of cytochrome c from mitochondria to activate the initiator caspase, caspase 9, in a macromolecular complex called the apoptosome [23, 24]. As with the extrinsic pathway, the initiator caspase then activates caspase 3 and the cell undergoes apoptosis [24-26]. The activation of caspase 8 can also lead to the release of cytochrome c due to the cleavage of the Bcl-2-family protein Bid [27, 28]. The importance of mitochondria for the apoptotic machinery is further underlined by the fact that several proteins of the Bcl-2 family with either anti-apoptotic (e.g. Bcl-2, Bcl-xL and Mcl-1) or pro-apoptotic (e.g. Bax, Bak and Bik) functions reside in the outer mitochondrial membrane [29].

In the case of TNF, this results in the activation of nuclear factor-kappa B (NF-κB) which directly regulates the expression of several families of genes with anti-apoptotic activities, including the IAPs which directly bind and inhibit caspase activation and activity [18, 30, 31], and members of the Bcl2 family involved in cytochrome c release from mitochondria [32]. In order to prevent the inappropriate activation of apoptosis, these pathways are regulated by multiple inhibitory or pro-survival mechanisms [33] (Fig. **2**). NF-κB is maintained in an inactive state in the cytoplasm of the cell by inhibitor of kappa B (I-κB) and is activated when I kappa kinase (IKK) is activated and phosphorylates I-κB [34, 35]. Phosphorylated I-κB is rapidly degraded by the proteasome [34] allowing NF-κB translocation to the nucleus [35]. In addition to inflammatory mediators, NF-κB induces the expression of genes such as Bcl-2, x-IAP and c-IAP which interfere with both the intrinsic and extrinsic apoptosis pathways [34, 36]. On the other hand, the activation of the phosphoinositide 3 kinase (PI3K) signaling pathway also inhibits apoptosis [37, 38]. Following growth factor binding, active PI3K phosphorylates the lipid phosphatidylinositol bisphosphate (PIP2) to form PIP3 which recruits protein kinase B (PKB)/Akt and phosphoinositide-dependent kinase 1 (PDK1) to cellular membranes [11]. PDK1 activates PKB/Akt [11]. Once activated, PKB/Akt phosphorylates the pro-apoptotic Bcl-2 family member, Bad, and inhibits the forkhead family of transcription factors, repressing the transcription of genes encoding pro-apoptotic proteins like Bim and FasL [11]. Other important classes of genes regulated by NF-κB include pro-inflammatory cytokines and their receptors as well as adhesion molecules and factors in involved in cell cycle regulation [39]. The combined interaction of these genes results generally in a pro-survival response induced by NF-κB. Furthermore, manipulation of NF-κB function by pathogenic agents plays a critical role in several infectious diseases [40].

Infection by the protozoan parasite, *T. gondii*, is often accompanied by the production and secretion of cytokines and other immune effectors that can induce apoptosis in host cells [41]. This response creates a hostile environment characterized by increased levels of FasL, TNF-α, interferon-gamma (IFN-γ) and various other cytokines which induce apoptosis, and the activities of immune effector cells [41]. Often, the resultant type 1 helper T cell (Th1) cytokine response induces apoptosis in uninfected cells during infection. However, this apoptosis is not observed in the cells infected by these pathogens, suggesting a strong selective pressure to block apoptosis [41]. Although the specific molecular mechanisms of the infected cells to apoptotic stimuli remain unknown in many cases, research concerning the regulation of apoptosis has suggested direct or indirect interference by *T. gondii*. First, the parasites may induce a pro-survival response such as the NF-κB or PI3K responses described above. Second, the parasites may produce and secrete factors that directly or indirectly inhibit or modulate these pathways. Third, the parasite may directly interact with the signaling effector molecules responsible for regulating the apoptotic pathway. To date, parasite modulation of apoptosis seems to be primarily the result of infection-dependent changes in host gene expression impacting genes involved in apoptosis.

Inhibition of Host-Cell Apoptosis by *T. Gondii* Nfection

T. gondii protects infected host cells against apoptosis. Treatment of several murine [42] and human [43] cell lines with a variety of pro-apoptotic signals, including Fas-dependent and perforin/granzyme-dependent T-cell cytotoxicity, growth factor deprivation, irradiation, and treatment with apoptosis-promoting agents indeed induced apoptosis in uninfected but not in *T. gondii*-infected cells, including monocytic/histiocytic, granulocytic, and T- and B-cell lines. The inhibitory effect correlated with the state of infection of the individual cell and required the presence of viable, but not necessarily replicating, parasites [42, 43], suggesting that the continuous secretion of a parasite-derived molecule(s) is involved. The fact that parasitized host cells are protected against treatment with such a diverse array of pro-apoptotic stimuli indicates that central components of the apoptosis-inducing machinery are targeted.

T. gondii infection is found to block both the activity and activation of caspase 3 implicating upstream events in the respective cascades [44-46]. Given that a profound blockade of caspase 3 and upstream caspase (8 and 9) is observed in cells infected with *T. gondii* [44, 46, 47], suggesting an inhibitory mechanism against apoptosis (Fig. **3**).

A potential direct mechanism could be the secretion of IAP proteins by *T. gondii* into the host cell effectively blocking caspase activation (Fig. **3**).

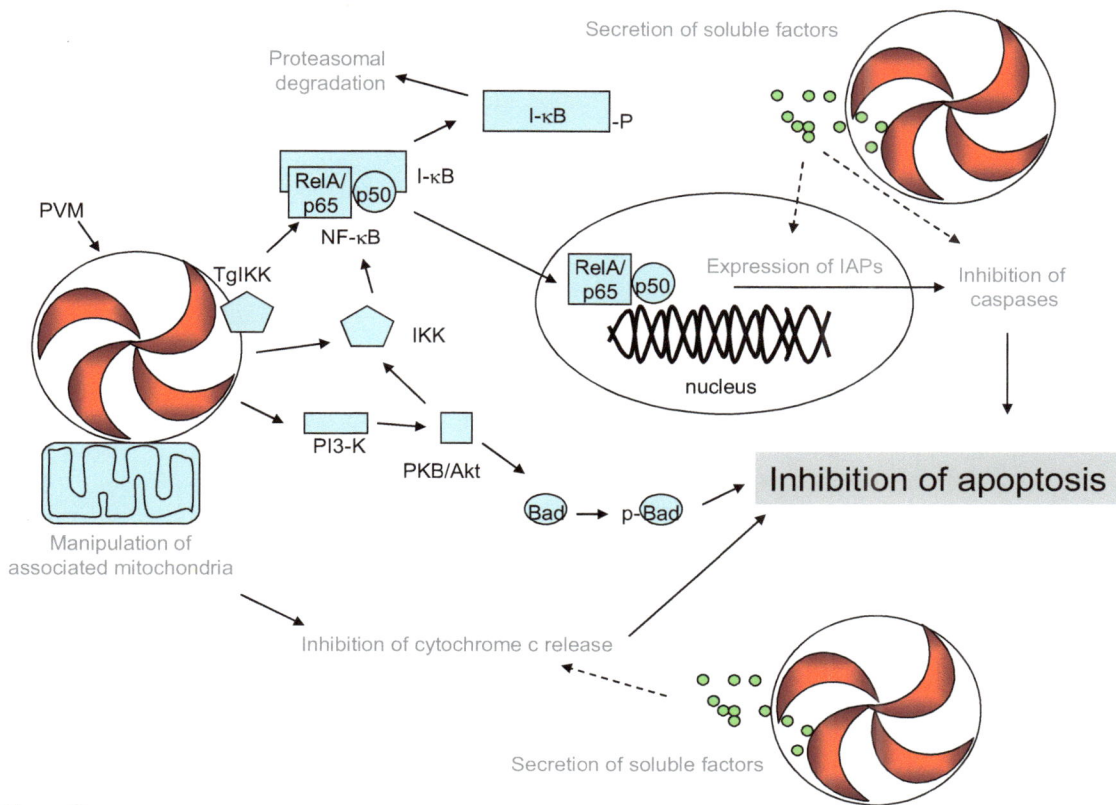

Fig. 3

Figure 3: Potential mechanisms for interference with apoptosis by *T. gondii*. The parasite may interfere directly or indirectly with the initiation, activation and signaling of the apoptosis cascade. Direct interference could include the manipulation of parasitophorous vacuole membrane (PVM)-associated mitochondria to inhibit cytochrome c release. In addition, the putative secretion of the parasite-derived soluble factors into the host cell cytoplasm may directly inhibit cytochrome c release, expression IAPs or caspases. The most important indirect method is the parasite-mediated activation of the host pro-survival/anti-apoptotic machinery. *T. gondii* infection induces the activation of NF-κB. The transcription factor, NF-κB, is maintained in the cytosol due to the binding of IκB. Activation of NF-κB occurs when Iκ kinase (IKK) or *T. gondii* IKK (TgIKK) is activated and phosphorylates IκB, targeting it for degradation. Following the degradation of IκB, NF-κB translocates to the nucleus and induces the transcription of multiple genes including anti-apoptotic genes. Infection with *T. gondii* also activates PI3K. Once active, PI3K phosphorylates PKB/Akt which then inactivates the pro-apoptotic Bcl-2 protein, Bad, blocking the transcription of pro-apoptotic genes. PKB/Akt also activates IKK resulting in the activation of the NF-κB response.

There are several facts arguing against a 'direct' inhibition of caspases by a parasite factor(s). An examination of the *T. gondii* genome yields no credible hits of the baculoviral IAP repeat (BIR) domain sequence, which is a marker for discovering IAP proteins [14, 48]. The *T. gondii* vacuolar membrane, while impermeable to molecules >1300 Da [49], would not permit diffusion of a potentially secreted IAP. While extravacuolar secretion into the host cytoplasm of parasite proteins has been reported [50], it is likely to be inefficient and energetically unfavorable. A critical requirement for a *T. gondii* IAP to be effective is its presence within the host cytoplasm at a level comparable to its target caspase. Such a high concentration would require massive expression and a high level of secretion into the cytoplasm. Therefore, *T. gondii* may block caspase activity by triggering the pro-survival and anti-apoptotic response in the host cell acting by an indirect mechanism (Fig. **3**). Such a mechanism would involve the parasite-directed activation of host cell functions resulting in the establishment of an anti-apoptotic state.

Molecular Mechanism of Apoptosis Inhibition by *T. Gondii*

The inhibition of apoptosis by *T. gondii* has been linked to the activation of PI3-K [51]. During the early stages of infection, cells exhibit increased levels of active PKB/Akt, Erk1/2 and p38 MAPK [51] (Fig. **3**). These results suggest that during the early stages of infection, the activation of PI3K is responsible for preventing apoptosis perhaps by countering an apoptotic response induced by invasion as a natural component of the host defense mechanism.

T. gondii activation of NF-κB in fibroblasts exhibits a distinct temporal dimension to its activation profile [52]. Host signaling events coincide with the extracellular phase, invasion and establishment of the PV result in NF-κB signaling that is completely dependent on the host IKK [52]. However, the delivery of parasite-derived IKK (TgIKK) to the PVM coincident with parasite replication ensures sustained activation [52]. It is important that the capacity of TgIKK to trigger NF-κB activation is critically dependent on the establishment of activation by the host IKK activity [52]. The early phases of *T. gondii* infection exhibit several signs of NF-κB activation (including the phosphorylation of IκBα) but in macrophages unlike fibroblasts [53], nuclear translocation of NF-κB is blocked [54, 55]. This blockade is transient and suggested to involve RelA/p65 phosphorylation [56]. Interestingly, this blockade in macrophages is lifted as the infection progresses and NF-κB localizes to the host nucleus [54-57] as reported following the infection of fibroblasts by *T. gondii* [52, 58]. The activation of NF-κB translocation from the cytoplasm to the nucleus by *T. gondii* is a topic of controversy. At least early in the infection process, *T. gondii* infection actually inhibits NF-κB translocation to the nucleus [54, 55, 59-61] while translocation is observed with more mature vacuoles [58]. This delay in NF-κB translocation occurs in spite of increased levels of phosphorylated-IκB in infected cells, an indication of activation, suggesting a parasite-directed mechanism to sequester NF-κB in the cytoplasm [54, 55, 57]. A phenotype accompanying this unexpected cytoplasmic localization is the failure of bacterial lipopolysaccharide to stimulate the production of the pro-inflammatory cytokines Interleukin-12 (IL-12) and TNF [54, 55]. The lack of responsiveness to a potent activator suggests parasite-directed interference with the signaling pathways in infected macrophages.

The critical role of NF-κB in pro-survival responses implicates whether this transcription factor plays a specific role in the *T. gondii* mediated blockade of apoptosis. The use of mouse embryonic fibroblasts derived from RelA/p65−/− murine embryos (homozygous null are embryonic lethal) [62] permitted a definitive assessment of the role of NF-κB in the parasite-mediated blockade. Infection did not protect host-cell apoptosis of p65−/− cells indicating an essential role for NF-κB in the inhibition of apoptosis [46]. Accordingly, unlike *T. gondii*-infected wild type cells, infected p65−/− cells exhibited apoptosis following activation by staurosporine or TNF [46]. These features, which include morphological changes as well as biochemical indicators, indicated a loss of infection-mediated protection from apoptosis. Consistent with the hypersensitivity of p65−/− cells to TNF-mediated apoptosis [62] a dramatic induction of caspase 3 activity was observed even with extremely low levels of this cytokine. The loss of protection from apoptosis in the p65−/− background strongly implicates NF-κB-regulated gene expression in the blockade of apoptosis.

NF-κB activation results in the transcriptional upregulation of anti-apoptotic genes [51, 58] and depends on both the host IKK and a novel parasite kinase activity, TgIKK, to phosphorylate IκBα at the PVM [52, 53]. Perhaps the most intriguing observation regarding phosphorylated IκB in the infected cell is its localization [58]. Remarkably, phosphorylated IκB is distributed on the PVM, the parasite modified 'organelle' delimiting the intracellular parasite from the host cell cytoplasm [63]. This suggests that parasite-directed events are recruiting the IκB–NF-κB complex to the PVM resulting in a highly active kinase activity and/or an inhibition of phosphorylated IκB degradation.

Mitochondrial release of cytochrome c from the intermembrane space is a triggering event in apoptosis [25, 64]. A *T. gondii* mediated blockade of cytochrome c release would inhibit the initiation of apoptosis. *T. gondii* infected cells resist the release of cytochrome c in response to diverse apoptogenic triggers [44]. This suggests parasite-directed events with regard to the Bcl2 family of proteins [58]. The parasite infection promotes the activation of anti-apoptotic Bcl2 family members, but not those on the pro-apoptotic arm to increase the resistance of mitochondria in infected cells to apoptogenic triggers that promote cytochrome c release [58, 65]. A high level of cytochrome c release is consistent with an increase in the relative level of anti-apoptotic Bcl2 members to their pro-apoptotic counterparts as suggested by transcriptional data [58].

The release of cytochrome c initiating apoptosis is believed to occur simultaneously for all mitochondria within the apoptotic cell [64]. PVM-associated mitochondria may not undergo the permeability transition retaining their cytochrome c. This indicates that PVM-associated mitochondria are physiologically distinct and are possibly under an additional level of direct control by the parasite. The release of cytochrome c from non-PVM-associated mitochondria should, on its own, activate apoptosis. However, in the presence of either endogenous or synthetic caspase inhibitors, induction of apoptosis is blocked, despite cytochrome c release [30]. Thus, by a combination of the caspase blockade [44, 46] and the higher threshold for cytochrome c release (enforced by the parasite-directed modulation of Bcl2 family members) [58], *T. gondii* blocks multiple steps in the mitochondrial arm of apoptosis.

In addition, *T. gondii* has been suggested to inhibit caspase 9 activation through direct inhibition of the apoptosome in *in vitro* reconstitution experiments [66] and by inhibiting the release of cytochrome c [44, 67]. The *T. gondii*-dependent inhibition of cytochrome c release also correlates with selective, parasite-dependent degradation of the pro-apoptotic proteins Bad and Bax [67] accompanied by the increased transcription of anti-apoptotic proteins such as Bfl-1 and Bcl-2 [58] and increased levels of Mcl-1 [44]. These changes suggest that *T. gondii* induces a shift, either through increased production, increased degradation, or both, in this regulatory family of proteins that results in an anti-apoptotic state in the host cell. *T. gondii*-infected HeLa cells also exhibit decreased phospho-c-Jun N-terminal kinase (JNK) levels following exposure to Ultraviolet (UV) [67]. As JNK is required for the induction of apoptosis by UV [68], this decrease may block the transmission of the apoptotic stimulus required to induce cytochrome c release in these cells [67]. However, recent study suggests that manipulation of the JNK pathway does not involve NF-κB and is not a central component of the parasite enforced block of apoptosis [69]

Other studies also mentioned apoptosis inhibition by *T. gondii* infection. The inhibition might be achieved at least partially by parasite-induced upregulation of Bcl-2 homologs, such as the murine anti-apoptotic protein A1, which is expressed in peritoneal exudate cells after intraperitoneal infection with *T. gondii* [70]. Poly(ADP-ribose) polymerase-1 (PARP-1) is an abundant nuclear protein that is involved in DNA repair, cell cycle control, programmed cell death and transcriptional regulation. *T. gondii* significantly decreased PARP expression in its host cells within 10 min of infection but that the amount of PARP normalized during prolonged infection. The blockade of host cell apoptosis by *T. gondii* occurs independently of the inhibition of PARP after infection [71]. In the presence of γδ T cells *in vivo* or after the addition of exogenous IFN-γ and TNF *in vitro*, the expression of heat shock protein 65 (HSP65) might also be involved in the protection of murine macrophages against host cell apoptosis [72].

Induction of Host-Cell Apoptosis by *T. Gondii* Infection

Acute infection with *T. gondii* induces a state of transient immunosuppression in both humans and mice, as determined by decreased levels of antibody production and T lymphocyte responses against homologous and heterologous antigens [73-76]. T lymphocyte apoptosis induced by *T. gondii* infection may downregulate the immune responses to the parasite [77-79]. In addition, high levels of apoptosis in hosts have been associated with unrestricted parasite multiplication leading to high parasite burdens in various tissues of the host [80-82]. The levels of host-cell apoptosis were markedly dependent on the genotype [83] and the virulence of the parasite [72, 82]. These results suggested that parasite-triggered apoptosis of host cells may not be a general phenomenon after *T. gondii* infection but rather represents a characteristic determinant of the cause of toxoplasmosis. Lymphocyte apoptosis may also influence local immunity after natural parasite transmission via the gut, because oral infection with *T. gondii* led to apoptosis in Peyer's patch T cells [78].

Acute maternal infection with *T. gondii* during pregnancy is associated with adverse pregnancy outcomes. *T. gondii* might result in abortion with or without direct transmission of the parasite to the foetus. CD4+CD25+-regulatory T cells are known to be involved in maternal tolerance toward the foetus-bearing alloantigens. With a model of pregnant mice infected with *T. gondii*, Foxp3 mRNA expression levels in both splenocytes and placenta were reduced markedly during the process of infection. Furthermore, the numbers of splenic CD4+CD25+-regulatory T cells and placental Foxp3+ cells decreased synchronously in the infected mice and the reduction of splenic CD4+CD25+-regulatory T cells were associated with apoptosis induced by the infection. Foetal loss caused by *T. gondii* could be independent of vertical infection and be dependent of inflammatory responses [84]. Furthermore, foetal resorption induced by *T. gondii* was accompanied by haemorrhage, spiral artery dilation, hypocellularity of the decidua basalis, apoptosis of placental cells, a decline in uterine mature natural killer cell numbers, increased indoleamine 2,3-dioxygenase mRNA levels and reduced IL-15 mRNA levels [61]. In mice, *T. gondii*-induced abortion in early gestation is not due to a direct action of the parasite at the maternofoetal interface but rather to massive IFN-γ release. These results suggest that apoptosis plays a crucial role for *T. gondii* infection during pregnancy.

CD4+ splenocytes undergo apoptosis during acute infection in mice, resulting in a state of transient unresponsiveness to mitogenic and antigenic stimulation [77]. Apoptosis in such cells might be initiated by Fas–FasL interaction because an increased expression of both molecules has been shown to induce apoptosis in murine Peyer's patch T cells following peroral infection [78] and in inflammatory cells and eye tissue after intraocular inoculation of *Toxoplasma* [85]. This form of apoptosis is counteracted by Bcl-2 or Bcl-X$_L$ [86]. Expression of Fas and Fas–FasL-mediated apoptosis in *T. gondii*-infected mice appears to be regulated by the secretion of proinflammatory cytokines, IL-12 and IFN-γ [87]. Moreover, recent evidence indicates that NF-κB2 plays a crucial role in the regulation of lymphocyte apoptosis and Fas–FasL interaction during chronic infection [87]. Although the impact of activation-induced cell death (AICD) of T cells in the course of toxoplasmosis has not yet been thoroughly investigated, it is thought that the elimination of T cells contributes to suppression of *Toxoplasma*-specific immune responses. Similarly, apoptosis in peritoneal macrophages after infection of mice with a highly virulent *Toxoplasma* strain has been supposed to inhibit the anti-parasitic activity of these cells [72, 82]. Furthermore, human dendritic cells infected by viable *T. gondii* have been shown to induce T lymphocyte apoptosis in a contact-dependent and Fas-dependent manner [79]. Fas-mediated apoptosis might, however, also help to limit overwhelming inflammatory responses and thus reduce immune-mediated clinical symptoms, at least in certain tissues [85], indicating that induction of apoptosis in the course of infection with *T. gondii* might be beneficial for the parasite and for the host.

Recent evidence has shown that death receptor ligation in *T. gondii*-infected cells leads to rapid egress of infectious parasites and lytic necrosis of the host cell, an active process mediated by the release of intracellular calcium as a consequence of caspase activation early in the apoptotic cascade [88]. Upon acting on infected cells via death receptor- or perforin-dependent pathways, T cells induce rapid egress of infectious parasites able to infect surrounding cells, including the antigen-specific effector cells. This result suggested that the induction of apoptosis in the course of infection with *T. gondii* might be beneficial for the parasite, but not for the hosts.

Molecular Mechanism of Apoptosis Induction

Two pathways of *T. gondii*-derived factors are thought to trigger apoptosis in host cells (Fig. **4**).

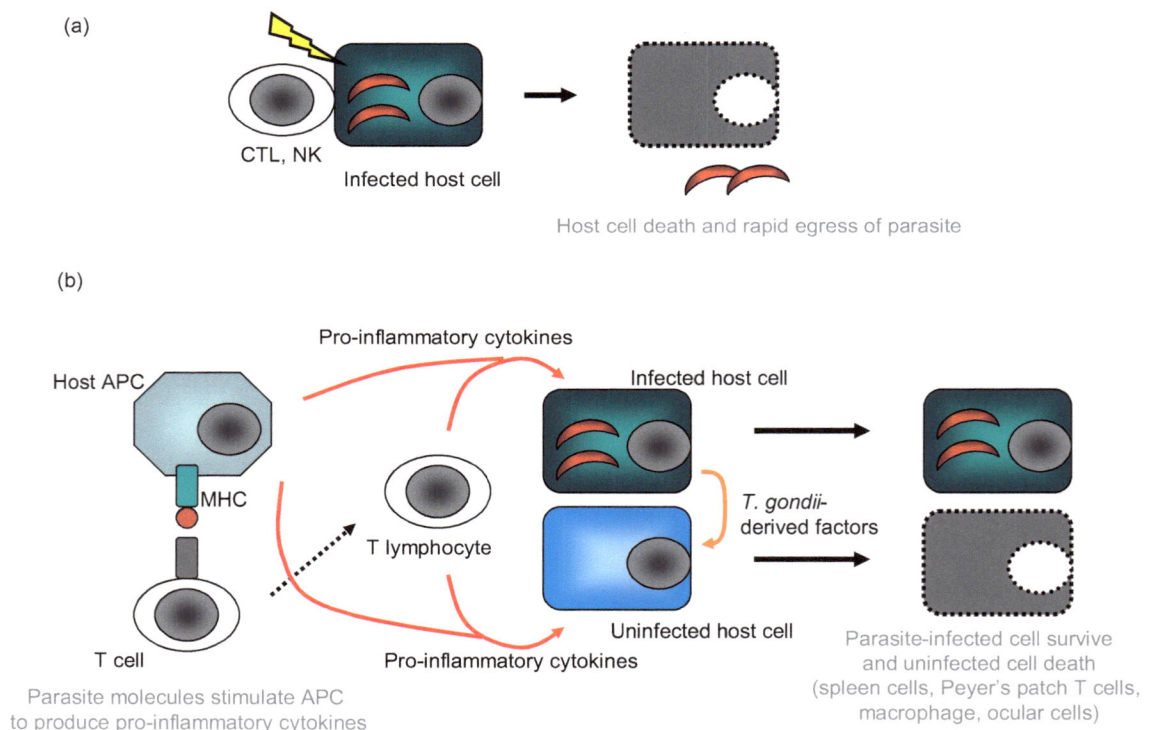

Fig. 4

Figure 4: Potential mechanisms for apoptosis induction by *T. gondii* infection. (a) CTL and NK cells attack the infected target cells, inducing host-cell apoptosis and rapid egress of the live parasites. (b) Parasite-derived molecules, such as profilin, HSP70, GPIs and cyclophilin 18, stimulate antigen-presenting cells (APC) to produce pro-inflammatory cytokines. Pro-inflammatory cytokines from T lymphocyte or APC trigger apoptosis in uninfected bystander cells, not in the infected cells. Moreover, *T. gondii*-derived factors could enhance apoptosis in uninfected cells.

First is that the parasite-derived factors induce or enhance host-cell apoptosis, second is that production of proinflammatory cytokines via the stimulation with parasite molecules trigger the apoptosis.

Although parasite-derived factors which direct activity of apoptosis induction have not been identified, the Programmed Cell Death 5 of *T. gondii* (TgPDCD5), a homologue of the human apoptosis-related molecule, enhanced host-cell apoptosis [89, 90]. TgPDCD5 was located in the cytosol and also detected in the secreted fraction. Furthermore, the addition of recombinant TgPDCD5 to culture medium resulted in the enhancement of host-cell apoptosis triggered by apoptosis-promising reagents in a macrophage cell line and leukemic cell line [89]. Additionally, recombinant TgPDCD5 and transgenic parasite overexpressed TgPDCD5 enhanced host-cell apoptosis in a macrophage cell line in the presence of IFN-γ [89, 90]. These results suggest that TgPDCD5 has a pro-apoptotic effect on host cells.

Still, other mechanisms may lead to an increase in host-cell apoptosis. Recent studies have shown that *T. gondii*-derived molecules could stimulate Toll-like receptors (TLRs) and regulate the production of pro-inflammatory cytokines such as IL-12, TNF-α or IL-6 [91]. These molecules might play a crucial role in modulating host-defense mechanisms and thus act as virulence factors. Profilin of *T. gondii* induces the production of IL-12, a cytokine necessary for the protective IFN-γ response via TLR11 dependent activation [92]. The parasite's heat shock protein 70 (TgHSP70) was shown to be a 'danger signal' during lethal acute *T. gondii* infection. Moreover, TgHSP70-induced nitric oxide (NO) release was dependent on TLR2 [93]. Glycosylphosphatidylinositols (GPIs) are involved in the pathogenicity of the protozoan parasites and are known to induce TNF-α production [94]. The equivalent molecules in *T. gondii* can both stimulate cytokine production in macrophages and serve as a TLR2 ligand [94]. Furthermore, *T. gondii* cyclophilin 18 can trigger IL-12 production via the CCR5-dependent pathway [95, 96]. Therefore, interaction of TLR with profilin, HSP70 and GPIs of *T. gondii*, and CCR5 with *T. gondii* cyclophilin 18 might contribute to host-cell apoptosis by overproduction of pro-inflammatory cytokines, resulting in a weakening of the host's resistance.

Apoptosis and Pathogenesis

T. gondii is auxotrophic with regard to critical metabolites including purines, certain amino acids [97] and cholesterol [98]. These nutrients have to be obtained from the host cell, scavenged either from the host's biosynthetic machinery or transport functions. Interestingly, cell metabolism and apoptosis itself are tightly linked particularly in the context of energy metabolism [99]. Starvation for specific nutrients serves as a potent apoptotic trigger, suggesting a nutritional reason for rapidly growing parasites to block apoptosis [99]. Furthermore, an apoptotic cell is likely to be a poor provider of critical components to the growing parasite. By blocking apoptosis, the parasite likely ensures a steady supply of metabolites for its growth.

The reduced levels of apoptosis in certain cell populations of the host may lead to an enhanced inflammatory response to the parasite [70, 72]. Inflammatory leukocytes limit parasite replication by T cell-independent effector mechanisms [100] but can also induce host mortality due to overwhelming immunopathology [3, 101]. After infection with *T. gondii*, the presence of CD8+ and CD4+ T lymphocytes with cytolytic activity against parasite-infected target cells have been observed [102, 103]. Because CD8+ T cells represent the more relevant effector cells in the effective control of *T. gondii* [104, 105], cytotoxicity via the induction of apoptosis has been thought to represent an important effector mechanism for restricting parasite growth. However, this is obscured by the fact that cytotoxic T-lymphocyte-mediated lysis of *T. gondii*-infected target cells does not lead to death of intracellular parasites [40] and enhances rapid egress of the parasite [88]. In perforin knockout mice, granule-mediated cytotoxicity of T lymphocytes and NK cells has indeed been shown to be dispensable in controlling parasite replication during the acute phase of infection [106]. The perforin-mediated target cell lysis partially restricted tissue cyst development within the brain and decreased susceptibility of mice during chronic *Toxoplasma* encephalitis [106]. These results suggested that cells harboring latent bradyzoite-containing tissue cysts are more susceptible to apoptosis induced by CTL-mediated cytotoxicity than tachyzoite-containing host cells. Bradyzoites and tachyzoites differ in their ability to interfere with signaling cascades of the host cells because of different metabolic systems and expressed proteins. Although apoptosis might play an important role in the innate and adaptive defense against acute infection with *T. gondii*, it would also contribute to parasite control during chronic toxoplasmic encephalitis.

Apoptosis plays a crucial role in the pathogenesis of *T. gondii* infection. Certain tissues maintain a condition of immune privilege through control of their populations of immune cells. Induction of high levels apoptosis in splenocytes [80, 81], Peyer's patch T cells [78], and peritoneal macrophages [72, 82] after infection of mice with *T. gondii* may lead to defective immune responses to the parasite. Importantly, extensive apoptosis was associated with high levels of parasite burden and increased susceptibility of mice to death after infection. T-cell and B-cell apoptosis can also be promoted by cells infected with *T. gondii* [79] through Fas–FasL interaction by a form of unilateral fratricide. The level of apoptosis in T lymphocytes and other leukocytes appears to correlate with the induction of pathology during toxoplasmosis. In the eye, the purpose of immune privilege is to prevent inflammatory cells from causing damage to the delicate structures required for vision [107]. To accomplish this, FasL and transforming growth factor (TGF)-β are produced by many ocular cells. FasL functions by engaging the death receptor pathways in activated T cells, and deleting T cells by apoptosis in a process similar to the AICD [108] seen during the stage of T-cell elimination at the end of an immune response [85]. CNS immune privilege was construed as CNS isolation from the immune system by the blood-brain barrier (BBB), the lack of draining lymphatics, and the apparent immunoincompetence of microglia, the resident CNS macrophage. The brain is limited in its capacity to deliver antigen to local lymph nodes and cause T-cell activation [109]. The skewing of the response to antigen from the brain towards a humoral response indicates the prevention of dangerous inflammatory T cell responses. It is unknown whether *T. gondii* penetrates the CNS selectively or whether these sites of immune privilege have limited capacity to eradicate the parasite. Progression of chronic toxoplasmosis in mice correlates with rising levels of IL-10 mRNA in the CNS [3]. Since the IL-10 modulates macrophage-mediated tachyzoite killing, production of anti-inflammatory mediators may contribute to toxoplasma encephalitis susceptibility [110]. Higher levels of IL-10 later during chronic infection could play a role in down-regulating the inflammatory response once the cyst burden has decreased and, in this way, could be beneficial for the host [111]. In addition, an early transient IL-4 response occurs in the brains of cyst-susceptible C57BL/10 mice [112, 113]. In the chronically infected brain, IL-4 (like IL-10) functions to down-regulate protective IFN-γ. The downside to immune privilege is that parasites such as *T. gondii* thrive in this environment. However, *T. gondii* expand this immunocompromised condition to other locations by regulating the transcriptional machinery of the host cells to produce FasL [114, 115], thereby encouraging removal of cells of the host immune system, and also by inhibiting expression of major histocompatibility class II molecules on antigen-presenting cells (APCs) by interfering with transcription pathways [116, 117].

The dual activity of *T. gondii* on host cell apoptosis might require an exquisitely balanced interplay between the parasite and the pro- and anti-apoptotic signals of the host. *T. gondii* relies on the integrity of its host cell and on a continuous supply of essential metabolites. Initiation of apoptosis in parasite-positive host cells might reduce the production of viable parasites, and *Toxoplasma* might thus rely on the inhibition of apoptosis of its host cell. Induction of apoptosis in certain immune cell populations might, however, be required to downregulate parasite-specific immune responses, thereby contributing to parasite survival but also to the prevention of immune-mediated pathology.

CONCLUDING REMARKS

Apoptosis has been established as a crucial modulator of host-parasite interactions. Apoptosis of *T. gondii*-infected host cells might exert parasiticidal activity, but this parasite has been shown to modulate host cell death via direct or indirect mechanisms. These are fascinating examples of how *T. gondii* evade potentially protective host responses, or even exploit host cell apoptosis, to establish and maintain parasitic infection. In order to distinguish between situations in which increased apoptosis functions as a host defense mechanism or represents an evasion strategy induced by the parasite, investigations of the inhibition of distinct apoptosis pathways are needed. The apoptotic cell itself plays a crucial role in the pathogenesis of parasitic infections by regulating activity of scavenger macrophages, parasite replication and host pathology. Furthermore, the discovery of *T. gondii* products which can both induce and inhibit host-cell apoptosis and the regulatory mechanisms between the parasite-derived factors and host factors help us to understand the pathogenesis of *T. gondii* infections and find new therapeutic approaches.

REFERENCES

[1]   Luft BJ, Remington JS. AIDS commentary. Toxoplasmic encephalitis. J Infect Dis 1988; 157: 1-6.
[2]   Denkers EY, Gazzinelli RT. Regulation and function of T-cell-mediated immunity during *Toxoplasma gondii* infection. Clin Microbiol Rev 1998; 11: 569-88.
[3]   Gazzinelli RT, Eltoum I, Wynn TA, Sher A. Acute cerebral toxoplasmosis is induced by *in vivo* neutralization of TNF-alpha and correlates with the down-regulated expression of inducible nitric oxide synthase and other markers of macrophage activation. J Immunol 1993; 151: 3672-81.
[4]   Carruthers VB, Suzuki Y. Effects of *Toxoplasma gondii* Infection on the Brain. Schizophr Bull 2007; 33: 745-51.
[5]   Dubey JP, Lindsay DS, Speer CA. Structures of *Toxoplasma gondii* tachyzoites, bradyzoites, and sporozoites and biology and development of tissue cysts. Clin Microbiol Rev 1998; 11: 267-99.

[6]   Vaux DL, Strasser A. The molecular biology of apoptosis. Proc Natl Acad Sci U S A 1996; 93: 2239-44.

[7]   Williams GT. Programmed cell death: a fundamental protective response to pathogens. Trends Microbiol 1994; 2: 463-4.

[8]   Barry M, Bleackley RC. Cytotoxic T lymphocytes: all roads lead to death. Nat Rev Immunol 2002; 2: 401-9.

[9]   Lüder CG, Gross U, Lopes MF. Intracellular protozoan parasites and apoptosis: diverse strategies to modulate parasite-host interactions. Trends Parasitol 2001; 17: 480-6.

[10] Roulston A, Marcellus RC, Branton PE. Viruses and apoptosis. Annu Rev Microbiol 1999; 53: 577-628.

[11] Engelman JA, Luo J, Cantley LC. The evolution of phosphatidylinositol 3-kinases as regulators of growth and metabolism. Nat Rev Genet 2006; 7: 606-19.

[12] Carmen JC, Sinai AP. Suicide prevention: disruption of apoptotic pathways by protozoan parasites. Mol Microbiol 2007; 64: 904-16.

[13] Schaumburg F, Hippe D, Vutova P, Lüder CG. Pro- and anti-apoptotic activities of protozoan parasites. Parasitology 2006; 132: 69-85.

[14] Sinai AP, Payne TM, Carmen JC, Hardi L, Watson SJ, Molestina RE. Mechanisms underlying the manipulation of host apoptotic pathways by *Toxoplasma gondii*. Int J Parasitol 2004; 34: 381-91

[15] Yuan J. Transducing signals of life and death. Curr Opin Cell Biol 1997; 9: 247-51.

[16] Trapani JA, Davis J, Sutton VR, Smyth MJ. Proapoptotic functions of cytotoxic lymphocyte granule constituents *in vitro* and *in vivo*. Curr Opin Immunol 2000; 12: 323-9.

[17] Thornberry NA, Lazebnik Y. Caspases: enemies within. Science 1998; 281: 1312-6.

[18] Deveraux QL, Stennicke HR, Salvesen GS, Reed JC. Endogenous inhibitors of caspases. J Clin Immunol 1999; 19: 388-98.

[19] Ekert PG, Silke J, Vaux DL. Caspase inhibitors. Cell Death Differ 1999; 6: 1081-6.

[20] Kischkel FC, Hellbardt S, Behrmann I, *et al*. Cytotoxicity-dependent APO-1 (Fas/CD95)-associated proteins form a death-inducing signaling complex (DISC) with the receptor. EMBO J 1995; 14: 5579-88.

[21] Muzio M, Chinnaiyan AM, Kischkel FC, *et al*. FLICE, a novel FADD-homologous ICE/CED-3-like protease, is recruited to the CD95 (Fas/APO-1) death--inducing signaling complex. Cell 1996; 85: 817-27.

[22] Peter ME, Krammer PH. The CD95(APO-1/Fas) DISC and beyond. Cell Death Differ 2003; 10: 26-35.

[23] Green DR. Apoptotic pathways: ten minutes to dead. Cell 2005; 121: 671-4.

[24] Opferman JT, Korsmeyer SJ. Apoptosis in the development and maintenance of the immune system. Nat Immunol 2003; 4: 410-5.

[25] Green DR, Reed JC. Mitochondria and apoptosis. Science 1998; 281: 1309-12.

[26] Saraste A, Pulkki K. Morphologic and biochemical hallmarks of apoptosis. Cardiovasc Res 2000; 45: 528-37.

[27] Kuwana T, Smith JJ, Muzio M, Dixit V, Newmeyer DD, Kornbluth S. Apoptosis induction by caspase-8 is amplified through the mitochondrial release of cytochrome c. J Biol Chem 1998; 273: 16589-94.

[28] Li H, Zhu H, Xu CJ, Yuan J. Cleavage of BID by caspase 8 mediates the mitochondrial damage in the Fas pathway of apoptosis. Cell 1998; 94: 491-501.

[29] Adams JM, Cory S. The Bcl-2 protein family: arbiters of cell survival. Science 1998; 281: 1322-6.

[30] Deveraux QL, Roy N, Stennicke HR, *et al*. IAPs block apoptotic events induced by caspase-8 and cytochrome c by direct inhibition of distinct caspases. EMBO J 1998; 17: 2215-23.

[31] Salvesen GS, Duckett CS. IAP proteins: blocking the road to death's door. Nat Rev Mol Cell Biol 2002; 3: 401-10.

[32] Korsmeyer SJ. BCL-2 gene family and the regulation of programmed cell death. Cancer Res 1999; 59: 1693-1700.

[33] Danial NN, Korsmeyer SJ. Cell death: critical control points. Cell 2004; 116: 205-19.

[34] Hayden MS, Ghosh S. Signaling to NF-kappaB. Genes Dev 2004; 18: 2195-224.

[35] Perkins ND. Integrating cell-signalling pathways with NF-kappaB and IKK function. Nat Rev Mol Cell Biol 2007; 8: 49-62.

[36] Karin M, Lin A. NF-kappaB at the crossroads of life and death. Nat Immunol 2002; 3: 221-7.

[37] Osaki M, Oshimura M, Ito H. PI3K-Akt pathway: its functions and alterations in human cancer. Apoptosis 2004; 9: 667-76.

[38] Yao R, Cooper GM. Requirement for phosphatidylinositol-3 kinase in the prevention of apoptosis by nerve growth factor. Science 1995; 267: 2003-6.

[39] Li Q, Verma IM. NF-kappaB regulation in the immune system. Nat Rev Immunol 2002; 2: 725-34

[40] Tato CM, Hunter CA. Host-pathogen interactions: subversion and utilization of the NF-kappa B pathway during infection. Infect Immun 2002; 70: 3311-7.

[41] Gazzinelli RT, Denkers EY. Protozoan encounters with Toll-like receptor signalling pathways: implications for host parasitism. Nat Rev Immunol 2006; 6: 895-906.

[42] Nash PB, Purner MB, Leon RP, Clarke P, Duke RC, Curiel TJ. *Toxoplasma gondii*-infected cells are resistant to multiple inducers of apoptosis. J Immunol 1998; 160: 1824-30.

[43] Goebel S, Lüder CG, Gross U. Invasion by *Toxoplasma gondii* protects human-derived HL-60 cells from actinomycin D-induced apoptosis. Med Microbiol Immunol 1999; 187: 221-6.

[44] Goebel S, Gross U, Lüder CG. Inhibition of host cell apoptosis by *Toxoplasma gondii* is accompanied by reduced activation of the caspase cascade and alterations of poly(ADP-ribose) polymerase expression. J Cell Sci 2001; 114: 3495-505.

[45]   Hippe D, Gais A, Gross U, Lüder CG. Modulation of caspase activation by *Toxoplasma gondii*. Methods Mol Biol 2009; 470: 275-88.

[46]   Payne TM, Molestina RE, Sinai AP. Inhibition of caspase activation and a requirement for NF-kappaB function in the *Toxoplasma gondii*-mediated blockade of host apoptosis. J Cell Sci 2003; 116: 4345-58.

[47]   Hippe D, Lytovchenko O, Schmitz I, Lüder CG. Fas/CD95-mediated apoptosis of type II cells is blocked by *Toxoplasma gondii* primarily via interference with the mitochondrial amplification loop. Infect Immun 2008; 76: 2905-12.

[48]   Hozak RR, Manji GA, Friesen PD. The BIR motifs mediate dominant interference and oligomerization of inhibitor of apoptosis Op-IAP. Mol Cell Biol 2000; 20: 1877-85.

[49]   Schwab JC, Beckers CJ, Joiner KA. The parasitophorous vacuole membrane surrounding intracellular *Toxoplasma gondii* functions as a molecular sieve. Proc Natl Acad Sci U S A 1994; 91: 509-13.

[50]   Fischer HG, Stachelhaus S, Sahm M, Meyer HE, Reichmann G. GRA7, an excretory 29 kDa *Toxoplasma gondii* dense granule antigen released by infected host cells. Mol Biochem Parasitol 1998; 91: 251-62.

[51]   Kim L, Denkers EY. *Toxoplasma gondii* triggers Gi-dependent PI 3-kinase signaling required for inhibition of host cell apoptosis. J Cell Sci 2006; 119: 2119-26.

[52]   Molestina RE, Sinai AP. Host and parasite-derived IKK activities direct distinct temporal phases of NF-kappaB activation and target gene expression following *Toxoplasma gondii* infection. J Cell Sci 2005; 118: 5785-96.

[53]   Molestina RE, Sinai AP. Detection of a novel parasite kinase activity at the *Toxoplasma gondii* parasitophorous vacuole membrane capable of phosphorylating host IkappaBalpha. Cell Microbiol 2005; 7: 351-62.

[54]   Butcher BA, Kim L, Johnson PF, Denkers EY. *Toxoplasma gondii* tachyzoites inhibit proinflammatory cytokine induction in infected macrophages by preventing nuclear translocation of the transcription factor NF-kappa B. J Immunol 2001; 167: 2193-201.

[55]   Butcher BA, Denkers EY. Mechanism of entry determines the ability of *Toxoplasma gondii* to inhibit macrophage proinflammatory cytokine production. Infect Immun 2002; 70: 5216-24.

[56]   Shapira S, Harb OS, Margarit J, *et al*. Initiation and termination of NF-kappaB signaling by the intracellular protozoan parasite *Toxoplasma gondii*. J Cell Sci 2005; 118: 3501-8.

[57]   Shapira S, Speirs K, Gerstein A, Caamano J, Hunter CA. Suppression of NF-kappaB activation by infection with *Toxoplasma gondii*.J Infect Dis 2002; 185: 66-72.

[58]   Molestina RE, Payne TM, Coppens I, Sinai AP. Activation of NF-kappaB by *Toxoplasma gondii* correlates with increased expression of antiapoptotic genes and localization of phosphorylated IkappaB to the parasitophorous vacuole membrane. J Cell Sci 2003; 116: 4359-71.

[59]   Denkers EY, Kim L, Butcher BA. In the belly of the beast: subversion of macrophage proinflammatory signalling cascades during *Toxoplasma gondii* infection. Cell Microbiol 2003; 5: 75-83.

[60]   Lieberman LA, Hunter CA. The role of cytokines and their signaling pathways in the regulation of immunity to *Toxoplasma gondii*. Int Rev Immunol 2002; 21: 373-403.

[61]   Senegas A, Villard O, Neuville A, *et al*. *Toxoplasma gondii*-induced foetal resorption in mice involves interferon-gamma-induced apoptosis and spiral artery dilation at the maternofoetal interface. Int J Parasitol 2009; 39: 481-7.

[62]   Beg AA, Baltimore D. An essential role for NF-kappaB in preventing TNF-alpha-induced cell death. Science 1996; 274: 782-4.

[63]   Lingelbach K, Joiner KA. The parasitophorous vacuole membrane surrounding *Plasmodium* and *Toxoplasma*: an unusual compartment in infected cells. J Cell Sci 1998; 111: 1467-75.

[64]   Goldstein JC, Waterhouse NJ, Juin P, Evan GI, Green DR. The coordinate release of cytochrome c during apoptosis is rapid, complete and kinetically invariant. Nat Cell Biol 2000; 2: 156-62.

[65]   Vander Heiden MG, Thompson CB. Bcl-2 proteins: regulators of apoptosis or of mitochondrial homeostasis? Nat Cell Biol 1999; 1: 209-16

[66]   Keller P, Schaumburg F, Fischer SF, Häcker G, Gross U, Lüder CG. Direct inhibition of cytochrome c-induced caspase activation *in vitro* by *Toxoplasma gondii* reveals novel mechanisms of interference with host cell apoptosis. FEMS Microbiol Lett 2006; 258: 312-9.

[67]   Carmen JC, Hardi L, Sinai AP. *Toxoplasma gondii* inhibits ultraviolet light-induced apoptosis through multiple interactions with the mitochondrion-dependent programmed cell death pathway. Cell Microbiol 2006; 8: 301-15.

[68]   Tournier C, Hess P, Yang DD, *et al*. Requirement of JNK for stress-induced activation of the cytochrome c-mediated death pathway. Science 2000; 288: 870-4.

[69]   Carmen JC, Southard RC, Sinai AP. The complexity of signaling in host-pathogen interactions revealed by the *Toxoplasma gondii*-dependent modulation of JNK phosphorylation. Exp Cell Res 2008; 314: 3724-36.

[70]   Orlofsky A, Weiss LM, Kawachi N, Prystowsky MB. Deficiency in the anti-apoptotic protein A1-a results in a diminished acute inflammatory response. J Immunol 2002; 168: 1840-6.

[71]   Gais A, Beinert N, Gross U, Lüder CG. Transient inhibition of poly(ADP-ribose) polymerase expression and activity by *Toxoplasma gondii* is dispensable for parasite-mediated blockade of host cell apoptosis and intracellular parasite replication. Microbes Infect 2008; 10: 358-66.

[72] Hisaeda H, Sakai T, Ishikawa H, *et al.* Heat shock protein 65 induced by gammadelta T cells prevents apoptosis of macrophages and contributes to host defense in mice infected with *Toxoplasma gondii*. J Immunol 1997; 159: 2375-81.

[73] Luft BJ, Kansas G, Engleman EG, Remington JS. Functional and quantitative alterations in T lymphocyte subpopulations in acute toxoplasmosis. J Infect Dis 1984; 150: 761-7.

[74] Strickland GT, Sayles PC. Depressed antibody responses to a thymus-dependent antigen in toxoplasmosis. Infect Immun 1977; 15: 184-90.

[75] Wing EJ, Boehmer SM, Christner LK. *Toxoplasma gondii*: decreased resistance to intracellular bacteria in mice. Exp Parasitol. 1983; 56: 1-8.

[76] Yano A, Norose K, Yamashita K, *et al.* Immune response to *Toxoplasma gondii*--analysis of suppressor T cells in a patient with symptomatic acute toxoplasmosis. J Parasitol. 1987; 73: 954-61.

[77] Khan IA, Matsuura T, Kasper LH. Activation-mediated CD4+ T cell unresponsiveness during acute *Toxoplasma gondii* infection in mice. Int Immunol 1996; 8: 887-96.

[78] Liesenfeld O, Kosek JC, Suzuki Y. Gamma interferon induces Fas-dependent apoptosis of Peyer's patch T cells in mice following peroral infection with *Toxoplasma gondii*. Infect Immun 1997; 65: 4682-9.

[79] Wei S, Marches F, Borvak J, *et al. Toxoplasma gondii*-infected human myeloid dendritic cells induce T-lymphocyte dysfunction and contact-dependent apoptosis. Infect Immun. 2002; 70: 1750-60.

[80] Gavrilescu LC, Denkers EY. IFN-gamma overproduction and high level apoptosis are associated with high but not low virulence *Toxoplasma gondii* infection. J Immunol 2001; 167: 902-9.

[81] Mordue DG, Monroy F, La Regina M, Dinarello CA, Sibley LD. Acute toxoplasmosis leads to lethal overproduction of Th1 cytokines. J Immunol 2001; 167: 4574-84.

[82] Nishikawa Y, Kawase O, Vielemeyer O, *et al. Toxoplasma gondii* infection induces apoptosis in noninfected macrophages: role of nitric oxide and other soluble factors. Parasite Immunol 2007; 29: 375-85.

[83] Grigg ME, Bonnefoy S, Hehl AB, Suzuki Y, Boothroyd JC. Success and virulence in *Toxoplasma* as the result of sexual recombination between two distinct ancestries. Science 2001; 294: 161-5.

[84] Ge YY, Zhang L, Zhang G, *et al.* In pregnant mice, the infection of *Toxoplasma gondii* causes the decrease of CD4+CD25+ -regulatory T cells. Parasite Immunol 2008; 30: 471-81.

[85] Hu MS, Schwartzman JD, Yeaman GR, *et al.* Fas-FasL interaction involved in pathogenesis of ocular toxoplasmosis in mice. Infect Immun 1999; 67: 928-35.

[86] Van Parijs L, Abbas AK. Role of Fas-mediated cell death in the regulation of immune responses. Curr Opin Immunol 1996; 8: 355-61

[87] Caamaño J, Tato C, Cai G, *et al.* Identification of a role for NF-kappa B2 in the regulation of apoptosis and in maintenance of T cell-mediated immunity to *Toxoplasma gondii*. J Immunol 2000; 165: 5720-8.

[88] Persson EK, Agnarson AM, Lambert H, *et al.* Death receptor ligation or exposure to perforin trigger rapid egress of the intracellular parasite *Toxoplasma gondii*. J Immunol 2007; 179: 8357-65.

[89] Bannai H, Nishikawa Y, Matsuo T, *et al.* Programmed Cell Death 5 from *Toxoplasma gondii*: a secreted molecule that exerts a pro-apoptotic effect on host cells. Mol Biochem Parasitol 2008; 159: 112-20.

[90] Bannai H, Nishikawa Y, Ibrahim HM, *et al.* Overproduction of the pro-apoptotic molecule, programmed cell death 5, in *Toxoplasma gondii* leads to increased apoptosis of host macrophages. J Vet Med Sci 2009; 71: 1183-89.

[91] Yarovinsky F, Sher A. Toll-like receptor recognition of *Toxoplasma gondii*. Int J Parasitol 2006; 36: 255-9.

[92] Yarovinsky F, Zhang D, Andersen JF, *et al.* TLR11 activation of dendritic cells by a protozoan profilin-like protein. Science 2005; 308: 1626-9.

[93] Mun HS, Aosai F, Norose K, *et al.* Toll-like receptor 4 mediates tolerance in macrophages stimulated with *Toxoplasma gondii*-derived heat shock protein 70. Infect Immun 2005; 73: 4634-42.

[94] Debierre-Grockiego F, Azzouz N, Schmidt J, *et al.* Roles of glycosylphosphatidylinositols of *Toxoplasma gondii*. Induction of tumor necrosis factor-alpha production in macrophages. J Biol Chem 2003; 278: 32987-93.

[95] Aliberti J, Valenzuela JG, Carruthers VB, *et al.* Molecular mimicry of a CCR5 binding-domain in the microbial activation of dendritic cells. Nat Immunol 2003; 4: 485-90.

[96] Yarovinsky F, Andersen JF, King LR, *et al.* Structural determinants of the anti-HIV activity of a CCR5 antagonist derived from *Toxoplasma gondii*. J Biol Chem 2004; 279: 53635-42.

[97] Sinai AP, Joiner KA. Safe haven: the cell biology of nonfusogenic pathogen vacuoles. Annu Rev Microbiol 1997; 51: 415-62.

[98] Coppens I, Sinai AP, Joiner KA. *Toxoplasma gondii* exploits host low-density lipoprotein receptor-mediated endocytosis for cholesterol acquisition. J Cell Biol 2000; 149: 167-80.

[99] Plas DR, Thompson CB. Cell metabolism in the regulation of programmed cell death. Trends Endocrinol Metab 2002; 13: 75-8.

[100] Sher A, Oswald IP, Hieny S, Gazzinelli RT. *Toxoplasma gondii* induces a T-independent IFN-gamma response in natural killer cells that requires both adherent accessory cells and tumor necrosis factor-alpha. J Immunol 1993; 150: 3982-9.

[101] Gazzinelli RT, Wysocka M, Hieny S, *et al*. In the absence of endogenous IL-10, mice acutely infected with *Toxoplasma gondii* succumb to a lethal immune response dependent on CD4+ T cells and accompanied by overproduction of IL-12, IFN-gamma and TNF-alpha. J Immunol 1996; 157: 798-805.

[102] Hakim FT, Gazzinelli RT, Denkers E, Hieny S, Shearer GM, Sher A. CD8+ T cells from mice vaccinated against *Toxoplasma gondii* are cytotoxic for parasite-infected or antigen-pulsed host cells. J Immunol 1991; 147: 2310-6.

[103] Montoya JG, Lowe KE, Clayberger C, *et al*. Human CD4+ and CD8+ T lymphocytes are both cytotoxic to *Toxoplasma gondii*-infected cells. Infect Immun 1996; 64: 176-81.

[104] Gazzinelli R, Xu Y, Hieny S, Cheever A, Sher A. Simultaneous depletion of CD4+ and CD8+ T lymphocytes is required to reactivate chronic infection with *Toxoplasma gondii*. J Immunol 1992; 149: 175-80.

[105] Suzuki Y, Remington JS. Dual regulation of resistance against *Toxoplasma gondii* infection by Lyt-2+ and Lyt-1+, L3T4+ T cells in mice. J Immunol 1988; 140: 3943-6.

[106] Denkers EY, Yap G, Scharton-Kersten T, *et al*. Perforin-mediated cytolysis plays a limited role in host resistance to *Toxoplasma gondii*. J Immunol 1997; 159: 1903-8.

[107] Streilein JW. Ocular immune privilege: the eye takes a dim but practical view of immunity and inflammation. J Leukoc Biol 2003; 74: 179-85.

[108] Ferguson TA, Stuart PM, Herndon JM, Griffith TS. Apoptosis, tolerance, and regulatory T cells--old wine, new wineskins. Immunol Rev 2003; 193: 111-23.

[109] Mendez-Fernandez YV, Hansen MJ, Rodriguez M, Pease LR. Anatomical and cellular requirements for the activation and migration of virus-specific CD8+ T cells to the brain during Theiler's virus infection. J Virol 2005; 79: 3063-70.

[110] Gazzinelli RT, Oswald IP, James S, Sher A. IL-10 inhibits parasite killing and nitrogen oxide production by IFN-γ activated macrophages. J Immunol 1992; 148: 1792-6.

[111] Burke JA, Roberts CW, Hunter CA, Murray M, Alexander J. Temporal differences in the expression of mRNA for IL-10 and IFN-γ in the brains and spleens of C57BL/6 mice infected with *Toxoplasma gondii*. Parasite Immunol 1994;16: 305-14

[112] Hunter CA., Roberts CW, Alexander J. Kinetics of cytokine mRNA production in the brains of mice with progressive toxoplasmic encephalitis. Eur J Immunol 1992; 22: 2317-22.

[113] Roberts CW, Ferguson DJP, Jebbari H, Satoskar A, Bluethmann H, Alexander J. 1996. Different roles for interleukin-4 during the course of *Toxoplasma gondii* infection. Infect Immun 1996; 64: 897-904.

[114] Eidsmo L, Wolday D, Berhe N, *et al*. Alteration of Fas and Fas ligand expression during human visceral leishmaniasis. Clin Exp Immunol 2002; 130: 307-13.

[115] Nishikawa Y, Makala L, Otsuka H, Mikami T, Nagasawa H. Mechanisms of apoptosis in murine fibroblasts by two intracellular protozoan parasites, *Toxoplasma gondii* and *Neospora caninum*. Parasite Immunol 2002; 24: 347-54.

[116] Lüder CG, Lang C, Giraldo-Velasquez M, Algner M, Gerdes J, Gross U. *Toxoplasma gondii* inhibits MHC class II expression in neural antigen-presenting cells by down-regulating the class II transactivator CIITA. J Neuroimmunol 2003; 134: 12-24.

[117] Lüder CG, Stanway RR, Chaussepied M, Langsley G, Heussler VT. Intracellular survival of apicomplexan parasites and host cell modification. Int J Parasitol 2009; 39: 163-73.

CHAPTER 9

Presentation of Skin-Derived *Leishmania* Antigen by Dendritic Cell Subtypes

Uwe Ritter*

Department of Immunology, University of Regensburg, Regensburg, Germany

Abstract: The tropical disease leishmaniasis is initiated by flagellated parasites of the genus *Leishmania (L.)*, which are inoculated into the skin during the blood meal of a sandfly vector. A broad spectrum of clinical manifestations in humans, ranging from a self-limiting cutaneous infection to disseminating visceral leishmaniasis, are described with respect to the transmitted *Leishmania* species. During the last decades the experimental model of leishmaniasis, in which mice are infected with stationary phase promastigote parasites, allowed the examination of many immunological details of the host-parasite interaction. For instance, it is shown that the obligatory intracellular *Leishmania* parasites need phagocytic cells for replication as soon as the parasites are located in the dermal compartment. In this regard, neutrophils and macrophages play a pivotal role as host cells for *Leishmania* replication. On the other hand, infected macrophages produce leishmanicidal molecules after appropriate activation by antigen-specific T helper (h) cells. Thus, healing of leishmaniasis is associated with a protective Th1-type response, characterized by an early interferon-γ production by CD4$^+$ T cells and the expression of inducible nitric oxide synthase by activated macrophages. In this context, it is generally accepted that professional antigen presenting cells are crucial for the induction of the protective Th1-type response in skin-draining lymph nodes. Due to the fact that *L. major* parasites enter the body via the skin, epidermal Langerhans Cells (LCs) were thought to be responsible for the initiation of the adaptive T cell-mediated immunity. More recent data indicate that dermal Dendritic Cells (DCs), rather than epidermal LCs, might be important for the initiation of the adaptive immune response. However, an indirect role for migratory skin-derived epidermal LCs in T cell-mediated immunity, possibly in delivering skin-derived antigens to cutaneous lymph node-resident DCs, could not be excluded in general. Based on the current knowledge about the role of DC subsets in experimental leishmaniasis, it is feasible that distinct DC subtypes interact with particular T cell populations: LCs with "regulatory" T cells, Langerin$^+$ DCs with CD8$^+$ T cells, and Langerin$^-$ DCs with CD4$^+$ T cells.

INTRODUCTION

The skin is one of the largest organs in humans and fulfils different physiological and immunological functions. The cutaneous compartment is the interface to the environment and faces chemical compounds and microorganisms, some of which are pathogens that should not enter the mammalian organism.

In this context, physical barriers such as the epidermis are crucial to protect the body from invading microorganisms (Fig. **1A**). Additionally, the uppermost part of the *Stratum corneum* is coated with lipids that inhibit the infiltration of microorganisms into deeper layers such as the dermis (Fig. **1B**). Further protection is mediated by a shield of dead keratinocytes, which first proliferate and die upon translocation to the surface of the epidermis (*Stratum lucidum*).

However, all particular strategies to prevent the skin from infections are futile once pathogens are incorporated into the dermal compartment; that happens when skin-barriers are damaged by injury or blood-sucking arthropods. In this case, different pathogens such as protozoans, viruses, and bacteria are transmitted directly into the dermis of mammalians. If this takes place, an efficient antigen-specific immune response against skin-invading pathogens needs to be mounted as soon as possible to prevent subsequent spreading of the microorganisms within the host.

Mammalians possess complex soluble and cellular defense mechanisms to combat invading pathogens such as *Leishmania* parasites. It is commonly accepted that professional antigen presenting cells (APCs), such as dendritic cells (DCs), are crucial for initiation of an efficient immune response against these parasites. However, the distinct subtypes of DCs mediating the initiation of that specific defense cascade are discussed controversially. In the following chapters, processes involved in the initiation of a T cell-mediated immune response will be presented in detail.

*Corresponding Author: Uwe Ritter, Dept. of Immunology, University of Regensburg, Franz-Josef-Strauss-Allee-11, Regensburg, Germany. Tel.: +49-941-944-5464. Fax: +49-941-944-5462; e-mail: uwe.ritter@klinik.uni-regensburg.de

Emilio Jirillo (Ed)
All rights reserved - © 2010 Bentham Science Publishers Ltd.

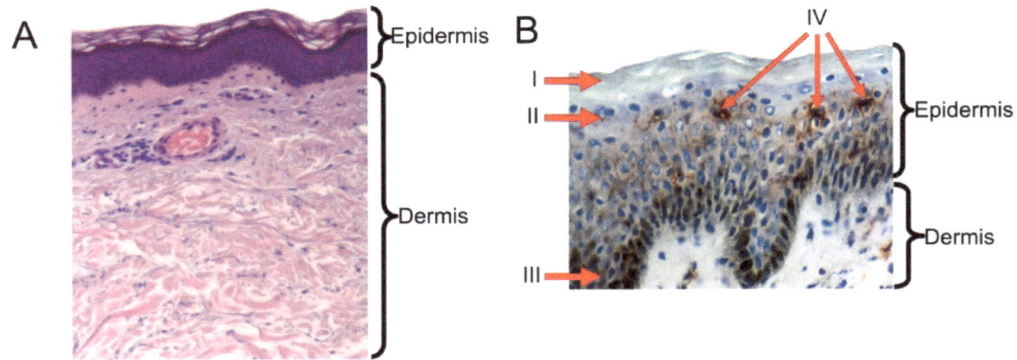

Figure 1: Bright field illuminations of human skin sections. A) Overview of the anatomical structures of the human skin. The epidermal and dermal compartments are shown (the paraffin section was kindly provided by Esther von Stebut, Department of Dermatology Mainz, Germany). Counterstaining was performed with Hematoxylin and Eosin. **B)** An immunohistochemstry staining performed with anti-CD1a monoclonal antibody, recognizing Langerhans cells, is shown. For visualization of CD1a-positive cells, a three-step streptavidin-peroxidase method with 3-amino-9-ethyl-carbazole as substrate was used [8]. Counterstaining was performed with Hematoxylin. (I = *Stratum corneum*, II = *Stratum lucidum*, III = Melanocytes, IV = Langerhans cells).

THE TROPICAL DISEASE LEISHMANIASIS

Leishmaniasis is a vector-borne parasitic infection encountered in tropical and subtropical regions of the world. The obligatory intracellular protozoan parasite, responsible for the disease, is a member of the Genus *Leishmania* (*L.*) (Family: *Trypanosomatidae,* Order: *Kinetoplastida*).

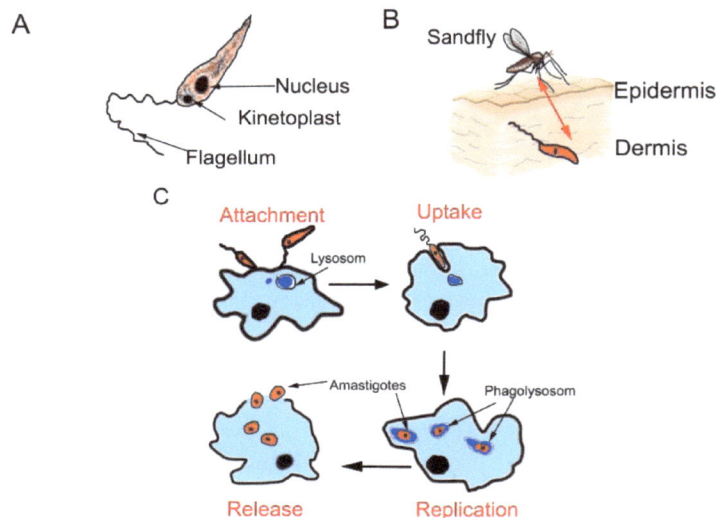

Figure 2: The live cycle of *Leishmania major* parasites. A) This schematic illustration shows the spindle-shaped form of a promastigote *L. major* parasite. The major characteristics of that parasite stage, such as *flagellum, kinetoplast*, and *nucleus* are indicated. **B)** The transmission of *Leishmania* parasites into the dermal compartment of the mammalian host is displayed. **C)** Transformation of promastigote parasites to amastigotes parasites. For phagocytosis, an attachment of parasites to phagocytic cells is necessary. Based on the specific milieu within the phagolysosome, the parasite modifies its protein biosynthesis to survive within that toxic environment. Furthermore, the parasite changes its morphology. It becomes compact and reduces the *flagellum*. Due to the intracellular parasite replication, the phagocytes burst. The released amastigote parasites are phagocytosed by other phagocytic cells. The parasite starts to spread and the clinical picture of leishmaniasis emerges.

One characteristic feature of the diploid parasites is the so-called flagella pocket, an invagination of the inner plasma membrane at the front part of the cell body that forms the exit site of the *flagellum* (Fig. **2A**) [1]. This *flagellum* adheres the parasite to the digestive tract of the invertebrate sandfly vectors. Furthermore, promastigote parasites use their *flagellum* to migrate to the sandfly's proboscis. This is a crucial event, because it allows between ten and one hundred parasites to be transferred to the mammalian host by subcutaneous injection during the blood meal (Fig. **2B**) [2].

Leishmania parasites have evolved a smart strategy to hide from the host immune response once they have entered the dermal compartment. As shown in (Fig. **2C**), the parasites allow themselves to be absorbed by host cells. This procedure is called phagocytosis and is generally defined as a process in which phagocytic cells (e.g. macrophages) engulf microorganisms and cellular debris. Specific surface molecules of the parasite facilitate the activation of the complement system, resulting in a coating of the parasite surface with complement fragment C3bi and C3b. Because macrophages express the corresponding complement receptor 3 (CR3) for C3bi and C3b, a contact between parasites and macrophages is induced and a complex program is started by the macrophages to engulf the parasite. After phagocytosis, the parasites are detectable within specialized compartments called phagolysosome (PV), in which promastigote parasites lose the external *flagellum* and transform into amastigotes which are adapted to the conditions within the PVs (Fig. **2C** and [3] for further reading). Besides macrophages, *Leishmania* parasites can also be detected within DCs, neutrophils, and fibroblasts [4, 5].

In contrast to extracellular promastigote parasites, which show just a short interaction with mammalian host cells, amastigotes can persist within their human host cells for years and are responsible for different clinical courses of the disease [6]. Both partners are responsible for the different clinical courses: *i*) the genus of *Leishmania* spp. and *ii*) the host-specific factors. In humans, diverse organs such as the skin, mucosa, and internal organs can be affected.

L. donovani and *L. infantum* cause **visceral leishmaniasis** that in the old world is mainly prevalent in India and to a lesser extent also in parts of southern Europe, the Middle East, and East and Central Africa. In visceral leishmaniasis, the infection is not confined to the entry site of the parasite but spreads to internal organs such as the liver, which enlarges due to an accumulation of Kupffer cells. Additionally, parasite clusters are detectable in the spleen and also in the bone marrow. The incubation period of this form of leishmaniasis lasts between two weeks and eighteen months. If it remains untreated, secondary infections such as pneumonia, tuberculosis, or dysentery can be lethal [7].

Cutaneous leishmaniasis in the old world is mostly restricted to the Middle East and the Mediterranean region (Fig. **3A**).

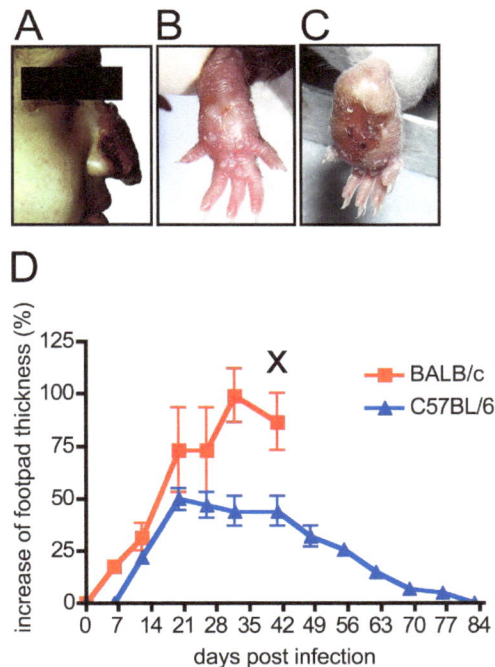

Figure 3: Leishmaniasis. A) The clinical manifestation of cutaneous leishmaniasis caused by *Leishmania tropica* is shown. One characteristic of that disease is the massive ulceration at the site of infection (the picture was kindly provided by PD Dr. J. Clos, Bernhard-Nocht-Institute for Tropical Medicine, Hamburg, Germany). **B)** Resistant C57BL/6 mice developed signs of inflammation at the site of infection. An infected footpad 23 days after infection is shown. C) Susceptible BALB/c mice show massive swelling and ulceration at the site of infection. A representative infected footpad 33 days after infection is shown. D) The increase in footpad swelling is monitored and represents an indicator for both the manifestation of the parasite and subsequently the efficiency of the host derived immune response against the parasites. As indicated in the figure, the course of leishmaniasis depends on the genetically background. In contrast to C57BL/6 mice (B), BALB/c mice develop a strong footpad swelling and ulceration at the site of infection (C and D). Experiment with BALB/c mice usually are terminated 40 days after infection (see C, "X").

Causative organisms of this form of leishmaniasis are *L. tropica, L. aethiopica, L. mexicana,* and *L. braziliensis* as well as *L. major,* which is used for most studies performed in the experimental model of leishmaniasis. Depending on the host immune response, two different clinical pictures can develop: in a cell-mediated immune response, a small knot forms at the entry site two to eight weeks after infection, which first ulcerates and then heals up within three to 24 months. This so-called localized cutaneous leishmaniasis (LCL) imparts protection against reinfection. Furthermore, most of the patients suffering with LCL develop a delayed type hypersensitivity reaction (after 24-72 hours) against *Leishmania* antigen when tested with the Montenegro Skin Test [8].

If no or no sufficient cell-mediated immune response takes place, extensive additional lesions develop, which lead to a leper like clinical picture that is called diffuse cutaneous leishmaniasis (DCL). This variant of leishmaniasis is rarely seen in infections with *L. mexicana* and can persist for years. In contrast to LCL, DCL patients do not develop a DTH reaction against *Leishmania* parasites [8, 9].

Mucocutaneous leishmaniasis is caused by *L. braziliensis, L. mexicana,* and the subspecies of *L. peruviana* and is predominantly spread in South and Central America. It initially resembles cutaneous leishmaniasis but soon metastasizes to the nasal and oropharyngeal mucosa, which leads to severe tissue damage and deformations. This can happen several weeks or even years after cure of the cutaneous lesion [10].

Leishmaniasis is mainly treated with Antimonial compounds, such as Glucantime, that blocks enzymes of the parasitic metabolism, and purine analogs and polyamines, which are toxic to the parasites. More recently additional therapeutic drugs came up like liposomal Amphotericin B, Miltefosine, and Paromomycin [11]. However, these treatments are known to induce side effects; therefore, prophylactic measures are currently in face of development. Among others, various devitalized or subunit vaccines have been tested as well as vaccines using attenuated *Leishmania* parasites [12]. Furthermore, DNA vaccines have been shown to promote immunity for a prolonged period of time in experimental models. However, an efficient vaccination is not available at the moment [13].

THE HOST IMMUNE RESPONSE AGAINST *LEISHMANIA MAJOR*

Adaptive Immunity

Invading a mammalian organism is risky for the parasite. It is important for the parasite that infected host cells as well as the host, survive as long as possible to provide a parasite reservoir for other sandflies not yet infected with *Leishmania spp.* In other words, parasites that kill their host before non-infected sandflies have a chance to get infected while soaking blood limit their own propagation. Thus it is not astonishing that *Leishmania* parasites show smart strategies to hide within distinct host cells such as myeloid cells for subsequent replication without killing their mammalian host organism.

In addition to humans, rodents are natural hosts for some *Leishmania* spp. Therefore, some pathological manifestations seen in humans have been successfully reproduced in rodents (Fig. **3B, C, D**). Consequently, the knowledge about the immune response against *Leishmania* parasites was predominantly generated within the experimental animal model of leishmaniasis.

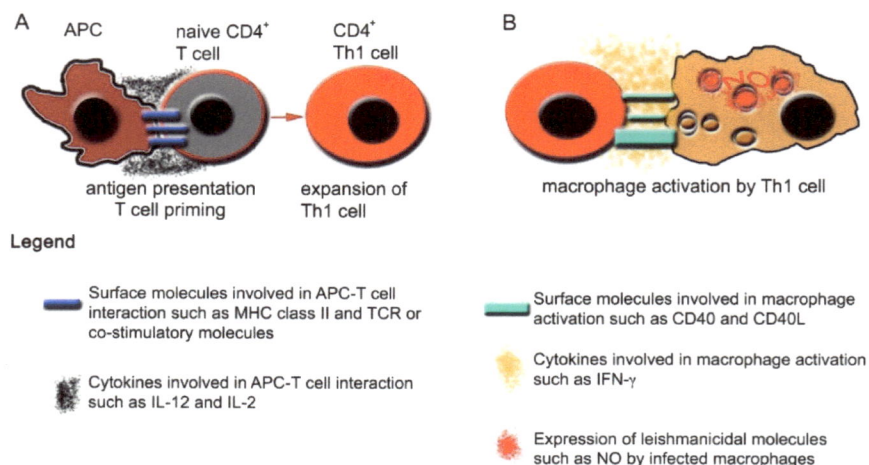

Figure 4: Simplified scheme of priming and function of Th1 type effector cells. A) Antigen presenting cells (APCs) present processed antigen via MHC class II molecules to CD4$^+$ T cells. The presence of costimulatory molecules on APCs results in the activation of naïve

antigen-specific Th1 cells. In the presence of soluble mediators such as IL-12 and IL-2, antigen-specific T cells start to proliferate and expand. Subsequently, Th1 effector cells are induced. **B)** One hallmark of Th1 type effector cells is the expression of the Th1 cytokine IFN-γ and the surface marker CD40L. This phenotype enables them to activate infected macrophages. After appropriate activation by Th1 cells, macrophages start to produce leishmanicidal molecules like NO that kill the parasite (indicated by NO radicals and red color within the macrophage).

Under laboratory conditions, inbred mice of different genetic backgrounds develop divergent immune responses following subcutaneous or intradermal infection with *L. major*. It is important to mention that beside the genetic background of the infected mice, the *L. major* strain used for infection experiments influences the course of disease [14].

The conventional *L. major* mouse model uses a high dose of parasites for infection (1-3×10^6) whereas other groups use lower numbers (10-1000) of parasites for infection. After parasite inoculation, soluble and cellular components of the innate immune response interact with the parasites [15]. Especially neutrophils are detectable within hours at the site of infection and dominate the cellular infiltrate [16]. Neutrophils are well known as traditional phagocytes contributing to the "first line of defense" against infectious agents or "non-self" substances that penetrate the body's physical barriers [17]. Paradoxically, the very same myeloid cells are involved in parasite survival and replication. Based on human neutrophils (and macrophages), some authors propose a "Trojan horse" function of neutrophils, in which *Leishmania* parasites within apoptotic neutrophils are transferred to macrophages, where the replication of parasites continues [5, 18, 19]. Consequently, both cell types, macrophages and neutrophils, are pivotal for initial parasite replication within the host. At the first glance, macrophages seem to be save havens for *Leishmania* parasites. However, macrophages change their "handling" of the parasites dramatically after the adaptive immune response is initiated.

Healing of leishmaniasis correlates with the ability to develop a protective CD4$^+$ T cell response also designated as T helper 1 (Th1) response – characterized by an early interferon-γ (IFN-γ) production by Th1 cells and the expression of inducible nitric oxide synthase by activated macrophages (Fig. **4B**) [20]. In contrast to Th1-competent C57BL/6 mice, susceptibility of BALB/c mice is associated with a diminished IFN-γ-, but increased IL-4-production (Fig. **3C**) [20]. Thus, CD4$^+$ T cells were shown to be the key players in the adaptive immune response against *L. major* ([21] for further reading).

Th1 and Th2 effector cells derive from a common CD4$^+$ T cell precursor [22]. Several stimuli have been reported to influence the pathway of maturation of CD4$^+$ T cell precursors [23]. Using CD4$^+$ T cells transgenic for a unique TCR alpha/beta receptor, it was demonstrated that certain cytokines such as IL-12 and IL-4 are crucial for the polarization of Th1 or Th2 cells, respectively [23]. But which antigen presenting cells produce these Th1- or Th2-driving cytokines?

One of the central processes in T cell activation is the cell-cell contact of T cells and professional antigen presenting cells such as DCs. In this context, it was proposed that different kinds of DC with different capacities to drive Th1 (DC1 cells) or Th2 T cells (DC2 cells) might exist [24]. Another quite attractive hypothesis postulates that distinct DCs of the epidermal compartment, so called Langerhans cells (LCs), are responsible for priming CD4$^+$ T cells [25]. However, the role of LCs in experimental leishmaniasis is discussed controversially [26-28]. The current view of their involvement in T cell-mediated immune response against *L. major* parasites will be presented in the following chapter.

It is commonly accepted that peptides need to be bound to MHC class II molecules for the induction of an antigen-specific Th1 response. Beside the contact between MHC class-II molecule and the T cell receptor (TCR), additional signals mediated by co-stimulatory molecules (e.g.CD28-CD80) and soluble cytokines (mainly IL-12, IL-2, IL-21) are necessary for clonal expansion of Th1 cells (Fig. **4A**).

The CD4$^+$ T cells are primed in skin-draining LNs (SDLNs) but must exit them and enter the site of infection to perform their effector functions [29]. After antigen-specific activation, effector T cells show distinct modification of their repertoires of trafficking ligands and receptors that restrict their ability to interact with different microvessels.

The expression of the LN-homing receptor CD62L on naïve T cells is important to facilitate migration into the SDLNs [30]. The density of CD62L molecules on T cells is substantially decreased after their activation and subsequent division *in vivo* [31]. Consequently, the properties to interact with the mucin-like ligands within the SDLNs are abrogated. Thus, activated T cells can start their passage to the periphery. Due to the fact that effector T cells that are primed in SDLNs show migratory selectivity for the skin, distinct zip codes were postulated responsible for that tissue-specific homing (for further reading [32]). Mainly the molecules P-/E-selectin ligands and the chemokine receptor (CCR) 4 and/or CCR10 are discussed to be crucial for efficient homing into the skin. Based on these distinct skin-homing patterns, Th1 cells migrate to the site of infection where they get the chance to activate infected macrophages by releasing IFN-γ and/or CD40-CD40L interaction. After activation, macrophages produce leishmanicidal molecules that kill the intracellular pathogens (Figure 4B) [33, 34].

Beside the protective CD4$^+$ T cell response, Belkaid *et al.* described *Leishmania*-specific CD8$^+$ T-cells [35]. The role of MHC class-I-dependent response in experimental leishmaniasis is differentially discussed. Erb *et al.* demonstrated that CD8-deficient mice control parasite replication as efficient as control mice, whereas Belkaid *et al.* argue for an adjuvant role of CD8$^+$ T cells in experimental leishmaniasis [36, 37].

In summary, professional antigen presenting cells (APCs) are crucial for the induction of an antigen-specific T cell (CD4 or CD8) response [38]. Based on their anatomical position, epidermal LCs were described to be crucial for antigen uptake and subsequent presentation of antigen to naïve T cells residing in SDLNs in experimental leishmaniasis [25, 39, 40]. In the next chapter these results will be put to question.

DENDRITIC CELL SUBTYPES FEASIBLE FOR PRESENTATION OF SKIN-DERIVED *LEISHMANIA-ANTIGEN*

DCs are highly mobile cells connecting the site of infection with the lymphoid and non-lymphoid organs. As shown in (Fig. **5**), DCs are subdivided into different subclasses according to the expression of distinct surface and cytoplasmatic antigens and their particular tissue localization ([41] for further reading). In general, murine DCs express MHC class II and class I molecules and are positive for the CD11c (for further reading [42]). Within the skin, different DC subclasses were identified (see Fig. **5B**).

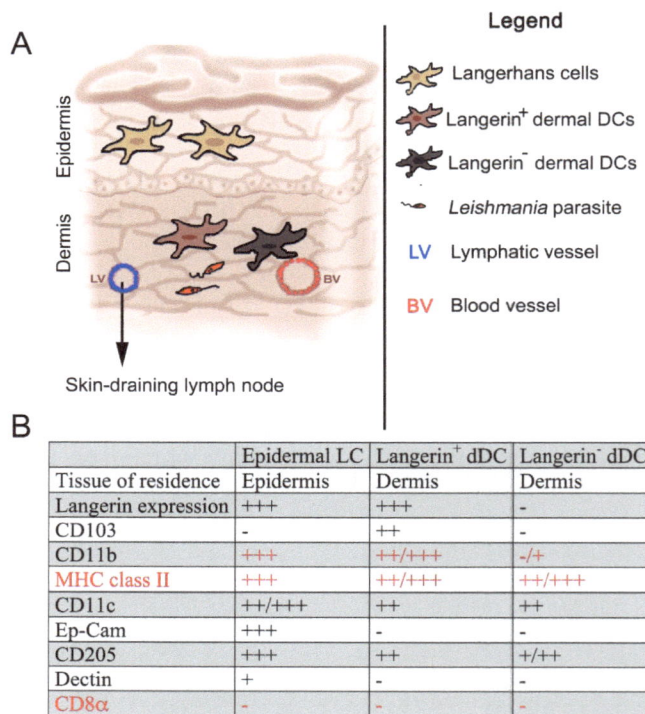

	Epidermal LC	Langerin$^+$ dDC	Langerin$^-$ dDC
Tissue of residence	Epidermis	Dermis	Dermis
Langerin expression	+++	+++	-
CD103	-	++	-
CD11b	+++	++/+++	-/+
MHC class II	+++	++/+++	++/+++
CD11c	++/+++	++	++
Ep-Cam	+++	-	-
CD205	+++	++	+/++
Dectin	+	-	-
CD8α	-	-	-

Figure 5: Dendritic cell subtypes within the skin. A) Dendritic cell subtypes within the skin are shown. **B)** The characteristics of cutaneous dendritic cell subtypes are summarized. The expression levels are indicated. (−) signifies no expression, (+) signifies low expression, (++) signifies intermediate expression, and (+++) signifies high expression [81, 93].

Langerhans cells are the most commonly known dendritic cells within the epidermis. They are positive for the C-type lectin Langerin (CD207) and a series of other surface molecules, such as MHC class II, CD11b, CD205, and epithelial cell adhesion molecule (Ep-CAM), that are summarized in Table **1** [43, 44]. Within the dermis, a new Langerin$^+$ DC subtype was identified recently ([45, 46] for further reading). According to their location, they are termed dermal DCs (dDCs).

Based on the expression of Ep-CAM, CD103, and dendritic cell-associated C-type lectin (Dectin), it is possible to differentiate Langerin$^+$ dermal DCs (dDCs) from Langerin$^+$ epidermal LCs. In contrast to LCs, Langerin$^+$ dDCs do not express Ep-CAM or Dectin. Furthermore, CD103 is only expressed on Langerin$^+$ dDCs but not on LCs. Other molecules like MHC class II, MHC class I, CD205, CD11c are expressed comparably on epidermal LCs and Langerin$^+$ dDCs. Last but not least, Langerin$^-$ dDCs were described to transport skin-derived antigen to the SDLNs. These Langerin$^-$ dDCs are MHC-class II^{high}, CD11c$^+$, CD11b$^+$, CD8α$^-$ and CD205$^{low\ to\ inter}$[42]. Therefore, at least three different skin-derived DCs such as LCs$^{Langerin+}$, dDCs$^{Langerin+}$, and dDC$^{Langerin-}$ might offer an interface between the cutaneous compartment and the SDLNs.

DCS PRESENTING SKIN-DERIVED *LEISHMANIA* ANTIGEN ARE RESPONSIBLE FOR T CELL ACTIVATION

It is generally accepted that professional antigen presenting cells are crucial for the induction of an antigen-specific T cell response in SDLNs. All cutaneous DC subtypes described above have the potential to present skin-derived antigen to naïve T cells in SDLNs.

However, if one particular DC subtype fulfils all three important tasks necessary for efficient T cell-priming *in vivo*, namely *i*) antigen uptake within the skin, *ii*) migration to the skin-draining lymph node, and *iii*) processing and subsequent presentation to antigen-specific T cells, is not known in detail. Different scenarios are generally conceivable.

Previous work has shown that subcutaneously injected *L. major*-pulsed LCs migrate to SDLNs, where they stimulate antigen-specific T cells [40]. Other reports demonstrated that the population of *L. major*-presenting cells does not express Langerin or other LC-associated molecules like CD205 and gp40 [27, 47]. Consequently, during the past few years it has become more and more confusing which kind of DC subpopulation is responsible for the priming of T cells. One reason for this controversy is the differences in experimental protocols, mouse models, parasite strains, and kinetics that were used to determine the impact of DCs in experimental leishmaniasis.

Nevertheless, based on genetically engineered mice suitable for transient depletion of Langerin$^+$ DCs by diphtheria toxin (DT), the interpretation of DCs in experimental leishmaniasis was revisited. Based on these novel data, possible early-phase scenarios will be discussed in the following chapter

FIRST HOURS AFTER INFECTION

L. major parasites developed several immune escape mechanisms to avoid early elimination by the host innate immune systems. One of the most efficient escape mechanisms is to hide within host cells for subsequent replication. Rapidly after infection, promastigote *L. major* parasites are taken up by skin-resident phagocytic cells (e.g. neutrophils and macrophages) and transform into the replicative amastigote form. Several surface molecules, such as complement receptor 3 (CR3), CD11b, C-type lectins, and Fcγ receptors, on phagocytic cells are thought to mediate the uptake of promastigote *Leishmania* parasites [48-50].

Although LCs and dermal DCs express some of these surface molecules and should therefore be sufficiently equipped for *Leishmania* phagocytosis, they might have different capacities in engulfing parasites [51]. Concerning this matter, it is important to mention that LCs are less efficient in the uptake of promastigote *L. major* parasites compared to other DCs [52]. This might be due to the fact that LCs do not express the complement receptor 3 (CR3) known to be involved in phagocytosis of *Leishmania* parasites [53-56]. Thus, it is doubtful that LCs get infected by promastigote parasites via CR3- or Fcγ-mediated phagocytosis during the early hours after infection. This is confirmed by other studies demonstrating that infection of LC-containing epidermal cell suspensions did not result in an uptake of promastigote parasites at all [57].

It is commonly accepted that APCs have the molecular machinery to "digest" intact parasites prior to processing parasite-derived protein and binding peptides to MHC class I or II molecules. However, it is feasible that APCs engulf parasite-derived components from the extracellular space for further processing and antigen presentation. Consequently, epidermal LCs might be involved in capturing *Leishmania*-antigen for subsequent transport to the SDLNs. In this context, the work of Kissenpfennig *et al.* is of outstanding interest. After epicutaneous application of Tetramethylrhodamine-5-(and-6)-isothiocyanate (TRITC) on the dorsal site of both ears of mice expressing the enhanced green fluorescent protein (EGFP) under the control of the Langerin promotor, the authors were able to distinguish between EGFP$^+$ LC-derived DCs and

EGFP⁻ dermal-derived DCs harboring TRITC⁺ within the SDLNs. Due to this experimental design, it was possible to demonstrate for the first time that Langerin⁻ DCs (EGFP⁻ but TRITC⁺) emerge within 24 to 48 hours after TRITC application, whereas the percentage of epidermal LCs (EGFP⁺ and TRITC⁺) increases substantially after 72 to 96 hours. Thus, dermal DCs seem to migrate much faster to the SDLN than LCs [58]. Transferring these results to the experimental model of leishmaniasis, it is most likely that the candidates mediating the presentation of *Leishmania* antigen during the early hours are dDCs [58].

To address the important question, whether T-cell priming is mediated by skin-derived dDCs during the very early hours after infection, mice were infected into the ear, which was removed 5 hours after infection [47]. One day later, DCs were isolated from SDLN and co-cultivated with *Leishmania*-antigen specific T cells. Interestingly, the DCs were capable of activating the T cells proving the DCs carried parasite antigen. Further characterization of the DC subtype responsible for the T cell-priming revealed that these DCs are CD11c^{high}, CD11b^{high}, Gr.1⁻, Langerin⁻, and CD8α⁻. Based on these experiments, neither LCs nor dDCs serve as vehicles for *L. major*-antigen [47]. Surprisingly, this model revealed that soluble antigen is swept into the draining lymph node and presented by lymph node-resident DCs. However, the biological relevance of that phenomenon, in the sense of induction of an effector/memory T cell response against *L. major* parasites, was not shown [47]. Based on vaccination studies, it is known that application of soluble *Leishmania* antigen alone without additional stimuli is not sufficient to induce a long term protection [59]. Hence, antigen that is passively swept to the SDLN might not induce an adaptive immune reaction that is typically characterized by the induction of an effector/memory T cell response. Consequently, migratory DCs with the capacity to polarize a Th1 response might be necessary.

Several Days after Infection

As described so far, DCs are crucial for the induction of an adaptive T cell-mediated immune response. Thus, it is likely that the probability to engulf *Leishmania* parasites or *Leishmania*-derived antigen within the dermal compartments correlates with the density of DCs within the infected tissue. Certainly, the number of DCs is marginal under steady state conditions but increases during the first few days after infection because of inflammatory signals, such as TNF [60]. Beside inflammation-supporting features, TNF additionally stimulates DCs to express costimulatory molecules, such as CD80 and CD86, and the chemokine receptor (CCR) 7 [61-63]. This process, also known as "DC maturation", is crucial for the emigration of DCs out of the skin to SDLNs [64].

In this context, the chemokine CCL21 needs to be mentioned. CCL21 is one of the ligands of CCR7 and is expressed by lymphatic endothelial cells (LECs) within the skin and high endothelial venules within the SDLNs [65]. Consequently, the combination of CCR7 on DCs and CCL21 expression by dermal LECs orchestrates the navigation of CCR7⁺ DCs from the dermal compartment to the lymphatic vessels and subsequently to the SDLNs [66, 67]. Thus, maturation of DCs that is accompanied by the enhanced expression of CCR7 and costimulatory molecules is crucial for both *i*) DC migration and *ii*) subsequent priming of naïve T cells within the SDLNs.

In further agreement with this concept, it was shown that CCR7 is also expressed during LC maturation [68]. Accordingly, both DCs subtypes - epidermal LCs and dermal DCs - show the potential to capture dermal antigen when passing the site of infection. It was hypothesized that LCs are pivotal for T cell immunity in experimental leishmaniasis [69, 70]. Furthermore, it was demonstrated that LCs are involved in priming of CD4⁺ T cells using a transgenic mouse model where MHC class II-expression is restricted to LCs [71]. Additionally, a correlation between impaired migration of LCs and a non-healing phenotype was determined in CCR2⁻/⁻ mice [72, 73].

Contradictory to these data, other groups clearly demonstrated that DCs other than LCs (e.g. dermal DCs) are responsible for priming of CD4⁺ T cells [27, 74]. Thus, the biological role of LCs in the adaptive immunity against cutaneous pathogens remained enigmatic. The development of a technique using DT *in vivo* to deplete distinct cell populations made it possible to revise the role of LCs in T cell-mediated immunology.

DT consists out of two different subunits "A (DTA)" and "B (DTB)" that fulfill different functions. DTB is necessary for the attachment on the cell surface mediated by the corresponding receptor (a subunit of heparin-binding EGF-like growth factor (HB-EGF) precursor). This binding of the B subunit to HB-EGF precursor facilitates the entry of DTA into the cell. Within the cell, DTA inhibits protein biosynthesis and induces rapid cell death. Due to the fact that the rodent homologue of HB-EGF precursor does not bind to DTB, the heterodimer is not internalized. Subsequently, mice are resistant to DT [75]. This can be changed by transgenic expression of the high-affinity human HB-EGF precursor (hereafter referred as DTR).

However, for DT-induced depletion of distinct cells, the expression of DTR must be subtype-specific. The transient DT-induced depletion of LCs was achieved by cloning the human DTR into the langerin locus. These genetically engineered mice (hereafter referred as Lang-DTR) changed the view on LCs in T cell-mediated immunity.

For example, LCs are dispensable for mounting a viral-specific effector T cell-response in a mouse model of HSV infection (for a review see [76]). Furthermore, gene gun immunization experiments revealed that LCs are not crucial for the induction of humoral or cell-mediated immunity [77]. Regarding the role of LCs in priming hapten-specific effector T cells through skin immunization, conflicting reports have been published [58, 78-80]. Last but not least, recently it was documented that LCs are not involved in priming of CD8$^+$ T cells against self-antigen [81].

Coming back to the experimental model of leishmaniasis, DT-induced ablation of Langerin$^+$ DCs *in vivo* proved that an efficient adaptive immune response is generated in the absence of LCs [82]. These data favor the concept that LCs might be in general dispensable for inducing any T cell-mediated immune response.

Searching for alternative functions of LCs in experimental leishmaniasis, Weiss *et al.* demonstrated that exposition of epidermal LCs with *Leishmania* antigen prior infection changes the course of leishmaniasis dramatically. Compared to control mice, antigen-exposed animals developed a chronic course of leishmaniasis [83]. The mechanism of LC-induced pathology was not analyzed in that study. However, using a clinical isolate of *L. major* (NIH/Sd strain) that causes "non-healing" lesions, Anderson *et al.* showed that IFN-γ-secreting Th1 cells that also produce IL-10 simultaneously are responsible for the development of non-healing lesions [84]. Analyzing the potential of LCs in immune modulation, Brewig *et al.* demonstrated that LCs are dispensable for the induction of a protective immune response against *L. major* [82]. However, the authors demonstrated that LCs take part in the generation of IL-10-producing Th1 cells [82]. Consequently, LC-induced IL-10-producing Th1 cells might be responsible for the chronic course of leishmaniasis induced by epidermal inoculation of *Leishmania* antigen. Therefore, it is feasible that LCs are more involved in immunopathology than in initiation of adaptive immunity as already postulated in references [28, 82].

Thus, the initiation of the protective Th1 response might be induced by other DC subtypes such as lymph node resident DCs, Langerin$^+$ dDCs, and Langerin$^-$ dDCs. Analyzing the phenotype responsible for priming naïve T cells within the SDLN, Brewig *et al.* chose the Lang-DTR mouse model. By modulation of the DT-application protocol, it is possible to eliminate LCs and Langerin$^+$ DCs simultaneously or LCs exclusively [43, 45, 46]. Mice depleted for LCs and other Langerin$^+$ DCs showed the same priming efficiency of CD4 T cells as control mice. Analyzing the number of activated CD4$^+$ cells at the site of infection, no difference was detectable between mice depleted for LCs and Langerin$^+$ DCs and control mice. The same result was obtained by selective depletion of Langerin$^+$ DCs. Consequently, Langerin$^+$ DCs (cutaneous DCs or lymph node resident DCs) are not involved in the priming and expansion of Th1 cells [82].

Acquired resistance in the experimental model relies on the activation and expansion of Th1 cells whereas *Leishmania*-specific CD8$^+$ T cells potentiate the clearance of parasites but are dispensable for the control of primary infections with *L. major* [21, 36, 85].

The ability to process pathogen-derived antigens is crucial for the induction of an adaptive immune response. For a long period, it was postulated that antigens within the cytoplasm are loaded in the endoplasmatic reticulum and presented at the cell surface on major histocompatibility complex (MHC) class I molecules. In contrast to those "endogeneous antigens", exogenous antigens present in endo/phagocytic compartments are presented on MHC class II molecules [86, 87]. In contrast to that paradigm, it is of interest that *Leishmania* parasites that enter the phagolysosomal pathway can elicit an MHC class I-dependent CD8$^+$ T cell response [35].

As mentioned above, it has generally been accepted that MHC class I molecules present peptides derived from proteins endogenously synthesized. This involves the proteloytic digestion of cytosolic antigens by the proteasome and subsequent transport of the peptides to the ER by the transporter associated with antigen processing (TAP) complex [88]. In 1976, Bevan showed that MHC class I mediated T- cell response is induced by antigens derived from exogenous source [89]. He showed that MHC antigens are transferred from donor cells to recipient antigen presenting cells and termed the process "cross-priming".

Beside this "indirect" antigen presentation, cells have additionally developed an intracellular machinery that transfers exogenous antigens into the MHC class I pathway. Different pathways for presentation of exogenous antigen via MHC class I have been described so far. Due to the fact that antigen must be degraded, two principle pathways exists: *i*) lysosomal degradation within the phagosome, and *ii*) proteasomal degeneration of peptides within the cytoslol (cytosolic pathaway, ref. [90] for further reading). TAPs are required for both processes to shuttle the peptides into the ER.

In the experimental model of leishmaniasis, it was demonstrated the *Leishmania* antigens are presented to CD8⁺ T cells by a TAP-independent pathway [91]. Consequently, parasite antigens are loaded to MHC class I molecules by an alternative vacuolar pathway. So far the exact mechanism of this vacuolar pathway is not known. However, it is tempting to speculate that *Leishmania*-proteins are directly degraded by endocytic proteases within the phagosome and are loaded to MHC class I molecules that are further on transported to the surface of antigen presenting cells (ref. [90] for further reading). The exact mechanism leading to presentation of parasite-derived antigen on MHC class I of APCs is not known so far (for further reading ref. [90]).

To address the question, whether Langerin⁺ or Langerin⁻ DCs differ in their capacity of cross-presentation, Brewig *et al.* depleted mice exclusively of Langerin⁺ DCs before infection with *L. major*. The experiments revealed that the proliferation of *L. major*-specific CD8⁺ T cells and subsequently the number of activated CD8⁺ T cells at the site of infection is reduced in the absence of Langerin⁺ DCs compared to control mice [82]. Consequently, antigen entry into the MHC class I pathway is reduced in Langerin⁻ DCs whereas Langerin⁺ DCs were capable of loading *Leishmania*-peptides onto MHC class I molecules.

Recently, it was shown by Savina *et al.*, that GTPases such as Rac2 controls cross-presentation in DC subpopulations [92]. Whether the Rac2 expression is reduced in Langerin⁻ DCs resulting in a diminished cross-presentation capacity needs to be analyzed in more detail.

Based on the current knowledge about the DCs in experimental leishmaniasis, it is feasible to assume that different DC subtypes interact with distinct types of T cells during the first days after infection: LCs with regulatory T cells, Langerin⁺ DCs with CD8⁺ T cells, and last but not least, Langerin⁻ DCs with CD4⁺ T cells (summarized in Fig. **6**) [26, 28, 82].

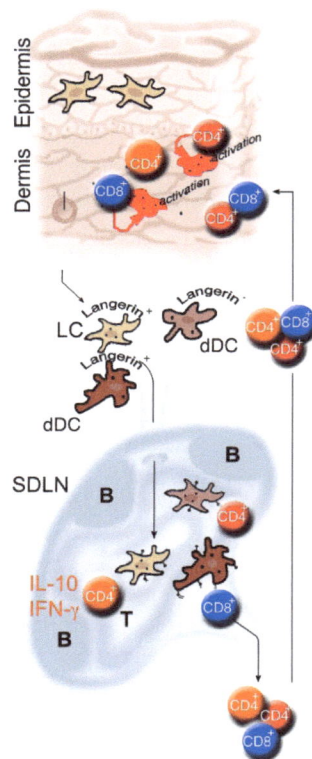

Figure 6: Current model of DC-mediated T cell- priming in experimental leishmaniasis. After infection, DC subtypes fulfill distinct functions within skin-draining lymph nodes: **Langerin⁺ Langerhans cells (LCs)** prime IFN-γ IL-10 double-producing CD4⁺ T cells.

Langerin$^+$ dermal DCs (dDCs) prime CD8$^+$ T cells. **Langerin$^-$ dDCs** prime CD4$^+$ T cells. At the site of infection, antigen-specific CD4$^+$ and CD8$^+$ activate infected macrophages to eliminate the intracellular *L. major* parasites.

CONCLUDING REMARKS

Antigen presentation of skin-derived antigen is a complex process. Based on genetically engineered mice and novel markers such as Langerin, an increasing body of evidence is provided that the function of Langerhans cells in experimental leishmaniasis was overemphasized. Contradictory to the formerly postulated role in adaptive immunity against *L. major,* mice depleted for LCs show no obvious phenotype regarding the development of an adaptive immune response whereas dermal DCs take part in an adaptive T cell response. However, the exact route of *Leishmania*-antigen to the skin-draining lymph node remains fragmentary. A full understanding of the cellular vehicles capturing antigen, together with a putative passive antigen passage to the skin-draining lymph node, would provide significant progress for appropriate development of cell-based vaccines and vaccination strategies in general.

ACKNOWLEDGEMENT

I thank Dr. Anja Wege and Dr. Sven Mostböck (University of Regensburg, Germany), and Dr. Andrea Horst (University Medical Center Hamburg Eppendorf, Germany) for critical review of the manuscript. This work was supported by the German Research Foundation (DFG, RI 1849/1-1).

REFERENCES

[1]　Pearson RD, Wheeler DA, Harrison LH, Kay HD. The immunobiology of leishmaniasis. Rev Infect Dis 1983; 5: 907-27.

[2]　Warburg A, Schlein Y. The effect of post-bloodmeal nutrition of Phlebotomus papatasi on the transmission of *Leishmania major*. Am J Trop Med Hyg 1986; 35: 926-30.

[3]　Bogdan C, Rollinghoff M. How do protozoan parasites survive inside macrophages? Parasitol Today. 1999; 15: 22-8.

[4]　Bogdan C, Donhauser N, Doring R, Rollinghoff M, Diefenbach A, Rittig MG. Fibroblasts as host cells in latent leishmaniosis. J Exp Med 2000; 191: 2121-30.

[5]　van Zandbergen G, Klinger M, Mueller A, *et al.* Cutting edge: neutrophil granulocyte serves as a vector for Leishmania entry into macrophages. J Immunol 2004;173: 6521-5.

[6]　Kima PE. The amastigote forms of Leishmania are experts at exploiting host cell processes to establish infection and persist. Int J Parasitol 2007; 37: 1087-96.

[7]　Andrade TM, Carvalho EM, Rocha H. Bacterial infections in patients with visceral *leishmaniasis*. J Infect Dis 1990;162:1354-9.

[8]　Ritter U, Moll H, Laskay T, , *et al.* Differential expression of chemokines in patients with localized and diffuse cutaneous American *leishmaniasis*. J Infect Dis. 1996;173: 699-709.

[9]　Mendes E. Transfer of delayed hypersensitivity to leishmanin (Montenegro reaction). Cell Immunol 1979; 42: 424-7.

[10]　Walton BC, Intermill RW, Hajduk ME. Differences in biological characteristics of three Leishmania isolates from patients with espundia. Am J Trop Med Hyg 1977; 26: 850-5.

[11]　Janvier F, Morillon M, Olliaro P. Visceral *leishmaniasis*: clinical sensitivity and resistance to various therapeutic agents. Med Trop (Mars) 2008; 68: 89-101.

[12]　Vanloubbeeck Y, Jones DE. The immunology of Leishmania infection and the implications for vaccine development. Ann N Y Acad Sci 2004;1026: 267-72.

[13]　Melby PC. Vaccination against cutaneous leishmaniasis: current status. Am J Clin Dermatol. 2002; 3: 557-70.

[14]　Ritter U, Mattner J, Rocha JS, Bogdan C, Korner H. The control of *Leishmania* (*Leishmania*) *major* by TNF in vivo is dependent on the parasite strain. Microbes Infect. 2004; 6: 559-65.

[15]　Liese J, Schleicher U, Bogdan C. The innate immune response against Leishmania parasites. Immunobiology 2008; 213: 377-87.

[16]　Peters NC, Egen JG, Secundino N, *et al. In vivo* imaging reveals an essential role for neutrophils in leishmaniasis transmitted by sand flies. Science 2008; 321:970-4.

[17]　Nathan C. Neutrophils and immunity: challenges and opportunities. Nat Rev Immunol 2006;6:173-82.

[18]　Laskay T, van Zandbergen G, Solbach W. Neutrophil granulocytes as host cells and transport vehicles for intracellular pathogens: apoptosis as infection-promoting factor. Immunobiology 2008; 213:183-91.

[19]　Laskay T, van Zandbergen G, Solbach W. Neutrophil granulocytes--Trojan horses for Leishmania major and other intracellular microbes? Trends Microbiol. 2003 ;11:210-4.

[20]　Alexander J, Bryson K. T helper (h)1/Th2 and *Leishmania*: paradox rather than paradigm. Immunol Lett 2005 ;15;99:17-23.

[21]　Sacks D, Noben-Trauth N. The immunology of susceptibility and resistance to *Leishmania major* in mice. Nat Rev Immunol 2002 ;2:845-58.

[22]   Rocken M, Saurat JH, Hauser C. A common precursor for CD4+ T cells producing IL-2 or IL-4. J Immunol 1992; 148: 1031-6.

[23]   Abbas AK, Murphy KM, Sher A. Functional diversity of helper T lymphocytes. Nature 1996; 383: 787-93.

[24]   Rissoan MC, Soumelis V, Kadowaki N,, *et al.* Reciprocal control of T helper cell and dendritic cell differentiation. Science 1999; 283:1183-6.

[25]   Moll H. Epidermal Langerhans cells are critical for immunoregulation of cutaneous leishmaniasis. Immunol Today 1993;14:383-7.

[26]   Ritter U, Osterloh A. A new view on cutaneous dendritic cell subsets in experimental leishmaniasis. Med Microbiol Immunol 2007; 196: 51-9.

[27]   Ritter U, Meissner A, Scheidig C, Korner H. CD8 alpha- and Langerin-negative dendritic cells, but not Langerhans cells, act as principal antigen-presenting cells in leishmaniasis. Eur J Immunol 2004; 34: 1542-50.

[28]   Moreno J. Changing views on Langerhans cell functions in leishmaniasis. Trends Parasitol 2007; 23: 86-8.

[29]   Scharton-Kersten T, Scott P. The role of the innate immune response in Th1 cell development following *Leishmania major* infection. J Leukoc Biol 1995; 57: 515-22.

[30]   Gallatin WM, Weissman IL, Butcher EC. A cell-surface molecule involved in organ-specific homing of lymphocytes. Nature 1983; 304: 30-4.

[31]   Oehen S, Brduscha-Riem K. Differentiation of naive CTL to effector and memory CTL: correlation of effector function with phenotype and cell division. J Immunol 1998; 161: 5338-46.

[32]   Mora JR, von Andrian UH. T-cell homing specificity and plasticity: new concepts and future challenges. Trends Immunol 2006; 27: 235-43.

[33]   Soong L, Xu JC, Grewal IS, *et al.* Disruption of CD40-CD40 ligand interactions results in an enhanced susceptibility to *Leishmania amazonensis* infection. Immunity 1996; 4: 263-73.

[34]   von Stebut E, Udey MC. Requirements for Th1-dependent immunity against infection with *Leishmania major.* Microbes Infect 2004; 6: 1102-9.

[35]   Belkaid Y, Von Stebut E, Mendez S, *et al.* CD8+ T cells are required for primary immunity in C57BL/6 mice following low-dose, intradermal challenge with *Leishmania major.* J Immunol 2002; 168: 3992-4000.

[36]   Erb K, Blank C, Ritter U, Bluethmann H, Moll H. *Leishmania major* infection in major histocompatibility complex class II-deficient mice: CD8+ T cells do not mediate a protective immune response. Immunobiology 1996; 195: 243-60.

[37]   von Stebut E. Cutaneous *Leishmania* infection: progress in pathogenesis research and experimental therapy. Exp Dermatol 2007; 16: 340-6.

[38]   Stingl G, Steiner G. Immunological host defense of the skin. Curr Probl Dermatol 1989;18: 22-30.

[39]   De Creus A, Van Beneden K, Taghon T, Stolz F, Debacker V, Plum J, et al. Langerhans cells that have matured in vivo in the absence of T cells are fully capable of inducing a helper CD4 as well as a cytotoxic CD8 response. J Immunol. 2000;165: 645-53.

[40]   Moll H, Fuchs H, Blank C, Rollinghoff M. Langerhans cells transport *Leishmania major* from the infected skin to the draining lymphonode for presentation to antigen-specific T cells. Eur J Immunol 1993; 23: 1595-601.

[41]   McLellan AD, Kapp M, Eggert A, *et al.* Anatomic location and T-cell stimulatory functions of mouse dendritic cell subsets defined by CD4 and CD8 expression. Blood 2002; 99: 2084-93.

[42]   Itano AA, Jenkins MK. Antigen presentation to naive CD4 T cells in the lymphonode. Nat Immunol 2003; 4: 733-9.

[43]   Bursch LS, Wang L, Igyarto B, *et al.* Identification of a novel population of Langerin+ dendritic cells. J Exp Med 2007; 204: 3147-56.

[44]   Borkowski TA, Nelson AJ, Farr AG, Udey MC. Expression of gp40, the murine homologue of human epithelial cell adhesion molecule (Ep-CAM), by murine dendritic cells. Eur J Immunol 1996; 26:110-4.

[45]   Ginhoux F, Collin MP, Bogunovic M, *et al.* Blood-derived dermal langerin+ dendritic cells survey the skin in the steady state. J Exp Med 2007; 204: 3133-46.

[46]   Poulin LF, Henri S, de Bovis B, Devilard E, Kissenpfennig A, Malissen B. The dermis contains langerin+ dendritic cells that develop and function independently of epidermal Langerhans cells. J Exp Med 2007; 204: 3119-31.

[47]   Iezzi G, Frohlich A, Ernst B, , *et al.* Lymphonode resident rather than skin-derived dendritic cells initiate specific T cell responses after *Leishmania major* infection. J Immunol 2006; 177: 1250-6.

[48]   Mosser DM, Edelson PJ. The mouse macrophage receptor for C3bi (CR3) is a major mechanism in the phagocytosis of *Leishmania promastigotes.* J Immunol 1985;135: 2785-9.

[49]   Colmenares M, Corbi AL, Turco SJ, Rivas L. The dendritic cell receptor DC-SIGN discriminates among species and life cycle forms of *Leishmania.* J Immunol 2004; 172: 1186-90.

[50]   Rosenthal LA, Sutterwala FS, Kehrli ME, Mosser DM. *Leishmania major*-human macrophage interactions: cooperation between Mac-1 (CD11b/CD18) and complement receptor type 1 (CD35) in promastigote adhesion. Infect Immun 1996; 64: 2206-15.

[51]   Reis e Sousa C, Stahl PD, Austyn JM. Phagocytosis of antigens by Langerhans cells *in vitro.* J Exp Med 1993;178: 509-19.

[52]   Soong L. Modulation of dendritic cell function by *Leishmania* parasites. J Immunol 2008; 180: 4355-60.

[53] Beckstead JH, Wood GS, Turner RR. Histiocytosis X cells and Langerhans cells: enzyme histochemical and immunologic similarities. Hum Pathol 1984;15: 826-33.

[54] Franklin WA, Mason DY, Pulford K, *et al.* Immunohistological analysis of human mononuclear phagocytes and dendritic cells by using monoclonal antibodies. Lab Invest 1986; 54: 322-35.

[55] Haines KA, Flotte TJ, Springer TA, Gigli I, Thorbecke GJ. Staining of Langerhans cells with monoclonal antibodies to macrophages and lymphoid cells. Proc Natl Acad Sci U S A 1983; 80: 3448-51.

[56] Sauder DN, Dinarello CA, Morhenn VB. Langerhans cell production of interleukin-1. J Invest Dermatol 1984; 82: 605-7.

[57] Locksley RM, Heinzel FP, Fankhauser JE, Nelson CS, Sadick MD. Cutaneous host defense in leishmaniasis: interaction of isolated dermal macrophages and epidermal Langerhans cells with the insect-stage promastigote. Infect Immun 1988; 56: 336-42.

[58] Kissenpfennig A, Henri S, Dubois B, *et al.* Dynamics and function of Langerhans cells in vivo: dermal dendritic cells colonize lymph node areas distinct from slower migrating Langerhans cells. Immunity 2005; 22: 643-54.

[59] Gurunathan S, Prussin C, Sacks DL, Seder RA. Vaccine requirements for sustained cellular immunity to an intracellular parasitic infection. Nat Med 1998; 4: 1409-15.

[60] Ritter U, Lechner A, Scharl K, Kiafard Z, Zwirner J, Korner H. TNF controls the infiltration of dendritic cells into the site of *Leishmania major* infection. Med Microbiol Immunol 2008; 197: 29-37.

[61] Ritter U, Wiede F, Mielenz D, Kiafard Z, Zwirner J, Korner H. Analysis of the CCR7 expression on murine bone marrow-derived and spleen dendritic cells. J Leukoc Biol 2004 ; 76: 472-6.

[62] Ritter U, Meissner A, Ott J, Korner H. Analysis of the maturation process of dendritic cells deficient for TNF and lymphotoxin-alpha reveals an essential role for TNF. J Leukoc Biol 2003; 74: 216-22.

[63] Banchereau J, Steinman RM. Dendritic cells and the control of immunity. Nature 1998; 392: 245-52.

[64] Forster R, Davalos-Misslitz AC, Rot A. CCR7 and its ligands: balancing immunity and tolerance. Nat Rev Immunol 2008; 8: 362-71.

[65] Kriehuber E, Breiteneder-Geleff S, Groeger M, *et al.* Isolation and characterization of dermal lymphatic and blood endothelial cells reveal stable and functionally specialized cell lineages. J Exp Med 2001; 194: 797-808.

[66] Schaerli P, Willimann K, Ebert LM, Walz A, Moser B. Cutaneous CXCL14 targets blood precursors to epidermal niches for Langerhans cell differentiation. Immunity 2005; 23: 331-42.

[67] Ohl L, Mohaupt M, Czeloth N, *et al.* CCR7 governs skin dendritic cell migration under inflammatory and steady-state conditions. Immunity 2004; 21: 279-88.

[68] Forster R, Schubel A, Breitfeld D, *et al.* CCR7 coordinates the primary immune response by establishing functional microenvironments in secondary lymphoid organs. Cell 1999; 99: 23-33.

[69] Will A, Blank C, Rollinghoff M, Moll H. Murine epidermal Langerhans cells are potent stimulators of an antigen-specific T cell response to *Leishmania major*, the cause of cutaneous leishmaniasis. Eur J Immunol 1992; 22: 1341-7.

[70] Blank C, Fuchs H, Rappersberger K, Rollinghoff M, Moll H. Parasitism of epidermal Langerhans cells in experimental cutaneous leishmaniasis with *Leishmania major*. J Infect Dis 1993; 67: 418-25.

[71] Lemos MP, Esquivel F, Scott P, Laufer TM. MHC class II expression restricted to CD8alpha+ and CD11b+ dendritic cells is sufficient for control of *Leishmania major*. J Exp Med 2004; 199: 725-30.

[72] Sato N, Kuziel WA, Melby PC, *et al.* Defects in the generation of IFN-gamma are overcome to control infection with *Leishmania donovani* in CC chemokine receptor (CCR) 5-, macrophage inflammatory protein-1 alpha-, or CCR2-deficient mice. J Immunol 1999; 163: 5519-25.

[73] Sato N, Ahuja SK, Quinones M, Kostecki V, Reddick RL, Melby PC, et al. CC chemokine receptor (CCR)2 is required for langerhans cell migration and localization of T helper cell type 1 (Th1)-inducing dendritic cells. Absence of CCR2 shifts the *Leishmania major*-resistant phenotype to a susceptible state dominated by Th2 cytokines, b cell outgrowth, and sustained neutrophilic inflammation. J Exp Med 2000;192: 205-18.

[74] Misslitz AC, Bonhagen K, Harbecke D, Lippuner C, Kamradt T, Aebischer T. Two waves of antigen-containing dendritic cells *in vivo* in experimental *Leishmania major* infection. Eur J Immunol 2004; 34: 715-25.

[75] Saito M, Iwawaki T, Taya C, *et al.* Diphtheria toxin receptor-mediated conditional and targeted cell ablation in transgenic mice. Nat Biotechnol 2001; 19: 746-50.

[76] Villadangos JA, Schnorrer P. Intrinsic and cooperative antigen-presenting functions of dendritic-cell subsets *in vivo*. Nat Rev Immunol 2007; 7: 543-55.

[77] Stoecklinger A, Grieshuber I, Scheiblhofer S, *et al.* Epidermal langerhans cells are dispensable for humoral and cell-mediated immunity elicited by gene gun immunization. J Immunol 2007; 179: 886-93.

[78] Fukunaga A, Khaskhely NM, Sreevidya CS, Byrne SN, Ullrich SE. Dermal dendritic cells, and not langerhans cells, play an essential role in inducing an immune response. J Immunol 2008; 180: 3057-64.

[79] Bennett CL, van Rijn E, Jung S, et al. Inducible ablation of mouse Langerhans cells diminishes but fails to abrogate contact hypersensitivity. J Cell Biol 2005; 169: 569-76.

[80]   Kaplan DH, Jenison MC, Saeland S, *et al*. Epidermal langerhans cell-deficient mice develop enhanced contact hypersensitivity. Immunity 2005; 23: 611-20.

[81]   Bursch LS, Rich BE, Hogquist KA. Langerhans cells are not required for the CD8 T cell response to epidermal self-antigens. J Immunol 2009; 182: 4657-64.

[82]   Brewig N, Kissenpfennig A, Malissen B, Veit A, Bickert T, Fleischer B, *et al*. Priming of CD8+ and CD4+ T cells in experimental leishmaniasis is initiated by different dendritic cell subtypes. J Immunol 2009;182: 774-83.

[83]   Weiss R, Scheiblhofer S, Thalhamer J, *et al*. Epidermal inoculation of *Leishmania*-antigen by gold bombardment results in a chronic form of leishmaniasis. Vaccine 2007; 25: 25-33.

[84]   Anderson CF, Oukka M, Kuchroo VJ, Sacks D. CD4(+)CD25(-)Foxp3(-) Th1 cells are the source of IL-10-mediated immune suppression in chronic cutaneous leishmaniasis. J Exp Med. 2007; 204: 285-97.

[85]   Uzonna JE, Joyce KL, Scott P. Low dose *Leishmania major* promotes a transient T helper cell type 2 response that is down-regulated by interferon gamma-producing CD8+ T cells. J Exp Med 2004; 199: 1559-66.

[86]   Watts C, Amigorena S. Phagocytosis and antigen presentation. Semin Immunol. 2001; 13: 373-9.

[87]   Heath WR, Carbone FR. Cross-presentation in viral immunity and self-tolerance. Nat Rev Immunol 2001; 1: 126-34.

[88]   Cresswell P. Intracellular surveillance: controlling the assembly of MHC class I-peptide complexes. Traffic 2000 ; 1: 301-5.

[89]   Bevan MJ. Cross-priming for a secondary cytotoxic response to minor H antigens with H-2 congenic cells which do not cross-react in the cytotoxic assay. J Exp Med 1976; 143: 1283-8.

[90]   Lin ML, Zhan Y, Villadangos JA, Lew AM. The cell biology of cross-presentation and the role of dendritic cell subsets. Immunol Cell Biol 2008; 86: 353-62.

[91]   Bertholet S, Goldszmid R, Morrot A, *et al. Leishmania* antigens are presented to CD8+ T cells by a transporter associated with antigen processing-independent pathway *in vitro* and *in vivo*. J Immunol 2006; 177: 3525-33.

[92]   Savina A, Peres A, Cebrian I, *et al*. The small GTPase Rac2 controls phagosomal alkalinization and antigen crosspresentation selectively in CD8(+) dendritic cells. Immunity 2009; 30: 544-55.

[93]   Merad M, Ginhoux F, Collin M. Origin, homeostasis and function of Langerhans cells and other langerin-expressing dendritic cells. Nat Rev Immunol 2008; 8: 935-47.

CHAPTER 10

Subversion of Host Cell Signalling by *Leishmania*: Role of Protein Tyrosine Phosphatases

Issa Abu-Dayyeh and Martin Olivier*

Centre for the Study of Host Resistance at the Research Institute of the McGill University Health Centre, and Departments of Microbiology and Immunology and Medicine, McGill University, Montréal, Québec, Canada

Abstract: In this chapter, we address the relationship between *Leishmania* and its host macrophage at the molecular level. Parasites of the genus *Leishmania* are able to secure their survival and propagation within their host by altering key signalling pathways involved in the ability of macrophages to directly kill pathogens or to activate cells of the adaptive immune system. One important step in this immune evasion process is the *Leishmania*-induced activation of host protein tyrosine phosphatase SHP-1. The latter has been shown to directly inactivate JAK2 and Erk1/2, and to play a role in the negative regulation of several transcription factors involved in macrophage activation such as: NF-κB, STAT-1α, and AP-1. These signalling alterations contribute to the inactivation of critical macrophage functions such as the production of IFN-γ-induced nitric oxide (NO), a free radical associated with parasite killing and clearance. In addition to interfering with IFN-γ receptor signalling, *Leishmania* is able to alter several LPS-mediated responses (e.g. IL-12, TNF-α, NO production) through mechanisms not yet fully understood. However, recent findings from our laboratory revealed a pivotal role for SHP-1 in the inhibition of TLR-induced macrophage activation through binding to and inactivating IL-1 receptor-associated kinase 1 (IRAK-1). Furthermore, we identified the binding site as an evolutionarily conserved ITIM-like motif, which we named Kinase Tyrosine-based Inhibitory Motif (KTIM). This accumulating knowledge helps us better understand evasion mechanisms employed by promastigotes and/or amastigotes of *Leishmania* which could help in the development of more efficient anti-leishmanial therapies in the near future.

INTRODUCTION

Apart from the impact of *Leishmania* on world health, leishmaniasis represents an elegant infection model that can teach us a lot about host-parasite interactions and immune evasion. This parasite has the ability to enter host macrophages (MØs) safely and replicate inside the very same phagocytes that were recruited to destroy it. The inability of MØs to kill the parasite and activate cells of the adaptive immune system is a product of the parasite's long-reported capacity to alter several key signalling pathways in the host. Many signalling alterations are seen early in the course of infection suggesting they start upon the initial contact between the parasite and the MØ. These rapid alterations of signalling pathways serve at least two main functions: Firstly, inhibition of MØ killing mechanisms that are triggered upon phagocytosis of foreign particles (e.g. production of reactive oxygen species) and secondly, inhibition of leishmanicidal functions that can be triggered in response to MØ activation in infected tissues in response to stimuli such as lipopolysaccharides (LPS) or interferon-γ (IFN-γ) (e.g. nitric oxide production). In this chapter, we will discuss the roles of promastigotes and amastigotes of *Leishmania* in disease establishment, focusing on the signalling pathways that they interfere with and the MØ functions that are affected by the alteration of these pathways.

INITIAL INTERACTION AND INTERNALIZATION

Leishmania Virulence Factors

In order to survive in the sandfly midgut and within the mammalian host, *Leishmania* requires a set of virulence factors that aid its survival. In this section, we will discuss the major ones.

Lipophosphoglycan (LPG)

Lipophosphoglycan (LPG) is one of the major surface glycoconjugate of promastigotes. It consists of a polymer of repeating Galβ1, 4Man-PO4 units attached to a glycan core that is inserted into the membrane via an inositol anchor. The

*Corresponding Author: Martin Olivier, Centre for the Study of Host Resistance at the Research Institute of the McGill University Health Centre, and Departments of Microbiology and Immunology and Medicine, McGill University, Montréal, Québec, Canada; Email: martin.olivier@mcgill.ca

Emilio Jirillo (Ed)
All rights reserved - © 2010 Bentham Science Publishers Ltd.

molecule is capped by a small oligosaccharide structure which varies among species [1]. Although the backbone of the repeating units, the glycan core, and the lipid anchor are conserved among *Leishmania* species, they differ in the additional oligosaccharide chains branching off the backbone sugars [1]. One important feature that draws the attention to LPG as a virulence factor is its ability to undergo several important modifications during the life cycle of the parasite. As the parasite changes from a non-infective procyclic to an infective metacyclic promastigote in the sandfly midgut, LPG doubles its length by increasing the number of its repeating units [2]. The structural changes of LPG are believed to protect the parasites from the gut's digestive enzymes and help the infectious ones detach from the sandfly's midgut and migrate to the foregut so they can be transported into the mammalian host during the fly's blood meal [3]. As promastigotes enter the mammalian host, LPG has been shown to play a key role in protecting the parasite against complement-mediated lysis [4] while maintaining the ability to bind members of the complement system [4, 5] and C-reactive protein [6] which helps in the opsonization of the parasite and its uptake by MØs through complement receptors (CRs) and C-reactive protein receptors (CRPRs), respectively. Interestingly, it has also been shown that LPG protects from the oxidative burst by blocking protein kinase C (PKC) activity [7] and scavenging hydroxyl radicals and superoxide anions [2]. Furthermore, this surface glycoconjugate was shown to inhibit phagosome maturation and phagolysosome formation in MØs [8, 9]. Other reported functions of LPG include its ability to inhibit IL-12 synthesis and release at the transcriptional level [10] and its ability to reduce inducible nitric oxide synthase (iNOS) mRNA expression and nitric oxide (NO) production when incubated with MØs prior to IFN-γ stimulation [11]. Although the requirement of LPG for virulence varies from one species of *Leishmania* to another, it was demonstrated that LPG-defective mutants of *L. donovani* and *L. major* are destroyed following phagocytosis and that they are able to survive following the restoration of LPG expression using genetic complementation of the LPG gene [12, 13]. Despite the many functions performed by LPG to help in the survival of promastigotes, this molecule is strongly down-regulated in amastigotes suggesting that it is dispensable for amastigote survival, most probably due to the presence of other mechanisms utilized by this form of the parasite to survive the harsh environment of MØs.

The next critical virulence factor is a zinc-dependent metalloprotease named **glycoprotein 63 (gp63)** found on the surface of the *Leishmania* parasite, that has a wide range of substrates including casein, gelatin, albumin, haemoglobin, and fibrinogen [14]. This protease belongs to the metzincin class [15] whose members include a sequence motif HExxHxxGxxH, and an N-terminal pro-peptide that renders the proenzyme inactive during translation, and is removed during maturation and activation [16]. Gp63 is abundant in promastigotes but has been shown to be down-regulated in amastigotes [17]. Nevertheless, the reduced expression of gp63 might be compensated for by the absence of LPG on the amastigote surface [18, 19] where gp63 is no longer buried in a sea of LPG and can therefore play an important role in the ability of amastigotes to modulate the host response despite its lower numbers compared to promastigotes.

Given its presence on both forms of the parasite, gp63 is likely to play different roles depending on the parasite stage. In promastigotes of *L. amazonensis and L. major*, gp63 is able to cleave C3b into iC3b and therefore help the parasite avoid complement-mediated lysis [20]. Generation of iC3b can also act as an opsonin aiding the parasite to interact with MØs through complement receptors 1 and 3 (CR1/CR3) [21, 22]. Gp63 also interacts with the fibronectin receptor (FR) and can thus help the parasite adhere to MØs that way [23]. Interestingly, incorporating gp63 into liposomes was able to protect intraliposomal serum bovine albumin from degradation. This observation can suggest a similar mechanism whereby gp63 can help amastigotes survive within the harsh environment of MØ phagolysosomes [24, 25]. Work in our laboratory has shown that gp63 plays an important role in the cleavage and activation of several MØ protein tyrosine phosphatases (PTPs) including the Src homology 2 domain-containing protein tyrosine phosphatase 1 (SHP-1) (M.A. Gomez and M. Olivier, manuscript under review). This novel role for gp63 can help explain the rapid ability of *Leishmania* to activate SHP-1 and negatively regulate several key signalling pathways in MØs [26].

More recently discovered, the **cysteine proteinases (CPs)** are mostly studied in *L. mexicana*, which was shown to exhibit high activity of CPs. This family includes: *L. mexicana* cysteine proteinase a (lmcpa), *L. mexicana* cysteine proteinase b (lmcpb), and *L. mexicana* cysteine proteinase c (lmcpc). lmcpb is a cathepsin L-like CP whose genes are multicopy and occur in a tandem array of 19 genes [27]. *lmcpa* (cathepsin L-like) and *lmcpc* (cathepsin C-like), on the other hand, are single copy genes [28, 29]. Although lmcpb is expressed in metacyclic promastigotes, which might indicate a role for these CPs in the virulence of this life-cycle stage [30], the expression of this cysteine proteinase is significantly increased in amastigotes [27]. The roles of lmcpa, lmcpb, and lmcpc in *Leishmania* virulence was studied through the generation of mutants deficient for the *cpa*, *cpb*, and *cpc* genes. Although lmcpc did not act as a virulence factor, lmcpa and lmcpb did. *L. mexicana* deficient in the multicopy *cpb* gene array had reduced virulence with poor lesion growth in BALB/c mice [31,

32]. The lmcpa was also implicated as a virulence factor based on the observation that *lmcpa/lmcpb* double null mutant parasites were less infective to BALB/c mice than *lmcpb* mutants only [30].

Several studies have suggested methods by which lmcpb can act as a virulence factor. In fact, a role for lmcpb was proposed in the degradation of inhibitory kappa B-alpha (IκB-α), inhibitory kappa B-beta (IκB-β), and nuclear factor kappa B (NF-κB) in MØs. This degradation was not seen with lmcpb mutants and was reversed when CP inhibitors were used [33]. The authors concluded that this could represent one mechanism by which *L. mexicana* can inhibit LPS-mediated IL-12 production in MØs. Another interesting report provided evidence that *L. amazonensis* amastigotes were able to internalize major histocompatibility complex (MHC) class II molecules found in the parasitophorous vacuoles of their host cells and degrade them within their megasomes in order to block antigen (Ag) presentation [34]. The role of CPs in the degradation of these molecules was confirmed when more MHC class II accumulation was observed inside amastigotes pre-treated with an irreversible CP inhibitor. In addition to the role of lmcpa and lmcpb as virulence factors, these proteinases can act as immunomodulators favoring a non-healing Th2 response during the course of infection. It has been shown that lmcpb inoculated into footpads of BALB/c mice increases IL-4 in the draining lymph nodes and polarizes splenocytes towards a Th2 response measured by their increased IL-5 production compared to controls [35]. This increase in IL-4 production was paralleled by an lmcpb-dependent reduction in the expression of both the IL-2R on activated T cells and the low-affinity IgER on mature resting B cells, and an increase in plasma IgE levels in mice injected with active recombinant lmcpb for two weeks [35]. It was also shown that wildtype (WT) but not *lmcpa/lmcpb* double mutants can induce IL-4 production in splenocytes cultured from BALB/c mice. The double mutants but not WT parasites, on the other hand, induced IL-2 production [32].

Finally, **acid phosphatases** are membrane-bound or secreted by pathogenic species of *Leishmania* and are also found to be constitutively released into the culture medium during *in vitro* growth [36]. One of the well-studied acid phosphatases is the histidine secretory acid phosphatase (SAcP) produced by *L. donovani* [37]. This acid phosphatase has been shown to dephosphorylate a wide range of substrates including glycerol phosphates, mono- and di- phosphorylated sugars, inositol phosphates and phosphorylated proteins [38-42]. Hydrolysis of such substrates by SAcP could generate essential nutrients and/or modify the host environment to the advantage of the parasite [43]. These modifications of host environment include the ability of acid phosphatases to inhibit toxic oxidative metabolite production by neutrophils [44].

Leishmania Modes of Entry to Macrophages

Phagocytosis by host MØs is a prerequisite to successful infections by promastigotes and amastigotes. Promastigotes have to do so upon entry to the mammalian host and amastigotes when they rupture infected MØs and go on to infect other ones. It is generally accepted that entry of *Leishmania* to host MØs is a receptor-mediated event, and several receptors have been shown to play a role in this process. We will hereby discuss the main ones whose involvement in parasite attachment and entry has been well established and supported by a respectable amount of previous work.

Complement Receptors (CRs):

Serum complement has been shown to improve parasite adhesion to MØs [21]. Importantly, the binding of the third component of complement to the parasite helps in its adhesion to host complement receptors [45]. Human MØs have two classes of complement receptors: CR1 (CD35) and CR3 (Mac-1, CD18/11b), which bind to C3b and iC3b, respectively [46]. The adhesion of parasites to CR1 is transient because of the factor I cofactor activity of CR1 and the parasite's gp63, which are both able to cleave C3b to iC3b [20, 47]. Based on this cleavage, the main complement receptor involved in the phagocytosis of *Leishmania* appears to be CR3 and not CR1. In addition to helping the parasite get phagocytosed, C3 fixation on parasites has been shown to aid in the intracellular survival of the parasite through enabling it to block the MØ respiratory burst [48].

Mannose-Fucose Receptor (MFR):

Sugar receptors play an important role in the recognition of pathogens due to their ability to detect carbohydrate moieties expressed on the surface of those organisms. One Important receptor implicated in the phagocytosis of *Leishmania* is the MFR. This receptor mediates the uptake of mannose- and fucose- terminated glycoproteins [49]. Further evidence regarding the ligand specificity of this receptor was obtained when rat fibroblasts transfected with mannose receptor c-DNA were rendered able to endocytose and degrade mannose-BSA in a specific manner [50]. The MFR was first identified in MØs [51], but was afterwards found to be expressed on other cell types such as dendritic cells (DCs) [52]. Upon binding of the ligand to the MFR, the receptor is rapidly internalized, the ligands are released into early endosomes and are quickly seen to co-localize with MHC class II-enriched compartments and lysosomes while the receptors recycle to the surface [53]. As LPG of *Leishmania* contains sugar moieties including mannose, it is not surprising to find out that the MFR can mediate the binding of the parasite to MØs [54]. This has been shown by reversing parasite binding (attachment and ingestion) through the use of soluble inhibitors of MFR activity, namely mannan and ribonuclease B [54]. It is noteworthy that this receptor plays a more important role in promastigote binding to MØs since it is this parasite stage that primarily expresses LPG on its surface.

C - Reactive Protein Receptor (CRPR):

C-Reactive Proteins (CRPs) are acute phase proteins mainly secreted by the liver. They are named so because they were initially discovered to be able to bind to and precipitate the C-polysaccharide of the *Streptococcus pneumonia* cell walls due to their ability to bind phosphorylcholine, a component of the C-polysaccharide, which they bind to in a calcium-dependent manner [55]. Indications that CRP can bind to *Leishmania* were supported by observations whereby CRP was found to bind some promastigotes in a calcium-dependent manner [56]. In fact, it was later found that the repeating phosphorylated disaccharides of LPG in metacyclic *L. donovani* promastigotes but not *L. major* promastigotes were responsible for the binding to CRP [6]. It has been suggested that the modifications of the LPG sugar backbone in the metacyclic stage might explain why CRP binds to metacyclic but not procyclic promastigotes. As for why CRPs bind to *L. donovani* but not *L. major* promastigotes, the substitutions that take place in the 3-position of the galactose of LPG of *L. major* that are known not to take place in *L. donovani* have been proposed to mediate the decreased binding affinity of CRP to LPG of *L. major* [6]. The discovery of LPG as a ligand of CRP directly implicated the CRP receptor in the binding and uptake of the *Leishmania* parasite. It is very interesting to note that although *Leishmania* is able to exploit CRP as an opsonin, the entry of the parasite via the CRPR does not trigger MØ activation as would normally happen in CRP-mediated uptake of other particles. It has been demonstrated that the CRP-mediated entry of *Leishmania* does not affect parasite survival in MØs and does not lead to the production of pro-inflammatory cytokines such as tumor necrosis factor alpha (TNF-α) and IL-12 [57].

Fibronectin Receptor (FR):

FRs belongs to the β1 integrin family, with two abundant members VLA-4 and VLA-5 [58, 59]. It has been shown that gp63 can exhibit fibronectin-like properties and interact with the FR [23]. This interaction suggests a role for the FR in the adhesion of *Leishmania* to MØs and in their uptake as seen by the slower and decreased parasite internalization upon the use of antibodies directed against β1 integrins [23]. The fact that parasites still manage to ultimately get internalized in the absence of functional fibronectin receptors suggests that these receptors might not be the primary mediators of parasite adhesion but can facilitate the process by stabilizing complement-mediated adhesion of parasites to MØs through the ability of the FR to bind to gp63 of *Leishmania* [23]. The binding of gp63 to integrins represents yet another mechanism by which gp63 can help in parasite adhesion and entry, the first being its ability to cleave complement components and use the cleaved forms as opsonins to adhere to MØs through CRs.

Fc Receptors (FcRs):

These are protein receptors found on several immune cells including MØs and have binding affinity to the Fc portion of immunoglobulins. Initial experiments showed that opsonizing *Leishmania* with parasite-specific IgG significantly enhanced the ability of promastigotes to enter MØs but did not have any enhancing effect on the ability of amastigotes derived from BALB/c mice to do so [60]. The initial conclusion was that the FcR might not play a role in amastigote infection. Further experiments revealed that the reason IgG opsonization did not augment the entry of amastigotes is the fact that amastigotes derived from mice lesions are already highly coated with immunoglobulins. Interestingly, amastigotes harvested from bone-marrow derived MØs (BMDMs) cultured *in vitro* or those collected from SCID mice, have enhanced entry to MØs in the presence of specific IgG due to the absence of immunoglobulins on the surface of these amastigotes prior to the opsonization step [60]. It is important to mention that amastigotes are still able to enter MØs in the absence of immunoglobulins as opsonins suggesting a role for other receptors including CRs. Based on receptor blocking experiments, it appears that amastigotes have the ability to switch binding receptors based on availability. Blocking the FcR or CR3 one at a time is not sufficient to observe a strong decrease in amastigote entry, and only when both receptors are blocked simultaneously that we observe a drastic decrease in amastigote entry to MØs [60]. It remains to be mentioned that entry by

FcR seems to be an important mechanism by which the already established amastigotes can enter and infect new cells, but most likely is not a mechanism utilized by promastigotes as when they first enter the host, no specific antibody response against the parasite is present.

Phosphatidylserine Receptor (PSR):

This is a receptor that detects phosphatidylserine (PS) on apoptotic cells, therefore enabling phagocytes to clear them in a non-inflammatory fashion. PS has been reported to be expressed on the surface of amastigotes in what is referred to as "apoptotic mimicry". By expressing PS, amastigotes of *L. amazonensis* have been shown to be able to bind to MØs through the PSR, mimicking apoptotic cells and therefore triggering an anti-inflammatory response by inhibiting NO production and increasing IL-10 and transforming growth factor-beta (TGF-β) secretion [61, 62]. By doing so, amastigotes are able to more readily attach to and infect MØs while avoiding any harmful inflammatory responses. It is worth mentioning that PS has been regarded as a contributor to amastigote virulence as it has been shown that amastigotes derived from susceptible BALB/c mice display more PS than those derived from resistant C57BL/6 mice [61].

ALTERATION OF MACROPHAGE SIGNALLING AND FUNCTIONS BY *LEISHMANIA*

Signalling Molecules Altered by Leishmania

Cells can control their physiology and function by activating and inhibiting their intracellular signalling pathways. A typical pathway is usually triggered by a ligand such as a cytokine or growth factor or pathogen-associated molecule. The binding of ligands to their receptors causes activation of the receptor via its phosphorylation and/or conformational change which in turn leads to the activation of second messengers in the cytosol. These second messengers ultimately lead to the activation of several transcription factors (TFs) that can translocate to the nucleus and bind to the promoters of their target genes generating a change in the cell's response. On the other hand, other signalling molecules like phosphatases are able to dephosphorylate molecules and can therefore counteract effects caused by protein phosphorylation. Using this negative feedback loop, the cell can establish a balance between activation and inhibition, and is able to return to the resting state following activation. Interestingly, many pathogens are able to alter the signalling of their target cells to their own advantage and *Leishmania* is no exception. *Leishmania* achieves this by either employing strategies to inhibit proteins that play a positive role in immune cell activation or by activating molecules known to play key roles in the negative regulation of immune cell signalling and function [26]. We will discuss below the main signalling molecules altered by *Leishmania* in an effort of the parasite to survive inside host MØs.

Protein Kinase C (PKC):

It is a family that comprises 10 serine/threonine kinases, first characterized as Ca^{+2} and phospholipid-dependent [63, 64]. The PKC family consists of three sub-families: conventional, novel, and atypical isoforms. Conventional isoforms include: PKC-alpha, -beta I, -beta II, and –gamma and these isoforms require Ca^{+2} and diacylglycerol (DAG) to function. Novel isoforms include: PKC-delta, -epsilon, -eta, and –theta and these isoforms require DAG but not Ca^{+2}. Atypical isoforms include: PKC-zeta and –lambda and these require neither DAG nor Ca^{+2} [65]. PKC signalling plays a key role in the response of MØs to activating cytokines such as IFN-γ and TNF-α [66, 67], cytokines which have important roles in driving several MØ functions including NO production [66] and oxidative burst [68]. Given the leishmanicidal effect of these functions, it is remarkable that *Leishmania* is able to block PKC activity in infected MØs. Promastigote LPG has been described to be able to block PKC activity [7, 69, 70]. This inhibition is achieved through the binding of LPG to the regulatory domain of PKC which contains the DAG, Ca^{+2}, and phospholipid binding sites [2]. It is interesting to observe that amastigotes, which lack LPG, are also able to inhibit PKC activity in monocytes [71], suggesting that factors other than LPG can also mediate this inhibitory effect. Indeed, *Leishmania*-induced ceramide generation [72] and GIPLs [70] have been shown to be able to inhibit PKC, providing a possible mechanism by which amastigotes can inhibit the activity of this kinase.

Janus Kinase 2 (JAK2):

It is one of four members of the Janus family of tyrosine kinases (JAK1, JAK2, JAK3, TYK2). As with the other members of the JAK family, JAK2 has two kinase-homologous domains at its C-terminus, the first is non-catalytic and has a regulatory function and the second exhibits kinase activity. JAK activation plays an important role in cell proliferation, differentiation, migration, apoptosis, as well as immune activation [73]. The JAK signalling pathway is initiated when a ligand (cytokine or growth factor) binds to its receptor inducing receptor multimerization. This process brings the cytoplasmic domains of the receptor subunits -which are associated with JAKs- into close proximity to each other, allowing the JAKs to transphosphorylate and therefore activate each other. Activated JAKs are then able to phosphorylate the receptors themselves on a conserved tyrosine residue (Tyr-440 in the case of IFNγRI) providing a docking site for the TF signal transducer and activator of transcription (STAT). JAKs then phosphorylate the docked STATs on a conserved tyrosine near their C-terminus. Phosphorylated STATs are then able to dimerize with the help of their conserved SH2 domains and proceed to translocate to the nucleus to bind their target regulatory sequences to activate or repress transcription [73, 74].

The promoter of the iNOS gene responsible for NO production has binding sites for several TFs including STAT-1 [75, 76]. Given the leishmanicidal effect of NO as a free radical, it is not surprising that *Leishmania* has the ability to block the JAK/STAT signalling pathway in response to IFN-γ stimulation. Indeed, it has been reported that infection with *L. donovani* amastigotes was able to block IFN-γ-induced JAK1, JAK2, and STAT-1 phosphorylation in PMA-differentiated U-937 promoncytic cells and human monocytes [77]. Our laboratory has gone further in studying the effect of *Leishmania* on JAK2 phosphorylation by reporting that *L. donovani* promastigotes were able to rapidly activate host SHP-1 and that this activation was associated with increased binding of SHP-1 to JAK2 and the subsequent inhibition of the phosphorylation of this kinase in response to IFN-γ stimulation [78]. Another study suggested that the *Leishmania*-induced unresponsiveness to IFN-γ stimulation can be due to the inhibition of the IFN-γ receptor (IFN-γR) complex formation. The authors observed decreased phosphorylation of IFN-γR-α and decreased association of the receptor with JAK2 caused by a downregulation of the receptor expression itself, but provided no clues on how the parasite could do so [79]. Another complication with this report is that the authors infected cells for 24 hours to see an appreciable effect on receptor expression and phosphorylation, which cannot explain the rapid dephosphorylation of JAK2 seen when BMDMs are infected with *Leishmania* promastigotes [78]. This supports the notion that early JAK/STAT inhibition must depend on parasite-induced alterations of existing signalling molecules of the host and not on alterations at the transcriptional level.

Mitogen-Activated Protein Kinases (MAPKs):

These are serine/threonine kinases activated by phosphorylation on two residues (threonine and tyrosine) in their kinase activation loop. These two residues are separated by a single residue unique for each group of MAPKs: glutamate for the extracellular signal-regulated kinase1/2 (Erk1/2), proline for Jun N-terminal kinase (JNK), and glycine for p38 [80]. The signalling cascade usually starts by an external stimulus causing the activation of a MAPK kinase kinase (MAPKKK) which is a serine/threonine kinase. The MAPKKK in turn phosphorylates a MAPK kinase (MAPKK) which is a dual specificity kinase that can phosphorylate both the threonine and tyrosine found in the T-X-Y motif found in the activation loop of MAPKs. Phosphorylation of the threonine and tyrosine causes a conformational change in the activation loop allowing it to clear the ATP binding site of MAPKs which it obstructs in the inactive state thus activating the kinase [81]. Upon their activation, MAPKs can phosphorylate cytosolic targets or translocate to the nucleus to phosphorylate TFs and thus can directly affect gene expression. We will hereby discuss the three main MAPKs in terms of their signalling roles and then review some of the mechanisms by which *Leishmania* can interfere with their activity.

Erk1/2:

Upon its activation by a MAPKK such as MEK1/2, Erk1/2 is able to phosphorylate more than 70 different substrates including TFs [82]. Erk1/2 has the ability to translocate to the nucleus where it is able to phosphorylate several members of the Ets family of proteins in the transactivation domain [83]. Activated Ets1/2, for example, interact with activating protein-1 (AP-1) and NF-κB in binding to gene promoters therefore enhancing transcription [80]. Other substrates of Erk1/2 from the Ets family include Elk-1 and the SRF accessory protein-1 (SAP-1) which play an important role in the regulation of c-fos (a subunit of AP-1) transcription [84]. Erk1/2 can also activate Fra1/2 [85], therefore having yet another way to activate AP-1.

JNK:

JNK was first cloned as a kinase that phosphorylates and activates the Jun AP-1 subunit [86], but was soon found to have a wider range of substrates. There are three JNK genes that can give rise to several splice variants [87]: JNK1 and JNK2 which are widely expressed, and JNK3 which is found only in brain tissue. JNK is activated by MAPKKs such as MKK4 and MKK7 [80] and activated JNK can phosphorylate c-Jun in addition to its ability to phosphorylate activating transcription factor-2 (ATF-2) on threonines 69 and 71 preventing its ubiquitination and degradation [88]. The phosphorylation of c-Jun has a direct effect on AP-1 activation while phosphorylation of ATF-2 enhances its ability to dimerize with c-Jun to drive c-Jun expression [89], or dimerize with ATF-6 to mediate signal transduction of stress signals associated with protein misfolding [80].

p38:

This MAPK contains at least four members: p38α and p38β which are ubiquitously expressed, p38γ found in skeletal muscles, and p38δ found in the prostate, testes, pancreas, and salivary, pituitary, and adrenal glands [90]. One of the main targets of p38 is the MAPK-activated protein kinase 2 (MAPKAP-K2) [91] which is a kinase able to phosphorylate several TFs such as: ATF-2 and ATF-1/cAMP response element binding (CREB) [80] which is a TF that binds to c-AMP-regulated enhancer (CRE) regions in cAMP-inducible genes like c-fos [92]. Notably, MAPKAP-K2 is also able to phosphorylate the SRE-binding TF serum response factor (SRF) that forms a complex with Elk-1 and regulates c-fos gene expression [80, 93].

In addition to playing important roles in the proliferation and differentiation of cells, MAPKs play a crucial role in the activation of immune cells including MØs through their ability to activate several TFs that control pro-inflammatory mediators [94]. As was the case with the JAK family, it is remarkable, though not unexpected, that the *Leishmania* parasite developed tactics to render several MAPK members inactive in response to parasite entry to MØs or to activating stimuli that follow infection.

Indeed, it was reported that the phagocytosis of *L. donovani* promastigotes by naive MØs does not lead to the activation of any of the three MAPKs (Erk1/2, JNK, p38) [95]. Additionally, several MAPKs have been shown to be inhibited in infected cells in response to activating stimuli such as LPS. For example, *L. amazonensis* amastigotes are able to block LPS-mediated Erk1 phosphorylation in infected MØs [96] and *L. donovani* amastigotes can block PMA-induced Erk1/2 phosphorylation in RAW264 MØs leading to the inhibition of Elk-1 and c-fos expression [97]. The authors of the latter study suggested a role for host PTPs in Erk1/2 inactivation, a hypothesis supported and more deeply explored by our laboratory where we provided evidence that PTP-SHP-1 is able to dephosphorylate and inactivate Erk1/2 through demonstrating that this MAPK was still able to be activated in *Leishmania*-infected SHP-1-deficient MØs in response to IFN-γ stimulation [98]. Furthermore, it has been suggested that the increased ceramide production in *L. donovani*-infected MØs can lead to reduced Erk1/2 phosphorylation ultimately leading to enhanced parasite survival [99]. Interestingly, amastigotes of *L. mexicana* were also reported to inhibit Erk1/2 signalling not by inhibiting their phosphorylation but rather by degrading them using the parasite's cysteine proteinases. Similar cysteine proteinase-dependent degradation was observed for JNK [33].

Regarding p38, it has been shown that this MAPK is non-responsive when MØs infected with *L. major* are stimulated with a CD40 antibody to mimic the MØ-T cell interaction. p38 inactivation correlated with impaired iNOS2 expression and NO production and therefore impaired leishmanicidal functions [100]. In fact, this inactivation makes sense in the light of experiments showing the importance of p38 activation in the control of *Leishmania* infection. The use of anisomycin, a p38 activator, enhanced parasite killing in MØs by triggering p38-dependent anti-leishmanial effects [100, 101].

Transcription Factors (TFs)

In order to inhibit gene expression of pro-inflammatory cytokines and microbicidal molecules, *Leishmania* developed several strategies to interfere with TFs that bind to the promoters of those genes. Several TFs are involved in this process including: NF-κB, STAT-1α, and AP-1, all of which have been shown to be modulated by the parasite. We will hereby discuss the role of each of these TFs in signalling and describe the known mechanisms by which the parasite is able to interfere with their functions.

NF-κB:

This TF is composed of five subunits: p65 (RelA), RelB, c-Rel, p50 (NF-κB1), and p52 (NF-κB2). These subunits associate together as homo- or heterodimers forming NF-κB [102]. Each subunit has three distinct structures: a Rel homology domain used for DNA binding, a dimerization domain, and a nuclear localization signal [103]. In addition to these structures p65, Rel B, and c-Rel have a transactivation domain suggesting their role in transcription activation [102]. NF-κB is held in an inactive state by binding to inhibitory kappa B (IκB) [104]. NF-κB is released from its inhibitor when IκB gets phosphorylated by IκB kinases (IKK), which are a family of three proteins: IKK-α and IKK-β, which phosphorylate IκB, and IKK-γ, which serves as a regulatory subunit of the IKK complex [102].

There exist two distinct pathways for NF-κB signalling: the classical pathway and the alternative pathway [103]. The classical pathway involves activation of receptors such as p55TNFR, IL-1R, or TLR. This results in the activation of IKK-β which in turn phosphorylates IκBα and leads to its polyubiquitination by an E3-ubiquitin ligase causing its degradation and the release of p65/p50 dimers that are now free to translocate to the nucleus to drive gene expression [105]. The alternative pathway, on the other hand, involves the activation of receptors such as B cell-activating factor receptor (BAFFR), CD40, and lymphotoxin beta receptor (LTBR) [106]. This activates NF-κB-inducing kinase (NIK) which phosphorylates IKK-α which in turn phosphorylates p100 that gets processed to a p52 subunit. This pathway leads to the accumulation of RelB/p52 dimers in the nucleus that drive gene expression [102].

NF-κB has more than 150 target genes, many of them code for inflammatory cytokines, chemokines, immunoreceptors, and cell adhesion molecules. Examples of these genes include: IFN-γ, IL-1, IL-6, IL-12, MIP-1α, MIP-1β, MIP-2, MCP-1, RANTES, and MHC class I [107]. It is therefore no surprise that this transcription factor is referred to as a "central mediator of the human immune response" [107].

Several groups have reported different strategies employed by *Leishmania* to alter NF-κB. *Leishmania*-induced ceramide generation by MØs was shown to play a role in NF-κB inhibition [99]. One study provided evidence that *L. major* amastigotes blocked the nuclear translocation of the p65/p50 complex selectively favoring the c-Rel/p50 complex that they proposed plays a role in the gene expression of immunosuppressive cytokines in MØs such as IL-10 [108]. Another study showed that cysteine proteinases of *L. mexicana* mediated NF-κB degradation and caused its inability to bind its DNA consensus sequence, thus partially explaining how the parasite can inhibit LPS-mediated IL-12 production [33]. Work from our laboratory showed that promastigotes of several pathogenic *Leishmania* species were able to cleave the p65 RelA subunit to generate a p35 RelA fragment that is able to translocate to the nucleus and bind DNA. This p35 fragment was suggested to be involved in the parasite's ability to drive NF-κB-mediated chemokine gene expression in infected MØs [109].

STAT: The STAT family consists of STAT-1, STAT-2, STAT-3, STAT-4, STAT-5α, STAT-5β, and STAT-6 [110]. These STATs are activated by distinct cytokines, for example, STAT-1 mediates responses to IFN-γ, STAT-3 to IL-10, STAT-4 to IL-12, and STAT-6 to IL-13 [111]. The signalling cascade involving STATs has been discussed previously in the JAK section. Briefly, upon the binding of the appropriate ligand to its receptor, JAKs associated to the cytoplasmic portion of the receptor will get activated and phosphorylate the receptor on a conserved tyrosine residue. This phosphorylation provides a docking site for STATs, which bind via their SH2 domains. STATs are phosphorylated by JAKs and are able to dimerize and translocate to the nucleus where they can activate gene expression [110].

We have previously described the ability of *Leishmania* to inhibit the JAK/STAT pathway through SHP-1-mediated JAK2 dephosphorylation [78]. Interestingly, our laboratory has also reported that the parasite is able to repress IFN-γ-mediated signalling in MØs through its ability to interfere with STATs. *L. donovani* promastigotes were shown to be able to cause proteasome-dependent STAT-1 degradation in infected MØs. However, whereas STAT-1 degradation was reversed using proteasome inhibitors [112], its capacity to respond to IFN-γ was still altered due to JAK2 inactivation (unpublished data).

AP-1: AP-1 is a structurally complex TF whose dimers are principally made of proteins belonging to the Jun (c-Jun, JunB, JunD) and fos (c-fos, fosB, Fra-1, Fra-2) subfamilies, although proteins of the Maf and ATF families can also participate in the formation of the AP-1 complex [113]. While members of the Jun subfamily can homodimerize, members of the fos subfamily have to dimerize with members of other subfamilies, mainly the Jun subfamily [113].

AP-1 can be activated by many kinds of stimuli such as growth factors, cytokines, hormones, and pathogens, which do so using several signalling molecules. PKC has been shown to play a role in c-fos expression [114]. Furthermore, MAPKs play a key role in AP-1 activation. Erk1/2 for example, can activate AP-1 either by activating elk which binds to and activate the c-fos gene [84] or by directly phosphorylating Fra1 and Fra2 enhancing their binding to c-Jun [115]. JNK can activate AP-1 by either phosphorylating c-Jun or ATF2 which dimerizes with c-Jun [116]. In addition, p38 is also able to phosphorylate c-Jun [117].

Keeping these AP-1 activators in mind, we can see that the previously mentioned tactics employed by *Leishmania* to interfere with PKC, Erk1/2, JNK, and p38 activities have a direct impact on the ability of the parasite to block AP-1 signalling in MØs. In addition, work from our group demonstrated a role for SHP-1 in AP-1 inhibition [98, 118] and a key role for the parasite's surface protease gp63 in the cleavage and degradation of key AP-1 subunits (I. Contreras and M. Olivier, manuscript in preparation). The latter finding provides the first demonstration that a parasite-derived molecule can directly interfere with AP-1 in host MØs in order to block its downstream functions.

NEGATIVE REGULATORS OF SIGNAL TRANSDUCTION

Protein Tyrosine Phosphatases (PTPs)

PTPs are proteins that have the ability to dephosphorylate substrates and are divided into receptor-like and non-receptor PTPs. Non-receptor PTPs can either dephosphorylate tyrosines only or can possess dual specificity dephosphorylating tyrosines as well as serines/threonines [119]. One common feature of PTPs is the presence of a PTP catalytic domain in which a critical cysteine is found within a conserved signature motif (I/V)HCxxGxxR(S/T) and mediates the hydrolysis via the formation of a thio-phosphate intermediate [120]. Receptor-like PTPs include: RPTP-α, CD45, and CD148 and the functions of some like CD45 in immune cell signalling is well-known [121]. We will however focus on a selected group of soluble PTPs who have been shown to play a role in *Leishmania* host evasion mechanisms namely: PTP-1B, TC (T cell)-PTP, PTP-PEST, and most importantly SHP-1.

PTP-1B and TC-PTP:

They are two ubiquitously expressed PTPs that have more than 73% identity in their catalytic domain [122]. PTP-1B is known to play important regulatory functions in metabolism, as demonstrated by the insulin hypersensitivity of PTP-1B$^{-/-}$ mice and their resistance to high fat diet-induced obesity [123, 124]. This insulin hypersensitivity was shown to be due to the ability of PTP-1B to dephosphorylate the insulin receptor [125]. PTP-1B also seems to play a role in the regulation of cytokine signalling through its ability to interact with and dephosphorylate members of the JAK family namely: JAK2 and TYK2 [126]. In addition to PTP-1B's role in the regulation of JAK/STAT signalling, a role for this phosphatase in the regulation of TLR4 signalling was proposed. PTP1B$^{-/-}$ MØs had increased LPS-induced iNOS expression and NO production compared to WT MØs and were more susceptible to endotoxic shock following low-dose LPS injection [121]. Given the ability of PTP-1B to regulate several cellular processes including signalling pathways of high importance in MØ function, it is rather surprising that no work has been published on the role that PTP-1B plays during *Leishmania* infection. In fact, very recent work from our laboratory showed that *Leishmania* gp63 was able to enhance PTP-1B activation by cleaving it. PTP-1B activity seems to inhibit MØ activation and help in parasite survival as seen in the delayed onset of footpad swelling and reduced parasite burden in PTP-1B$^{-/-}$ mice infected with *L. major* (M.A. Gomez and M. Olivier, manuscript under review).

TC-PTP$^{-/-}$ mice suffer from multiple immunological defects and die within five weeks of birth [127]. This observation and the findings that TC-PTP plays important roles in the negative regulation of JAK1, JAK3 [128], and nuclear STAT-1 [129] suggest the important role of this PTP in the regulation of immune responses. As is the case with PTP-1B, it is equally surprising that data is lacking regarding the role of TC-PTP during *Leishmania* infection. Our laboratory has shown that gp63 of *Leishmania* was able to enhance TC-PTP activation by cleaving it in host MØs (M.A. Gomez and M. Olivier, manuscript under review). This gp63-mediated TC-PTP cleavage along with the cleavage of PTP-PEST were very recently reported, by our group and M.L. Tremblay's group, to occur in fibroblasts infected with *Leishmania* and were suggested to enhance the catalytic activity of the PTPs in question and/or allow them to access additional substrates that might help the parasite establish itself [130].

SHP-1:

It is a PTP that contains two N-terminal SH2 domains (N-SH2, C-SH2), followed by a PTP domain responsible for dephosphorylating substrates, and a C-terminal tail [121]. This phosphatase is mostly expressed in hematopoietic cells [131, 132], but is also expressed at lower levels in epithelial [132], endothelial [133, 134], and central nervous system cells [135]. The SH2 domains have two main functions: Firstly, the N-SH2 domain plays an important auto-inhibitory role by interacting intramolecularly with the PTP domain keeping the PTP in the inactive state. Secondly, both SH2 domains have the ability to bind to phospho-tyrosine (p-Y) residues usually found within immunoreceptor tyrosine-based inhibitory motifs

(ITIMs) whose consensus sequence is (I/V/L/S)xYxx(L/V) [136]. This second feature of SH2-domains is thought to play a role in the detachment of the N-SH2 from the PTP domain once the C-SH2 domain binds to a target p-Y, therefore opening up and activating the PTP [121].

SHP-1 plays a key role in immune cell signalling, this is supported by the autoimmune and immunodeficiency syndrome exhibited by SHP-1$^{-/-}$ mice (motheaten mice). These mice are named so because of the patchy hair loss that they suffer from due to displacement of hair follicles by MØs and neutrophils that infiltrate the subepidermal tissue. These myeloid cells also migrate to several other sites causing severe inflammation and tissue damage [121, 137]. In addition to its role in BCR [138] and TCR [139-141] signalling, SHP-1 has been shown to be able to interact with non-receptor targets such as JAK2, JAK3 [142], several MAPKs [143, 144], and transcription factors such as STAT [145]. It is therefore an elegant tactic that *Leishmania* activates SHP-1 in infected MØs in order to inhibit several signalling pathways that can otherwise be deadly to the parasite.

At the signalling level, our laboratory have clearly demonstrated that *Leishmania* was able to rapidly activate host SHP-1 causing SHP-1-mediated JAK2 inactivation in MØs [78]. Additionally, we and others have implicated SHP-1 in the negative regulation of Erk1/2 activity [97, 98] and in the regulation of the downstream TFs NF-κB and AP-1 [98] during *Leishmania* infection. At the functional level, our laboratory showed that the injection of PTP inhibitors (bis-peroxovanadium compounds) to mice infected with *L. major* or *L. donovani* helped control the infection [146] in a manner dependent on iNOS expression and NO production [147]. Furthermore, we demonstrated that SHP-1-deficient viable motheaten mice, infected with *L. major*, did not develop footpad swelling and had significantly reduced parasitic loads [148]. This decreased pathology was associated with more neutrophil recruitment to the footpad and more iNOS mRNA expression [148].

As to how *Leishmania* is able to activate SHP-1, it has been proposed that *Leishmania*'s elongation factor-1α (EF-1α) is responsible for the activation of host SHP-1 seen 16 hours post-infection [149]. This report cannot explain; however, how SHP-1 is activated in earlier infection times nor does it explain how EF-1α of the parasite can shuttle from the phagolysosome where the parasite is to the cytosol where SHP-1 is found. A more plausible mechanism has been recently suggested by our group, where SHP-1 was shown to be activated via cleavage by the parasite's protease gp63, which gains access to the cytosol by going through the lipid raft of host MØs (M.A. Gomez and M. Olivier, manuscript under review). In conclusion, it appears that the rapid activation of SHP-1 by *Leishmania* is a key host evasion step whereby the parasite is able to utilize this phosphatase to negatively regulate several key MØ pathways and render it unresponsive to activating stimuli such as: IFN-γ and LPS. By doing so, the parasite is able to block several MØ functions such as NO production and the synthesis of many pro-inflammatory cytokines that can be deadly to the parasite if allowed to be produced.

Suppressors of Cytokine Signalling (SOCS)

This family is made of eight members: cytokine-inducible SH2-containing protein (CIS) and suppressors of cytokine signalling 1 to 7 (SOCS1-7). These proteins have a central SH2 domain and a SOCS box motif in their C-terminal and have been shown to play an important role in the regulation of over 30 cytokines including IL-6 and IFN-γ [150]. Both SOCS1 and SOCS3 are involved in the negative regulation of JAK/STAT signalling through the ability of both proteins to interact with Y1007 in the catalytic loop of JAK2 [151, 152]. SOCS1 and SOCS3 not only bind JAK2 but also have strong binding affinities to phosphotyrosines located within several receptor subunits such as the IFNγR1 [153] and the IL-12 Rβ2 [154]. SOCS gene expression is driven by JAK/STAT signalling where SOCS can inhibit this pathway in a negative feedback loop. This negative regulation can occur either by direct binding and inhibition of JAK (e.g. SOCS1), SH2-mediated binding of SOCS to the cytoplasmic domain of the receptor, followed by JAK inactivation (e.g. SOCS3), or by competing with STAT SH2 domains in the binding to critical phosphotyrsoines in the cytoplasmic domains of receptors (e.g. SOCS2). An additional regulation mechanism is the ability of the E3 ubiquitin-ligase complex to bind to the SOCS box motif targeting receptors or receptor-associated proteins to proteasome-mediated degradation [150].

The involvement of SOCS in *Leishmania* infection remains unclear due to the paucity of published research in that subject. One study reported the ability of live and heat-killed *L. donovani*, but not purified LPG, to transiently induce SOCS3 expression in MØs. This expression was independent of phagocytosis and cytokine release by the infected MØs [155]. This report does not explain which parasite component is able to induce SOCS3 expression nor does it demonstrate any downstream functional consequences of this induction. Further work is certainly required to explore the role of SOCS proteins in the inhibition of cytokine signalling in *Leishmania*-infected MØs.

MACROPHAGE FUNCTIONS ALTERED BY *LEISHMANIA*

Modulation of signalling pathways by *Leishmania* are intended to alter critical MØ functions to the advantage of the parasite. Upon the initial contact of *Leishmania* with the MØ, certain functions such as the production of chemokines and chemokine receptors are induced whereas others are inhibited. Among the functions inhibited by the parasite are those related to MØ activation and to their ability to present Ag and communicate with cells of the adaptive immune system. Hereby, we will discuss the main functions that *Leishmania* can interfere with upon initial interaction (0-6 h) or chronic infection (> 6 h) of host MØs.

Induction of Chemokine Expression

One of the important early challenges confronted by *Leishmania* is the ability to preferentially recruit cells of the immune system to the site of inoculation in order to infect them and establish disease in the host without getting killed. One key mechanism by which the parasite is able to do so is the induction of chemokine expression and production by host immune cells. One study showed that infection of mice with *L. major* upregulated the gene expression of several chemokines in cells collected from the footpad and their draining lymph nodes. These chemokines were measured by quantitative PCR and RNAase Protection Assay (RPA) and include: RANTES/CCL5, MIP-1α/CCL3, IP-10/CXCL10, and MCP-1/CCL2 [156]. In addition, our laboratory has clearly shown that *L. major* infection caused an upregulation in the expression of several chemokines in cells recruited to the air pouch of infected mice. These chemokines include: RANTES, MIP-1α, MIP-1β/CCL4, IP-10, MCP-1, and MIP-2/CXCL1) [157]. It is interesting to see that most of these chemokines are in part monocyte chemoattractants, recruiting MØs to infected tissues and helping the parasite get installed. It is equally interesting to see that none of these chemokines, with the exception of MIP-2, attract neutrophils. This is in accordance with our previous finding that neutrophil recruitment to infection sites is associated with parasite killing in SHP-1 deficient viable motheaten mice [148]. In addition, our laboratory has shown that cells recruited to the air pouch in *L. major*-infected mice not only upregulate chemokine expression but also the expression of chemokine receptors including: CCR1, CCR2, CCR3, and CCR5 [157].

So far, we have considered chemokine upregulation as beneficial to the parasite, yet it is important to bear in mind that secreted chemokines during leishmaniasis can act as a double-edged sword. While early selective activation of monocyte-chemotactic factors can help the parasite recruit MØs that they can infect, treatment of susceptible BALB/c mice infected with *L. major* with recombinant IP-10 in the early course of infection, for example, has been shown to increase NK cell cytotoxic activity in the draining lymph nodes and can drive a healing IFN-γ-mediated Th1 response [158]. In chronic infections, chemokine types, amounts, and duration of chemotactic effect have been implicated in parasite clearance or persistence. For instance, in visceral leishmaniasis, clearance of parasites from the liver is strongly associated with increased late phase IP-10 production and the Th1 effects associated with its presence [158]. Parasite persistence in the spleen, on the other hand, has been correlated with sustained MCP-1 but not IP-10 levels [159].

Inhibition of Microbicidal Free Radical Production

One of the dangers that *Leishmania* encounters recruiting and entering MØs is the ability of these cells to produce free radicals that are deadly to the parasite. Two main free radical molecules have been shown to have leishmanicidal effects: NO [160] and reactive oxygen intermediates (ROIs) [161].

NO is produced by NOS which converts one of the terminal nitrogens of the guanidino group of L-arginine to NO producing L-citrulline [162, 163]. The importance of this free radical in leishmaniasis was demonstrated by several groups. An early study showed the ability of activated MØs to kill *L. major* amastigotes by an L-arginine-dependent mechanism [164]. Another study confirmed this observation by showing that L-N-monomethyl arginine (L-NMMA), an L-arginine analogue and inhibitor of the NO pathway, was able to inhibit the leishmanicidal effect of MØs activated *in vitro* with IFN-γ or LPS. The authors also showed the ability of NO in cell-free suspensions to kill the parasite. Importantly, the same group demonstrated the importance of NO *in vivo* by rendering resistant CBA mice susceptible to *L. major* infection upon local administration of L-NMMA [160].

The question that comes to mind next is: how can NO contribute to parasite killing? Modes of action seem to include the ability of NO to cause modifications of proteins, injury to mitochondria, oxidation of membranes, DNA damage (e.g. depurination), modulation of cytokine production, and interference with maturation of immune cells [165]. Examples of *Leishmania* proteins inactivated by NO include the glycolytic enzyme glyceraldehyde 3-phosphate dehydrogenase (GAPDH) [166] and the Krebs cycle enzyme, aconitase, which NO can inhibit through triggering iron loss from its iron-sulfur prosthetic group [167].

Having discussed the detrimental effects of NO on *Leishmania*, it is comprehensible that the parasite is able to block its synthesis in response to stimuli such as IFN-γ [11], but how can *Leishmania* achieve this inhibition? A critical role for host SHP-1 has been proposed. As previously stated, *Leishmania* has the ability to rapidly activate SHP-1 in infected MØs and by doing so can interfere with several molecules involved in NO production including: JAK2, Erk1/2, and the TFs NF-κB and AP-1. Indeed, SHP-1 deficient MØs infected with *L. donovani* are still able to produce NO in response to IFN-γ stimulation unlike infected WT MØs which are refractory to a similar stimulation [98]. Expectedly, the IFN-γ-mediated NO production in infected SHP-1 deficient MØs correlated with successful phosphorylation of JAK2 and Erk1/2, and the activation of NF-κB and AP-1. These findings further elucidate the role of SHP-1 activation in parasite survival and propagation through its ability to contribute to NO inhibition [98].

We have previously mentioned that the iNOS promoter contains binding sites for NF-κB, STAT-1α, and AP-1. It therefore follows that all *Leishmania*-mediated signalling alterations of these TFs or of signalling molecules that activate them may contribute to NO inhibition in response to activating stimuli. We have discussed many of these alterations in the previous section, but will reiterate the ones of direct relevance to NO inhibition. These include: the ability of the parasite to inhibit PKC activity, inhibit MAPK activation, inhibit LPS-mediated NF-κB activation, induce ceramide formation, and cause proteasome-mediated STAT-1α degradation. Additionally, the *Leishmania*-induced production of the immunosuppressive molecules IL-10 and TGF-β by MØs may contribute to the ability of the parasite to inhibit NO [168, 169].

ROIs represent another source of danger to *Leishmania*. These intermediates include the superoxide radical and hydrogen peroxide produced by cells of the immune system such as: neutrophils and MØs in response to phagocytosis of foreign particles. Although important in parasite killing, the activity of the respiratory burst in mice was shown to have an early and transient effect only. This conclusion is based on the delayed granuloma formation and resolution of infection seen in respiratory burst-deficient X-CGD mice infected with *L. donovani* compared to WT [170]. Despite the critical role that NO seems to play in *Leishmania* killing [170], ROIs do contribute to parasite clearance and are therefore a target to be inhibited by the parasite. Indeed, *L. donovani* has been shown to inhibit the oxidative burst in infected MØs [71, 171, 172], and this inhibition was mediated by the parasite surface molecules LPG and gp63 [2, 173] and involve PKC inactivation [71]. Interestingly, it was later shown that LPG of *L. donovani* promastigotes is able to block NADPH oxidase assembly at the phagosome membrane without interfering with p47(phox) phosphorylation and its ability to form complexes with p67(phox) [174]. *L. donovani* amastigotes, on the other hand, were shown to effectively block superoxide release through inhibiting the phosphorylation of the NADPH oxidase component p47(phox), leading to defective recruitment of p47(phox) and p67(phox) to the phagosome [175]. The inhibition of p47(phox) phosphorylation could be a result of the previously reported ability of *Leishmania* amastigotes to inhibit PKC activity [71], which is reported to be required for p47(phox) phosphorylation [176].

Inhibition of Pro-Inflammatory Cytokine Production

IL-1 and TNF-α have been correlated with antimicrobial activities against bacteria and parasites *in vitro* and *in vivo* [177-180], and IL-12 is well-known for its ability to promote Th1 differentiation and to activate NK cells [181]. Concerning IL-1 and TNF-α, it has been shown that these molecules are not produced upon a 12 h *in vitro* infection of human monocytes with *L. donovani* amastigotes [182]. Interestingly, preinfection of those cells diminished LPS-mediated IL-1 production but not IL-1 m-RNA, suggesting inhibition at the translational level [182]. Another study showed that pre-incubation of human monocytes with purified LPG was able to cause inhibition of LPS-mediated IL-1β secretion [183]. The role of LPG in IL-1β inhibition was later shown to involve the ability of LPG to inhibit the transcription of the IL-1β gene in a manner dependent on the nucleotide region -310 to -57 of the promoter region [184]. This inhibitory effect of LPG on IL-1β gene transcription was suggested to involve an inhibition of the binding of an activation factor or an induction of an unknown transcription repressor [184]. Interestingly, an *in vivo* study using the mouse air pouch system showed that *L. major* was able to cause production of IL-1, IL-6, and TNF-α in the early stage of infection, an event that was less notable with *L. donovani* [185]. These findings could help explain the different pathologies caused by both species including the ability of *L. donovani* to visceralize and the restriction of *L. major* to the inoculation site. A later study by our laboratory clearly demonstrated that SHP-1 deficient mice stimulated with LPS or infected with *L. major* produced significantly higher amounts of IL-1, IL-6, and TNF-α compared to their littermates [157]. This suggests that SHP-1, activated by *Leishmania*, plays a pivotal role in the attenuation of the inflammatory response via repressing the production of these pro-inflammatory cytokines possibly contributing to parasite survival and pathogenesis.

IL-12 is another key cytokine inhibited by *Leishmania*. This inhibitory effect is necessary for parasite survival given the established role of this molecule in driving Th1 differentiation and production of IFN-γ by T cells and NK cells, which in turn can activate MØs to kill the parasite. It has been reported that infection of BMDMs with promastigotes of *L. major* or *L. donovani* fails to induce IL-12 production both following infection alone and upon subsequent LPS or heat-killed bacterial stimulation of MØs [186]. Similar observations were seen when murine MØs were infected with amastigotes of *L. major* and *L. mexicana* [187]. Furthermore, incubation of activated murine MØs with LPG led to the inhibition of IL-12 production by these cells, with the inhibition occurring at the transcriptional level [10]. The mechanism by which IL-12 is inhibited by *Leishmania* remains not fully understood. Roles for the MØ CR3 [188] and Fc-γR [189] have been proposed. Additionally, we have described in the previous section the role of *L. mexicana*'s cysteine proteinases in the cleavage of NF-κB and the possible involvement of this process in the inhibition of LPS-induced IL-12 production by infected MØs [33]. Very recently, our laboratory arrived to new findings that helped advance our knowledge of the mechanism by which *Leishmania* can inhibit LPS-mediated pro-inflammatory functions such as: IL-12 and TNF-α production. We have demonstrated that *Leishmania*-induced SHP-1 is able to bind to an evolutionarily conserved immunoreceptor tyrosine-based inhibitory motif (ITIM)-like motif (which we renamed kinase tyrosine-based inhibitory motif (KTIM)) found in the kinase domain of IL-1 receptor-associated kinase 1 (IRAK-1) causing its inactivation. SHP-1-bound IRAK-1 is no longer able to detach from Myeloid differentiation factor 88 (MyD88) to bind TNF receptor-associated factor 6 (TRAF6) and activate downstream signalling pathways, therefore explaining in part how the parasite is able to block LPS-mediated MyD88-dependent pro-inflammatory functions in host macrophages [190].

Production of Immunosuppressive Molecules

In addition to being able to suppress pro-inflammatory molecules like IL-1, IL-6, IL-12, and TNF-α, *Leishmania* is also able to induce the production of immunosuppressive molecules that can help further the survival and propagation of the parasite. Three immunosuppressive molecules have been reported to play important roles in disease establishment: prostaglandin E2 (PGE2), TGF-β, and IL-10.

PGE2 is produced from arachidonic acid with the help of enzymes known as cyclooxygenases (COXs). COXs have two isoforms: the constitutive COX-1 and the inducible COX-2 [191]. PGE2 has been demonstrated to inhibit MØ activation through interfering with several functions including generation of oxygen radicals, expression and release of LPS-induced TNF-α, and response to several pro-inflammatory cytokines [192]. It is therefore understandable why *Leishmania* has been reported to induce PGE2 production in infected MØs [193-195]. Following this line of thought, our laboratory showed that *Leishmania* was able to increase PGE2 production in infected MØs through its ability to induce COX-2 expression in a PKC-dependent manner [196]. This finding raises the interesting notion that PKC seems to be rapidly and transiently activated upon *L. donovani* infection resulting in increased PGE2 synthesis, and then gets inactivated afterwards to inhibit some of the PKC-dependent leishmanicidal functions described earlier in this chapter under the PKC section. Another interesting report correlated PGE2 production with increased visceralization of *L. donovani* in malnourished mice [197].

TGF-β is a potent suppressor of the immune system, with effects on a wide range of immune cells including: MØs, DCs, NK, and T cells [198]. Given the important role of these cells in the progression of *Leishmania* infections, it is not surprising to find out that several species of the parasite are able to induce TGF-β production and promote an anti-inflammatory environment [199]. This *Leishmania*-induced increase in TGF-β production has been correlated with reduced iNOS expression in immune cell infiltrates found in the skin lesion and draining lymph nodes of infected mice [169] and with impaired IL-12-driven IFN-γ production and cytotoxic abilities of NK cells derived from mice infected with *L. major* [200]. In support of the previous roles of TGF-β in suppressing various innate and adaptive immune functions during leishmaniasis, one study reported high levels of TGF-β in the local environment surrounding *L. chagasi*-infected MØs [201]. Furthermore, the same group showed that *in vitro* infection of human MØs with *L. chagasi* was associated with an increase in the biologically active form of TGF-β rather than an increase in m-RNA or total protein levels [201]. *L. chagasi*'s cysteine proteinase cathepsin B was implicated in the production of active TGF-β from the latent form [201], a mechanism reported to be shared by the *L. donovani* complex [202]. Additionally, as previously described under the phosphatidylserine receptor section, interaction of PS-expressing amastigotes with the PSR has been shown to trigger TGF-β production in infected MØs [62].

IL-10 is yet another anti-inflammatory cytokine induced by *Leishmania*. This cytokine has established roles in the inhibition of effector functions of key immune cells, importantly: T cells and monocytes/MØs. The principal function of this cytokine is to control and ultimately terminate inflammatory responses [203], making the induction of this cytokine of clear benefit to *Leishmania*. Ligation of the Fc-γR seems to play a role in the induction of IL-10 in MØs [204]. The binding of amastigote PS to its receptor can also trigger IL-10 production [62] as previously mentioned in the PSR section. The production of IL-10 leads to some similar consequences as those encountered by TGF-β production, importantly the ability to inhibit MØ activation and NO production [168]. In addition, IL-10 suppresses the production of pro-inflammatory cytokines such as: IL-1, IL-12, and TNF, and the expression of costimulatory molecules such as B7-1 and B7-2 [168]. The role of IL-10 in the progression of leishmaniasis *in vivo* is established based on reports where resistant mice were rendered more susceptible to *L. major* infection when they were designed to express an IL-10 transgene [205], and other reports where susceptible BALB/c mice were rendered more resistant to infection when their IL-10 gene was knocked-out [206]. All this accumulating data suggest IL-10 induction to be one effective mechanism used by *Leishmania* to evade MØ activation and killing.

Interference with Antigen Presentation

MØs are antigen presenting cells (APCs) that can link innate and adaptive immunity by phagocytosing foreign objects, digesting them in lysosomes, and coupling pathogen-associated Ags to MHC II molecules and presenting them on their surface to CD4+ T cells (T helper cells). The activation of T helper cells causes activation of other immune cells including B cells, cytotoxic CD8+ T cells, and MØs. Therefore, and in order to persist inside MØs and cause chronic infections, *Leishmania* had to develop ways to interfere with the ability of these cells to present foreign Ags.

One remarkable tactic the parasite utilizes is its ability to inhibit IFN-γ-induced MHC class II expression in infected MØs. Indeed, *L. chagasi* and *L. donovani* were both shown to inhibit MHC II expression in response to IFN-γ stimulation [207-209]. Surprisingly, MØs infected with *L. major* or *L. amazonensis* showed normal phagocytosis, Ag processing, and MHC II production, yet these cells failed to present parasitic Ags to T cell hybridomas [210, 211]. Authors of both studies concluded that the failure to present Ags to T cells is due to the parasite's ability to interfere with the loading of Ags onto MHC II molecules. Another interesting mechanism to control Ag presentation was presented previously in the section related to cysteine proteinases of *Leishmania*. Briefly, amastigotes of *L. amazonensis* have been shown to be able to internalize MHC II molecules and to degrade them using their cysteine proteinases [34].

Activation of CD4+ T cells involves a "two-signal model" whereby two signals are required to activate the T helper cell. The first signal is triggered by the binding of the T-cell receptor (TCR) to the MHC II-Ag complex on the APC, and the second is provided by the binding of CD28 or CD40L on T cells to costimulatory molecules of APCs such as those of the B7 family or CD40. Interestingly, apart from interfering with the first signal by inhibiting MHC II presentation, *Leishmania* has been demonstrated to interfere with MØ costimulatory signals. *L. donovani* infection was reported to block LPS-mediated B7-1 expression in infected MØs [212], a mechanism that seems to be mediated by prostaglandins [213]. Furthermore, *L. major* was reported to interfere with CD40 signalling in infected MØs in a p38-dependent manner [100]. This result is very interesting, especially that previous studies have established a protective role for CD40 in *Leishmania major* infections [214, 215], while others have reported that the disruption of CD40/CD40L ligation results in increased susceptibility to *L. amazonensis* infection [216]. The increased susceptibility caused by the disruption of CD40/CD40L ligation was in part due to the inhibition of iNOS expression [214, 216] and IL-12 production [217] by infected MØs.

So far in the previous paragraph, we have discussed several mechanisms by which *Leishmania* can interfere with key signalling pathways involved in MØ activation such as the JAK/STAT pathway. We also discussed alterations that occur to signalling molecules involved in TLR signalling such as MAPKs and the TFs NF-κB and AP-1. However, this does not give justice to TLR signalling, given its extremely important role in the activation of APCs to kill invading pathogens and/or activate cells of the adaptive immune system. Equally important are the strategies developed by pathogens to block TLR signalling pathways that can lead to undesirable activation of immune functions. We will therefore dedicate the rest of this chapter to discuss TLR signalling and what is known about its modulation by pathogens, with special emphasis on parasites including *Leishmania*, the subject of this chapter.

MODULATION OF TOLL-LIKE RECEPTOR (TLR) SIGNALLING BY *LEISHMANIA* AND OTHER PARASITES

TLR family members are known for their critical role in bridging the innate immune response to the adaptive one through recognizing pathogen-associated molecular patterns (PAMPs). In the light of the ongoing host-pathogen arms race, the detection of parasite PAMPs by TLRs has two main implications: First, the ability of cells of the immune system to detect parasites and eliminate them when favorable conditions are present. Second, the ability of parasites to counteract TLR detection by interfering with TLR signalling keeping immune cells in an inactive state and rendering them refractory to subsequent TLR stimulation.

One of the main parasite-derived molecules involved in TLR binding and activation are GPI-anchored proteins. *Trypanosoma cruzi*-derived GPI-anchors were shown to be detected by TLR2/TLR6 and CD14 and to activate NF-κB [218, 219], while GIPLs of *T. cruzi* activated Chinese hamster ovary (CHO) cells in a TLR4/CD14-dependent manner [220]. It has been also shown that GPI-mucin of *T. cruzi* is able activate TLR signalling on first exposure and induce tolerance to secondary TLR stimulation [221]. This was later shown to be mediated by the ability of GPI-mucin to induce the expression and activation of the serine/threonine phosphatase PP2A that acts on cellular IRAK-1, MAPKs, and IκB causing their inhibition and leading to tolerance [222]. The induction of PP2A was shown to require p38 and NF-κB, the very same molecules PP2A is induced to inhibit therefore giving rise to an autoregulatory loop [222]. LPG of *Leishmania* is another GPI-anchored protein detected by TLRs. It has been shown that LPG of *L. major* directly binds to TLR2 of MØs and NK cells [223, 224] and that LPG of *L. donovani* is also detected by TLR2 of activated MØs [225]. Interestingly, GPI-anchors derived from *Plasmodium falciparum* merozoites can induce TNF production in human monocytes and mouse MØs through interacting with TLR1/TLR2 and to a lesser extent TLR4 [226, 227]. Moreover, GPI- anchors of *Toxoplasma gondii* are detected by TLR2 and TLR4, which can thus play an important role in host defense against *T. gondii* infections [228].

Although less numerous than GPI-anchored ligands, non-GPI-related ligands represent an important group of parasite-related molecules detected by TLRs. An example is the *T. cruzi*-derived protein Tc52, which is able to induce pro-inflammatory cytokine production in DCs in a TLR2-dependent manner [229]. Other important non-GPI ligands include the DNA of *T. cruzi*, *T. brucei*, and *Babesia bovis*, which are able to activate MØs and DCs [230, 231], possibly through unmethylated CpG motifs [232] detected by TLR9 [233, 234]. TLR3 was recently shown to be upregulated in IFN-γ-primed MØs and to play a role in their leishmanicidal activity. The silencing of TLR3 led to impaired NO and TNF-α production in IFN-γ-primed MØs in response to *L. donovani* infection and increased parasite survival [225]. Given that the only known ligand of TLR3 is dsRNA, the parasite component that activates TLR3 remains unclear. The authors ruled out the presence of dsRNA *leishmania*virus infection in their parasite strain and also failed to detect natural *Leishmania*-derived double-stranded RNA structures such as rRNA or tRNA [225]. As far as apicomplexans are concerned, *Plasmodium*-derived hemozoin crystals were shown to induce pro-inflammatory cytokines in MØs [235, 236]. Initially, TLR9 was proposed as the binding receptor of hemozoin [237], this remains controversial as it has been later shown that TLR9 activation by hemozoin in DCs is mediated by malaria DNA attached to the crystal and that the activation of TLR9 by hemozoin was abolished upon treatment with nucleases [238]. In fact, recent data from our laboratory show that the pro-inflammatory cytokine IL-1β is induced by hemozoin through the Nod-like receptor family, pyrin domain containing 3 (Nlrp3) and the adaptor protein Asc, which lead to caspase 1 activation (Shio et al., *PLoS pathogens*, E-pub, 21st August, 2009). Concerning *Toxoplasma*, a profilin-like protein from *T. gondii* (PFTG) activates TLR11 in mouse cells [239], and heat shock proteins and partially purified preparations isolated from tachyzoites activate TLR4 and TLR2, respectively [240, 241].

The many parasite-related molecules that are detected by TLRs suggest an important role for TLR-related signalling molecules in the resistance to parasitic infections [242]. Given the fact that Th1-driving pro-inflammatory responses are beneficial to the host in several types of parasitic infections, it is not surprising that the activation of the MyD88-dependent pathway is crucial in the resistance to many protozoan diseases. Indeed, MyD88-deficient mice are highly susceptible to *T. cruzi* [243], *T. brucei* [234], *L. major* [244], and *T. gondii* [245] infections due to the decreased inflammatory response and the impaired production of Th1-associated cytokines such as IL-12 and IFN-γ in these mice. It is important to mention that MyD88-driven pro-inflammatory events are not always favorable to the host in the fight against protozoans. The decreased inflammatory and Th1 responses in MyD88-deficient mice were seen to improve pathology and outcome of *P. berghei* infection in mice. This suggests that *Plasmodium*, in this case, utilizes the MyD88-dependent pathway to cause tissue injury and worsen disease symptoms [246].

It is quite remarkable that the amount of susceptibility to several protozoan infections conferred by the absence of MyD88 is significantly higher than that observed when mice lacking a single TLR are used. This strongly suggests that several TLRs are simultaneously involved in the recognition of parasites, thus explaining why the loss of MyD88 can have a bigger impact on susceptibility compared to the loss of a single TLR [242]. Nevertheless, deficiency of relevant TLRs increases susceptibility to certain infections. For example, TLR9-deficient mice have higher parasitemia and mortality when infected with *T. cruzi* [233] or *T. brucei* [234]. TLR4-deficient mice are more susceptible to *L. major* infection with bigger lesion size and parasite loads compared to WT mice [247, 248], and TLR11-deficient mice are more susceptible to *T. gondii* infection manifesting increased cyst formation in the central nervous system and decreased IL-12 and IFN-γ production compared to WT mice [239].

The ability of TLRs to detect parasite PAMPs put together with the fact that many successful infections are associated with silent entry to target cells suggests that parasites must have evasion tactics to block TLR signalling and functions. Some of these mechanisms have been already described while others are still to be discovered. We will hereby discuss some evasion strategies employed by *Leishmania, Plasmodium,* and *Toxoplasma.*

The ability of *Leishmania* to interfere with TLR signalling components has been already discussed in this chapter under the "signalling pathways altered by *Leishmania*" section. These evasion mechanisms include the previously discussed ability of the parasite to interfere with the activation of all three MAPKs (Erk1/2, JNK, p38) (see MAPK section), and its ability to interfere with IκB, NF-κB, and AP-1 (see TF section). There is also evidence that signalling through CR1 and CR3, which *Leishmania* is known to bind to, can inhibit LPS- and IFN-γ-induced IL-12 production through impaired STAT-1 phosphorylation [188]. A similar role for Fc-γR ligation has been proposed [189, 249]. Nevertheless, very little is known about how the parasite can interfere with critical upstream proteins unique to IL-1/TLR signalling such as members of the IRAK family. Our laboratory has been interested for many years in exploring mechanisms utilized by *Leishmania* to block TLR signalling in MØs, and to evaluate the role of host SHP-1 in this process. Importantly, microarray experiments performed by our laboratory showed that the expression of many genes involved in immune cell signalling and functions was significantly higher in SHP-1 deficient compared to WT mice infected with *L. donovani* over the period of 2 weeks. (Fig. **1**). This finding supports a key role for SHP-1 in the negative regulation of MØ signalling pathways.

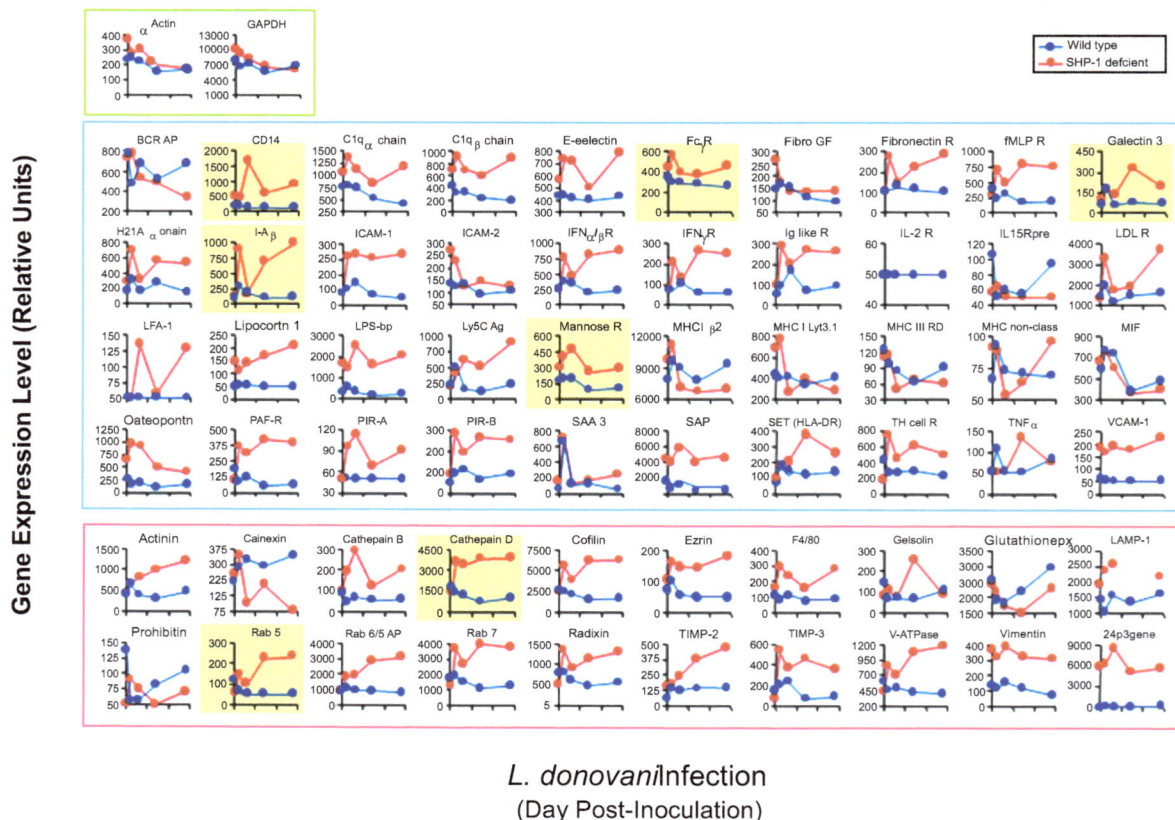

Figure 1: Impact of *L. donovani* infection on macrophage gene expression *in vivo.*

Furthermore, a specific role for SHP-1 in the negative regulation of TLR4 signalling was suggested when we observed that *L. donovani* infection caused an increase in the gene expression of CD14, the co-receptor of TLR4, in SHP-1 deficient mice seen *in vivo* by microarray analysis and northern blot, and in SHP-1 deficient MØs *in vitro* by northern blot and FACS analysis (Fig. **2**).

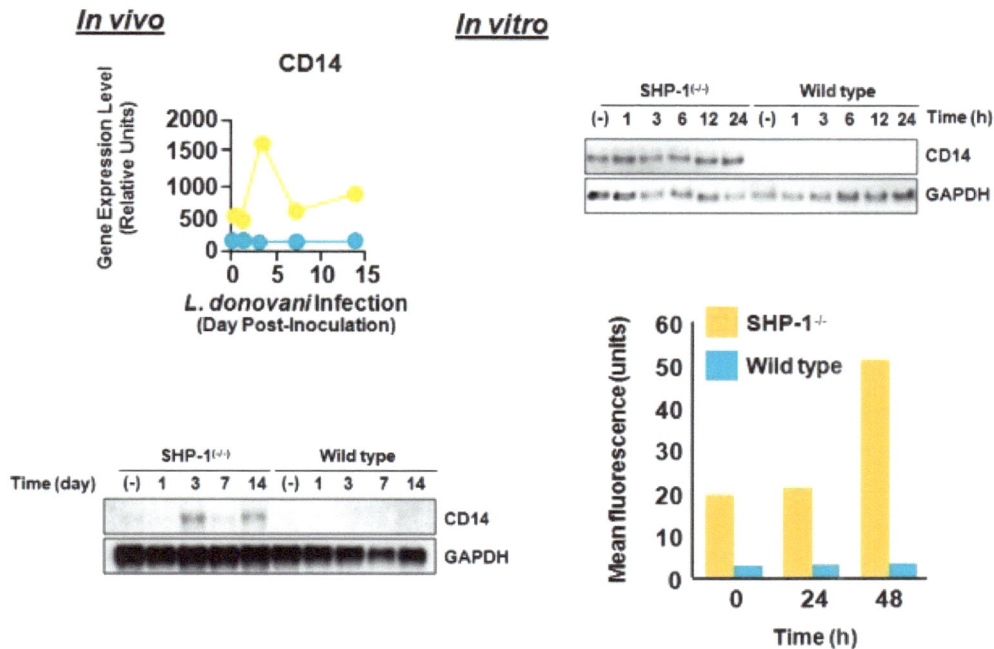

Figure 2: SHP-1-mediated CD14 inactivation.

Of utmost interest, we have recently established SHP-1 as a central regulator of TLR signalling which can be exploited by *Leishmania* to inhibit IRAK-1 leading to the inability of MØs to respond to a wide range of TLR ligand stimulation including LPS, favoring parasite survival [190].

Other pathogen evasion tactics include the ability of *P. falciparum* to cause infected erythrocytes to express *P. falciparum* erythrocyte membrane protein 1 (PfEMP1) which was shown to interact with the scavenger receptor CD36 on the surface of DCs [250] making the cells that phagocytose these infected erythrocytes become unresponsive to LPS stimulation, ultimately leading to defects in T cell activation [251-253] .

T. gondii is yet another parasite able to block LPS-mediated IL-12 and TNF-α production, the upregulation of co-stimulatory molecules, and the activation of T cells [254-257]. One way the parasite is able to do so is by activating STAT3 in IL-10-dependent and –independent manners [258, 259]. Although this *T. gondii*-induced inhibition of subsequent LPS stimulation might somehow resemble LPS tolerance in that it inhibits MAPKs like p38 [260], important differences between infection and LPS tolerance exist. Unlike LPS tolerance, *T. gondii* infection followed by LPS stimulation resulted in the activation of MKK3 and MKK6 (upstream activators of p38) and in the degradation of IκB [260]. This suggests that the inactivation of p38 observed when LPS stimulation is preceded by *Toxoplasma* infection is either due to the inhibition of another p38-activating kinase such as MKK4, or is mediated by a *T. gondii*-induced MAPK phosphatase that prevents the phosphorylation-dependent activation of p38 [242]. It is interesting to note that although *T. gondii* infection followed by LPS stimulation causes IκB activation, the liberated NF-κB fails to translocate to the nucleus [261, 262]. Later studies suggested that the lack of NF-κB translocation might actually be due to increased nuclear export of this TF rather than inhibition of nuclear import [263].

Based on the previous sections describing the importance of TLR signalling in fighting disease and the many tactics developed by pathogens to circumvent this, it is rather tempting to hope that by using TLR ligands in vaccination or treatment regiments, we can activate the immune system to fight pathogens and clear them more efficiently. For example, monophosphoryl lipid A (TLR4 ligand) is in an advanced stage of development for use in vaccines in combination with antigens of *P. falciparum* [264] and *Leishmania* species [265]. Other TLR ligands that demonstrated promising results in vaccination experiments include imiquimod and R848 (resiquimod) (TLR7/TLR8 ligands) which mounted a protective Th1 response against *L. major* antigens [266], and CpG-containing oligodeoxynucleotides (TLR9 ligand), which induced protective immunity against *T. cruzi, Leishmania, Plasmodium,* and *T. gondii* [242, 267-271]. Additionally, flagellin (TLR5 ligand) was successfully used to stimulate mucosal immunity [272], and might turn out to be important in developing vaccines that target pathogens of mucosal tissue such as *T. gondii* which infects the intestinal tract.

As far as treatment is concerned, the use of imiquimod and CpG-containing oligodeoxynucleotides as immunomodulators, for example, has been proven effective in the treatment of leishmaniasis in experimental models [273-275].

Collectively, it is clear that TLRs play a crucial role in mounting innate and adaptive immunity against invading pathogens. Alteration of TLR signalling by pathogens or by clinical drugs can play a key role in the outcome of infections. We have discussed in good detail strategies used by pathogens or by the clinic to alter TLR signalling. The activation of MyD88-dependent signalling and Th1 responses can turn out very useful in the elimination of many pathogens including *Leishmania*. However, these efforts must always be perceived with caution as exaggerated activation of inflammation can cause edema, pain, tissue injury, and in severe conditions could be deadly. In addition, certain infectious models like malaria seem to benefit from MyD88-dependent signalling and inflammation in their pathology and thus a completely different approach should be used when trying to fight *Plasmodium*. As opposed to using TLR ligands which can worsen the disease, TLR agonists could prove clinically effective in treating malaria. Nevertheless, the effects of blocking TLR-TLR-L interactions on the ability of the immune system to fight off other pathogens that can be/become present have to be taken into serious consideration.

CONCLUSIONS

Over the last 15 years, research in our laboratory has accumulated strong evidence that the *Leishmania* parasite is able to establish itself and propagate within the mammalian host through its ability to alter several key signalling pathways in order to interfere with critical MØ functions that can otherwise threaten parasite survival. One key way *Leishmania* can do so is by exploiting host negative regulatory mechanisms such as PTPs. The ability of *Leishmania* to rapidly activate host PTPs such as SHP-1 is a central event contributing to the parasite's ability to inhibit several IFN-γ- and LPS-mediated functions that are crucial to MØ activation and to its ability to control and clear *Leishmania* parasites.

REFERENCES

[1]   Lodge R, Descoteaux A. Modulation of phagolysosome biogenesis by the lipophosphoglycan of *Leishmania*. Clin Immunol 2005; 114: 256-65.
[2]   Descoteaux A, Turco SJ. Glycoconjugates in *Leishmania* infectivity. Biochim Biophys Acta 1999; 1455: 341-52.
[3]   Sacks DL. *Leishmania*-sand fly interactions controlling species-specific vector competence. Cell Microbiol 2001; 3: 189-96.
[4]   Puentes SM, Sacks DL, da Silva RP, Joiner KA. Complement binding by two developmental stages of *Leishmania major* promastigotes varying in expression of a surface lipophosphoglycan. J Exp Med 1988; 167: 887-02.
[5]   Green PJ, Feizi T, Stoll MS, *et al*. Recognition of the major cell surface glycoconjugates of *Leishmania* parasites by the human serum mannan-binding protein. Mol Biochem Parasitol 1994; 66: 319-28.
[6]   Culley FJ, Harris RA, Kaye PM, *et al*. C-reactive protein binds to a novel ligand on *Leishmania donovani* and increases uptake into human macrophages. J Immunol 1996; 156: 4691-96.
[7]   Descoteaux A, Matlashewski G, Turco SJ. Inhibition of macrophage protein kinase C-mediated protein phosphorylation by *Leishmania donovani* lipophosphoglycan. J Immunol 1992; 149: 3008-15.
[8]   Desjardins M, Descoteaux A. Inhibition of phagolysosomal biogenesis by the *Leishmania* lipophosphoglycan. J Exp Med 1997; 185: 2061-68.
[9]   Scianimanico S, Desrosiers M, Dermine JF, *et al*. Impaired recruitment of the small GTPase rab7 correlates with the inhibition of phagosome maturation by *Leishmania donovani* promastigotes. Cell Microbiol 1999; 1: 19-32.
[10]   Piedrafita D, Proudfoot L, Nikolaev AV, *et al*. Regulation of macrophage IL-12 synthesis by *Leishmania* phosphoglycans. Eur J Immunol 1999; 29: 235-44.
[11]   Proudfoot L, Nikolaev AV, Feng GJ, *et al*. Regulation of the expression of nitric oxide synthase and leishmanicidal activity by glycoconjugates of *Leishmania* lipophosphoglycan in murine macrophages. Proc Natl Acad Sci USA 1996; 93: 10984-89.
[12]   Spath GF, Epstein L, Leader B, *et al*. Lipophosphoglycan is a virulence factor distinct from related glycoconjugates in the protozoan parasite *Leishmania major*. Proc Natl Acad Sci U S A 2000; 97: 9258-63.

[13] McNeely TB, Turco SJ. Requirement of lipophosphoglycan for intracellular survival of *Leishmania donovani* within human monocytes. J Immunol 1990; 144: 2745-50.

[14] McMaster WR, Morrison CJ, MacDonald MH, Joshi PB. Mutational and functional analysis of the *Leishmania* surface metalloproteinase GP63: similarities to matrix metalloproteinases. Parasitology 1994; 108: 29-36.

[15] Schlagenhauf E, Etges R, Metcalf P. The crystal structure of the *Leishmania major* surface proteinase leishmanolysin (gp63). Structure 1998; 6: 1035-46.

[16] Yiallouros I, Kappelhoff R, Schilling O, *et al.* Activation mechanism of pro-astacin: role of the pro-peptide, tryptic and autoproteolytic cleavage and importance of precise amino-terminal processing. J Mol Biol 2002; 324: 237-46.

[17] Schneider P, Rosat JP, Bouvier J, *et al. Leishmania major* - Differential Regulation of the Surface Metalloprotease in Amastigote and Promastigote Stages. Exp Parasitol 1992; 75: 196-06.

[18] McConville MJ, Schnur LF, Jaffe C, Schneider P. Structure of *Leishmania* lipophosphoglycan: inter- and intra-specific polymorphism in Old World species. Biochem J 1995; 310: 807-18.

[19] Pimenta PFP, Saraiva EMB, Sacks DL. The Comparative Fine-Structure and Surface Glycoconjugate Expression of 3 Life Stages of *Leishmania major*. Exp Parasitol 1991; 72: 191-204.

[20] Brittingham A, Morrison CJ, McMaster WR, *et al.* Role of the *Leishmania* surface protease gp63 in complement fixation, cell adhesion, and resistance to complement-mediated lysis. J Immunol 1995; 155: 3102-11.

[21] Mosser DM, Edelson PJ. The mouse macrophage receptor for C3bi (CR3) is a major mechanism in the phagocytosis of *Leishmania* promastigotes. J Immunol 1985; 135: 2785-89.

[22] Wozencraft AO, Blackwell JM. Increased infectivity of stationary-phase promastigotes of *Leishmania donovani*: correlation with enhanced C3 binding capacity and CR3-mediated attachment to host macrophages. Immunology 1987; 60: 559-63.

[23] Brittingham A, Chen G, McGwire BS, et al. Interaction of *Leishmania* gp63 with cellular receptors for fibronectin. Infect Immun 1999; 67: 4477-84.

[24] Chaudhuri G, Chaudhuri M, Pan A, Chang KP. Surface acid proteinase (gp63) of *Leishmania mexicana*. A metalloenzyme capable of protecting liposome-encapsulated proteins from phagolysosomal degradation by macrophages. J Biol Chem 1989; 264: 7483-89.

[25] Seay MB, Heard PL, Chaudhuri G. Surface Zn-proteinase as a molecule for defense of *Leishmania mexicana amazonensis* promastigotes against cytolysis inside macrophage phagolysosomes. Infect Immun 1996; 64: 5129-37.

[26] Olivier M, Gregory DJ, Forget G. Subversion Mechanisms by Which *Leishmania* Parasites Can Escape the Host Immune Response: a Signaling Point of View. Clin Microbiol Rev 2005; 18: 293-05.

[27] Souza AE, Waugh S, Coombs GH, Mottram JC. Characterization of a multicopy gene for a major stage-specific cysteine proteinase of *Leishmania mexicana*. FEBS Lett 1992; 311: 124-27.

[28] Mottram JC, Robertson CD, Coombs GH, Barry JD. A developmentally regulated cysteine proteinase gene of *Leishmania mexicana*. Mol Microbiol 1992; 6: 1925-32.

[29] Bart G, Coombs GH, Mottram JC. Isolation of lmcpc, a gene encoding a *Leishmania mexicana* cathepsin-B-like cysteine proteinase. Mol Biochem Parasitol 1995; 73: 271-74.

[30] Mottram JC, Coombs GH, Alexander J. Cysteine peptidases as virulence factors of *Leishmania*. Curr Opin Microbiol 2004; 7: 375-81.

[31] Mottram JC, Souza AE, Hutchison JE, *et al.* Evidence from disruption of the lmcpb gene array of *Leishmania mexicana* that cysteine proteinases are virulence factors. Proc Natl Acad Sci U S A 1996; 93: 6008-13.

[32] Alexander J, Coombs GH, Mottram JC. *Leishmania mexicana* cysteine proteinase-deficient mutants have attenuated virulence for mice and potentiate a Th1 response. J Immunol 1998; 161: 6794-01.

[33] Cameron P, McGachy A, Anderson M, *et al.* Inhibition of Lipopolysaccharide-Induced Macrophage IL-12 Production by *Leishmania mexicana* Amastigotes: The Role of Cysteine Peptidases and the NF-κB Signaling Pathway. J Immunol 2004; 173: 3297-04.

[34] De Souza Leao S, Lang T, Prina E, *et al.* Intracellular *Leishmania amazonensis* amastigotes internalize and degrade MHC class II molecules of their host cells. J Cell Sci 1995; 108: 3219-31.

[35] Pollock KGJ, McNeil KS, Mottram JC, *et al.* The *Leishmania mexicana* cysteine protease, CPB2.8, induces potent Th2 responses. J Immunol 2003; 170: 1746-53.

[36] Shakarian AM, Dwyer DM. Structurally conserved soluble acid phosphatases are synthesized and released by *Leishmania major* promastigotes. Exp Parasitol 2000; 95: 79-84.

[37] Shakarian AM, Ellis SL, Mallinson DJ, *et al.* Two tandemly arrayed genes encode the (histidine) secretory acid phosphatases of *Leishmania donovani* Gene 1997; 196: 127-37.

[38] Das S, Saha AK, Remaley AT, *et al.* Hydrolysis of phosphoproteins and inositol phosphates by cell surface phosphatase of *Leishmania donovani*. Mol Biochem Parasitol 1986; 20: 143-53.

[39] Gottlieb M, Dwyer DM. *Leishmania donovani*: surface membrane acid phosphatase activity of promastigotes. Exp Parasitol 1981; 52: 117-28.

[40] Gottlieb M, Dwyer DM. Identification and partial characterization of an extracellular acid phosphatase activity of *Leishmania donovani* promastigotes. Mol Cell Biol 1982; 2: 76-81.

[41] Lovelace JK, Dwyer DM, Gottlieb M. Purification and characterization of the extracellular acid phosphatase of *Leishmania donovani*. Mol Biochem Parasitol 1986; 20: 243-51.

[42] Remaley AT, Das S, Campbell PI, *et al.* Characterization of *Leishmania donovani* acid phosphatases. J Biol Chem 1985; 260: 880-86.

[43] Joshi MB, Mallinson DJ, Dwyer DM. The human pathogen *Leishmania donovani* secretes a histidine acid phosphatase activity that is resistant to proteolytic degradation. J Eukaryot Microbiol 2004; 51: 108-12.

[44] Remaley AT, Glew RH, Kuhns DB, *et al. Leishmania donovani*: surface membrane acid phosphatase blocks neutrophil oxidative metabolite production. Exp Parasitol 1985; 60: 331-41.

[45] Mosser DM, Springer TA, Diamond MS. *Leishmania* promastigotes require opsonic complement to bind to the human leukocyte integrin Mac-1 (CD11b/CD18). J Cell Biol 1992; 116: 511-20.

[46] Kane MM, Mosser DM. *Leishmania* parasites and their ploys to disrupt macrophage activation. Curr Opin Hematol 2000; 7: 26-31.

[47] Sutterwala FS, Rosenthal LA, Mosser DM. Cooperation between CR1 (CD35) and CR3 (CD 11b/CD18) in the binding of complement-opsonized particles. J Leukoc Biol 1996; 59: 883-90.

[48] Mosser DM, Edelson PJ. The third component of complement (C3) is responsible for the intracellular survival of *Leishmania major*. Nature 1987; 327: 329-31.

[49] Shepherd VL, Campbell EJ, Senior RM, Stahl PD. Characterization of the mannose/fucose receptor on human mononuclear phagocytes. J Reticuloendothel Soc 1982; 32: 423-31.

[50] Taylor ME, Conary JT, Lennartz MR, *et al.* Primary structure of the mannose receptor contains multiple motifs resembling carbohydrate-recognition domains. J Biol Chem 1990; 265: 12156-62.

[51] Stahl P, Schlesinger PH, Sigardson E, *et al.* Receptor-mediated pinocytosis of mannose glycoconjugates by macrophages: characterization and evidence for receptor recycling. Cell 1980; 19: 207-15.

[52] Sallusto F, Lanzavecchia A. Efficient presentation of soluble antigen by cultured human dendritic cells is maintained by granulocyte/macrophage colony-stimulating factor plus interleukin 4 and downregulated by tumor necrosis factor alpha. J Exp Med 1994; 179: 1109-18.

[53] Tan MC, Mommaas AM, Drijfhout JW, *et al.* Mannose receptor-mediated uptake of antigens strongly enhances HLA class II-restricted antigen presentation by cultured dendritic cells. Eur J Immunol 1997; 27: 2426-35.

[54] Blackwell JM, Ezekowitz RAB, Roberts MB, *et al.* Macrophage Complement and Lectin-Like Receptors Bind *Leishmania* in the Absence of Serum. J Exp Med 1985; 162: 324-31.

[55] Volanakis JE, Kaplan MH. Specificity of C-reactive protein for choline phosphate residues of pneumococcal C-polysaccharide. Proc Soc Exp Biol Med 1971; 136: 612-14.

[56] Raynes JG, Curry A, Harris RA. Binding of C-reactive protein to *Leishmania*. Biochem Soc Trans 1994; 22: 3S.

[57] Bodman-Smith KB, Mbuchi M, Culley FJ, *et al.* C-reactive protein-mediated phagocytosis of *Leishmania donovani* promastigotes does not alter parasite survival or macrophage responses. Parasite Immunol 2002; 24: 447-54.

[58] Ruoslahti E. Integrins. J Clin Invest 1991; 87: 1-5.

[59] Wayner EA, Garcia-Pardo A, Humphries MJ, *et al.* Identification and characterization of the T lymphocyte adhesion receptor for an alternative cell attachment domain (CS-1) in plasma fibronectin. J Cell Biol 1989; 109: 1321-30.

[60] Guy RA, Belosevic M. Comparison of receptors required for entry of *Leishmania major* amastigotes into macrophages. Infect Immun 1993; 61: 1553-58.

[61] Wanderley JLM, Moreira MEC, Benjamin A, *et al.* Mimicry of Apoptotic Cells by Exposing Phosphatidylserine Participates in the Establishment of Amastigotes of *Leishmania (L) amazonensis* in Mammalian Hosts. J Immunol 2006; 176: 1834-39.

[62] de Freitas Balanco JM, Moreira ME, Bonomo A, *et al.* Apoptotic mimicry by an obligate intracellular parasite downregulates macrophage microbicidal activity. Curr Biol 2001; 11:1870-03.

[63] Takai Y, Kishimoto A, Inoue M, Nishizuka Y. Studies on a cyclic nucleotide-independent protein kinase and its proenzyme in mammalian tissues. I. Purification and characterization of an active enzyme from bovine cerebellum. J Biol Chem 1977; 252: 7603-09.

[64] Inoue M, Kishimoto A, Takai Y, Nishizuka Y. Studies on a cyclic nucleotide-independent protein kinase and its proenzyme in mammalian tissues. II. Proenzyme and its activation by calcium-dependent protease from rat brain. J Biol Chem 1977; 252: 7610-06.

[65] Reyland ME. Protein kinase C isoforms: Multi-functional regulators of cell life and death. Front Biosci 2009; 14: 2386-99.

[66] Severn A, Wakelam MJ, Liew FY. The role of protein kinase C in the induction of nitric oxide synthesis by murine macrophages. Biochem Biophys Res Commun 1992; 188: 997-02.

[67] Warzocha K, Bienvenu J, Coiffier B, Salles G. Mechanisms of action of the tumor necrosis factor and lymphotoxin ligand-receptor system. Eur Cytokine Netw 1995; 6: 83-96.

[68]   Turco SJ, Descoteaux A. The lipophosphoglycan of *Leishmania* parasites. Annu Rev Microbiol 1992; 46: 65-94.

[69]   McNeely TB, Turco SJ. Inhibition of protein kinase C activity by the *Leishmania donovani* lipophosphoglycan. Biochem Biophys Res Commun 1987; 148: 653-57.

[70]   McNeely TB, Rosen G, Londner MV, Turco SJ. Inhibitory effects on protein kinase C activity by lipophosphoglycan fragments and glycosylphosphatidylinositol antigens of the protozoan parasite *Leishmania*. Biochem J 1989; 259: 601-04.

[71]   Olivier M, Brownsey RW, Reiner NE. Defective stimulus-response coupling in human monocytes infected with *Leishmania donovani* is associated with altered activation and translocation of protein kinase C. Proc Natl Acad Sci U S A 1992; 89: 7481-85.

[72]   Ghosh S, Bhattacharyya S, Das S, *et al*. Generation of ceramide in murine macrophages infected with *Leishmania donovani* alters macrophage signaling events and aids intracellular parasitic survival. Mol Cell Biochem 2001; 223: 47-60.

[73]   Rawlings JS, Rosler KM, Harrison DA. The JAK/STAT signaling pathway. J Cell Sci 2004; 117: 1281-83.

[74]   Woldman I, Varinou L, Ramsauer K, *et al*. The Stat1 binding motif of the interferon-gamma receptor is sufficient to mediate Stat5 activation and its repression by SOCS3. J Biol Chem 2001; 276: 45722-28.

[75]   Lowenstein CJ, Alley EW, Raval P, *et al*. Macrophage Nitric-Oxide Synthase Gene - 2 Upstream Regions Mediate Induction by Interferon-Gamma and Lipopolysaccharide. Proc Natl Acad Sci U S A 1993; 90: 9730-34.

[76]   Xie QW, Whisnant R, Nathan C. Promoter of the mouse gene encoding calcium-independent nitric-oxide synthase confers inducibility by interferon-gamma and bacterial lipopolysaccharide. J Exp Med 1993; 177: 1779-84.

[77]   Nandan D, Reiner NE. Attenuation of gamma-interferon-induced tyrosine phosphorylation in mononuclear phagocytes infected with *Leishmania-donovani* - selective-inhibition of signaling through Janus kinases and STAT1. Infect Immun 1995; 63: 4495-00.

[78]   Blanchette J, Racette N, Faure R, *et al*. *Leishmania*-induced increases in activation of macrophage SHP-1 tyrosine phosphatase are associated with impaired IFN-gamma-triggered JAK2 activation. Eur J Immunol 1999; 29: 3737-44.

[79]   Ray M, Gam AA, Boykins RA, Kenney RT. Inhibition of interferon-gamma signaling by *Leishmania donovani*. J Infect Dis 2000; 181: 1121-28.

[80]   Boldt S, Kolch W. Targeting MAPK signalling: Prometheus' fire or Pandora's box? Curr Pharm Des 2004; 10: 1885-05.

[81]   Chen Z, Gibson TB, Robinson F, *et al*. MAP kinases. Chem Rev 2001; 101: 2449-76.

[82]   Lewis TS, Shapiro PS, Ahn NG. Signal transduction through MAP kinase cascades. Adv Cancer Res 1998; 74: 49-139.

[83]   Chang F, Steelman LS, Lee JT, *et al*. Signal transduction mediated by the Ras/Raf/MEK/ERK pathway from cytokine receptors to transcription factors: potential targeting for therapeutic intervention. Leukemia 2003; 17: 1263-93.

[84]   Gille H, Sharrocks AD, Shaw PE. Phosphorylation of transcription factor p62TCF by MAP kinase stimulates ternary complex formation at c-fos promoter Nature 1992; 358: 414-17.

[85]   Treinies I, Paterson HF, Hooper S, *et al*. Activated MEK stimulates expression of AP-1 components independently of phosphatidylinositol 3-kinase (PI3-kinase) but requires a PI3-kinase signal To stimulate DNA synthesis. Mol Cell Biol 1999; 19: 321-29.

[86]   Hibi M, Lin A, Smeal T, *et al*. Identification of an oncoprotein- and UV-responsive protein kinase that binds and potentiates the c-Jun activation domain. Genes Dev 1993; 7: 2135-48.

[87]   Gupta S, Barrett T, Whitmarsh AJ, *et al*. Selective interaction of JNK protein kinase isoforms with transcription factors. EMBO J 1996; 15: 2760-70.

[88]   Fuchs SY, Tappin I, Ronai Z. Stability of the ATF2 transcription factor is regulated by phosphorylation and dephosphorylation. J Biol Chem 2000; 275: 12560-04.

[89]   van Dam H, Duyndam M, Rottier R, *et al*. Heterodimer formation of cJun and ATF-2 is responsible for induction of c-jun by the 243 amino acid adenovirus E1A protein. EMBO J 1993; 12: 479-87.

[90]   Lee JC, Kumar S, Griswold DE, Underwood DC, Votta BJ, Adams JL. Inhibition of p38 MAP kinase as a therapeutic strategy. Immunopharmacology 2000; 47: 185-01.

[91]   Rousseau S, Morrice N, Peggie M, *et al*. Inhibition of SAPK2a/p38 prevents hnRNP A0 phosphorylation by MAPKAP-K2 and its interaction with cytokine mRNAs. EMBO J 2002; 21: 6505-14.

[92]   Hunter T. Protein kinases and phosphatases: the yin and yang of protein phosphorylation and signaling Cell 1995; 80: 225-36.

[93]   Ling Y, West AG, Roberts EC, *et al*. Interaction of transcription factors with serum response factor. Identification of the Elk-1 binding surface. J Biol Chem 1998; 273: 10506-14.

[94]   Rao KM. MAP kinase activation in macrophages. J Leukoc Biol 2001; 69: 3-10.

[95]   Prive C, Descoteaux A. *Leishmania donovani* promastigotes evade the activation of mitogen-activated protein kinases p38, c-Jun N-terminal kinase, and extracellular signal-regulated kinase-1/2 during infection of naive macrophages. Eur J Immunol 2000; 30: 2235-44.

[96]   Martiny A, Meyer-Fernandes JR, de Souza W, Vannier-Santos MA. Altered tyrosine phosphorylation of ERK1 MAP kinase and other macrophage molecules caused by *Leishmania* amastigotes. Mol Biochem Parasitol 1999; 102: 1-12.

[97]   Nandan D, Lo R, Reiner NE. Activation of phosphotyrosine phosphatase activity attenuates mitogen-activated protein kinase signaling and inhibits c-FOS and nitric oxide synthase expression in macrophages infected with *Leishmania donovani*. Infect Immun 1999; 67: 4055-63.

[98] Forget G, Gregory DJ, Whitcombe LA, Olivier M. Role of host protein tyrosine phosphatase SHP-1 in *Leishmania donovani*-induced inhibition of nitric oxide production. Infect Immun 2006; 74: 6272-79.

[99] Ghosh S, Bhattacharyya S, Sirkar M, *et al*. *Leishmania donovani* suppresses activated protein 1 and NF-κB activation in host macrophages via ceramide generation: involvement of extracellular signal-regulated kinase. Infect Immun 2002; 70: 6828-38.

[100] Awasthi A, Mathur R, Khan A, *et al*. CD40 signaling is impaired in *L. major*-infected macrophages and is rescued by a p38MAPK activator establishing a host-protective memory T cell response. J Exp Med 2003; 197:1037-43.

[101] Junghae M, Raynes JG. Activation of p38 mitogen-activated protein kinase attenuates *Leishmania donovani* infection in macrophages. Infect Immun 2002; 70: 5026-35.

[102] Goetz CA, Baldwin AS. NF-kappaB pathways in the immune system: control of the germinal center reaction. Immunol Res 2008; 41: 233-47.

[103] Hayden MS, Ghosh S. Signaling to NF-kappaB. Genes Dev 2004; 18: 2195-24.

[104] Yamamoto Y, Gaynor RB. IkappaB kinases: key regulators of the NF-kappaB pathway. Trends Biochem Sci 2004; 29: 72-79.

[105] Viatour P, Merville MP, Bours V, Chariot A. Phosphorylation of NF-kappaB and IkappaB proteins: implications in cancer and inflammation. Trends Biochem Sci 2005; 30: 43-52.

[106] Siebenlist U, Brown K, Claudio E. Control of lymphocyte development by nuclear factor-kappaB. Nature Rev 2005; 5: 435-45.

[107] Pahl HL. Activators and target genes of Rel/NF-kappaB transcription factors. Oncogene 1999; 18: 6853-66.

[108] Guizani-Tabbane L, Ben-Aissa K, Belghith M, *et al*. *Leishmania major* amastigotes induce p50/c-Rel NF-kappa B transcription factor in human macrophages: involvement in cytokine synthesis. Infect Immun 2004 ; 72: 2582-89.

[109] Gregory DJ, Godbout M, Contreras I, *et al*. A novel form of NF-kappa B is induced by *Leishmania* infection: Involvement in macrophage gene expression. Eur J Immunol 2008; 38: 1071-81.

[110] Matsukawa A. STAT proteins in innate immunity during sepsis: lessons from gene knockout mice. Acta Med Okayama 2007; 61: 239-45.

[111] Reich NC, Liu L. Tracking STAT nuclear traffic. Nature Rev 2006; 6: 602-12.

[112] Forget G, Gregory DJ, Olivier M. Proteasome-mediated degradation of STAT1 alpha following infection of macrophages with *Leishmania donovani*. J Biol Chem 2005; 280: 30542-49.

[113] Shaulian E, Karin M. AP-1 as a regulator of cell life and death. Nature Cell Biol 2002; 4: 131-36.

[114] Kuo NT, Agani FH, Haxhiu MA, Chang CH. A possible role for protein kinase C in CO2/H+-induced c-fos mRNA expression in PC12 cells. Respir Physiol 1998; 111: 127-35.

[115] Gruda MC, Kovary K, Metz R, Bravo R. Regulation of Fra-1 and Fra-2 phosphorylation differs during the cell cycle of fibroblasts and phosphorylation in vitro by MAP kinase affects DNA binding activity. Oncogene 1994; 9: 2537-47.

[116] Gupta S, Campbell D, Derijard B, Davis RJ. Transcription factor ATF2 regulation by the JNK signal transduction pathway. Science 1995; 267: 389-93.

[117] Yamagishi S, Yamada M, Ishikawa Y, *et al*. p38 mitogen-activated protein kinase regulates low potassium-induced c-Jun phosphorylation and apoptosis in cultured cerebellar granule neurons. J Biol Chem 2001; 276: 5129-33.

[118] Blanchette J, Abu-Dayyeh I, Hassani K, *et al*. Regulation of macrophage nitric oxide production by the protein tyrosine phosphatase Src homology 2 domain phosphotyrosine phosphatase 1 (SHP-1). Immunology 2009; 127: 123-33.

[119] Larsen M, Tremblay ML, Yamada KM. Phosphatases in cell-matrix adhesion and migration. Nat Rev Mol Cell Biol 2003; 4: 700-11.

[120] Denu JM, Dixon JE. Protein tyrosine phosphatases: mechanisms of catalysis and regulation. Curr Opin Chem Biol 1998; 2: 633-41.

[121] Pao LI, Badour K, Siminovitch KA, Neel BG. Nonreceptor protein-tyrosine phosphatases in immune cell signaling. Annu Rev Immunol 2007; 25: 473-23.

[122] Bourdeau A, Dube N, Tremblay ML. Cytoplasmic protein tyrosine phosphatases, regulation and function: the roles of PTP1B and TC-PTP. Curr Opin Cell Biol 2005; 17: 203-09.

[123] Elchebly M, Payette P, Michaliszyn E, *et al*. Increased insulin sensitivity and obesity resistance in mice lacking the protein tyrosine phosphatase-1B gene. Science 1999; 283: 1544-48.

[124] Klaman LD, Boss O, Peroni OD, *et al*. Increased energy expenditure, decreased adiposity, and tissue-specific insulin sensitivity in protein-tyrosine phosphatase 1B-deficient mice. Mol Cell Biol 2000; 20: 5479-89.

[125] Elchebly M, Cheng A, Tremblay ML. Modulation of insulin signaling by protein tyrosine phosphatases. J Mol Med 2000; 78: 473-82.

[126] Myers MP, Andersen JN, Cheng A, *et al*. TYK2 and JAK2 Are Substrates of Protein-tyrosine Phosphatase 1B. J Biol Chem 2001; 276: 47771-74.

[127] You-Ten KE, Muise ES, Itie A, *et al*. Impaired bone marrow microenvironment and immune function in T cell protein tyrosine phosphatase-deficient mice. J Exp Med 1997; 186: 683-93.

[128] Simoncic PD, Lee-Loy A, Barber DL, *et al*. The T cell protein tyrosine phosphatase is a negative regulator of janus family kinases 1 and 3. Curr Biol 2002; 12: 446-53.

[129] ten Hoeve J, de Jesus Ibarra-Sanchez M, Fu Y, *et al*. Identification of a nuclear Stat1 protein tyrosine phosphatase. Mol Cell Biol 2002; 22: 5662-68.

[130] Halle M, Gomez MA, Stuible M, *et al*. The *Leishmania* surface protease GP63 cleaves multiple intracellular proteins and actively participates in p38 mitogen-activated protein kinase inactivation. J Biol Chem 2009; 284: 6893-08.

[131] Matthews RJ, Bowne DB, Flores E, Thomas ML. Characterization of hematopoietic intracellular protein tyrosine phosphatases: description of a phosphatase containing an SH2 domain and another enriched in proline-, glutamic acid-, serine-, and threonine-rich sequences. Mol Cell Biol 1992; 12: 2396-05.

[132] Plutzky J, Neel BG, Rosenberg RD. Isolation of a src homology 2-containing tyrosine phosphatase. Proc Natl Acad Sci U S A 1992; 89:1123-27.

[133] Kroll J, Waltenberger J. The vascular endothelial growth factor receptor KDR activates multiple signal transduction pathways in porcine aortic endothelial cells. J Biol Chem 1997; 272: 32521-27.

[134] Guo DQ, Wu LW, Dunbar JD, *et al*. Tumor necrosis factor employs a protein-tyrosine phosphatase to inhibit activation of KDR and vascular endothelial cell growth factor-induced endothelial cell proliferation. J Biol Chem 2000; 275: 11216-21.

[135] Massa PT, Saha S, Wu C, Jarosinski KW. Expression and function of the protein tyrosine phosphatase SHP-1 in oligodendrocytes. Glia 2000; 29: 376-85.

[136] Ravetch JV, Lanier LL. Immune inhibitory receptors. Science 2000; 290: 84-9.

[137] Shultz LD, Rajan TV, Greiner DL. Severe defects in immunity and hematopoiesis caused by SHP-1 protein-tyrosine-phosphatase deficiency. Trends Biotechnol 1997; 15: 302-07.

[138] Pani G, Kozlowski M, Cambier JC, *et al*. Identification of the tyrosine phosphatase PTP1c as a B-cell antigen receptor-associated protein involved in the regulation of B-cell signaling. J Exp Med 1995; 18: 2077-84.

[139] Carter JD, Neel BG, Lorenz U. The tyrosine phosphatase SHP-1 influences thymocyte selection by setting TCR signaling thresholds. Int Immunol 1999; 11: 1999-14.

[140] Chiang GG, Sefton BM. Specific dephosphorylation of the Lck tyrosine protein kinase at Tyr-394 by the SHP-1 protein-tyrosine phosphatase. J Biol Chem 2001; 276: 23173-78.

[141] Plas DR, Johnson R, Pingel JT, *et al*. Direct regulation of ZAP-70 by SHP-1 in T cell antigen receptor signaling. Science 1996; 272: 1173-76.

[142] Jiao H, Berrada K, Yang W, *et al*. Direct association with and dephosphorylation of Jak2 kinase by the SH2-domain-containing protein tyrosine phosphatase SHP-1. Mol Cell Biol 1996; 16: 6985-92.

[143] Bedecs K, Elbaz N, Sutren M, *et al*. Angiotensin II type 2 receptors mediate inhibition of mitogen-activated protein kinase cascade and functional activation of SHP-1 tyrosine phosphatase. Biochem J 1997; 325: 449-54.

[144] Matsubara H, Shibasaki Y, Okigaki M, *et al*. Effect of angiotensin II type 2 receptor on tyrosine kinase Pyk2 and c-Jun NH2-terminal kinase via SHP-1 tyrosine phosphatase activity: evidence from vascular-targeted transgenic mice of AT2 receptor. Biochem Biophys Res Commun 2001; 282: 1085-91.

[145] Ram PA, Waxman DJ. Interaction of growth hormone-activated STATs with SH2-containing phosphotyrosine phosphatase SHP-1 and nuclear JAK2 tyrosine kinase. J Biol Chem 1997; 272: 17694-02.

[146] Olivier M, Romero-Gallo BJ, Matte C, *et al*. Modulation of interferon-gamma-induced macrophage activation by phosphotyrosine phosphatases inhibition - Effect on murine Leishmaniasis progression. J Biol Chem 1998; 273: 13944-49.

[147] Matte C, Marquis JF, Blanchette J, *et al*. Peroxovanadium-mediated protection against murine leishmaniasis: role of the modulation of nitric oxide. Eur J Immunol 2000; 30: 2555-64.

[148] Forget G, Siminovitch KA, Brochu S, *et al*. Role of host phosphotyrosine phosphatase SHP-1 in the development of murine leishmaniasis. Eur J Immunol 2001; 31: 3185-96.

[149] Nandan D, Yi TL, Lopez M, *et al*. Leishmania EF-1 alpha activates the Src homology 2 domain containing tyrosine phosphatase SHP-1 leading to macrophage deactivation. J Biol Chem 2002; 277: 50190-07.

[150] Croker BA, Kiu H, Nicholson SE. SOCS regulation of the JAK/STAT signalling pathway. Semin Cell Dev Biol 2008; 19: 414-22.

[151] Yasukawa H, Misawa H, Sakamoto H, *et al*. The JAK-binding protein JAB inhibits Janus tyrosine kinase activity through binding in the activation loop. EMBO J 1999; 18:1309-20.

[152] Sasaki A, Yasukawa H, Suzuki A, *et al*. Cytokine-inducible SH2 protein-3 (CIS3/SOCS3) inhibits Janus tyrosine kinase by binding through the N-terminal kinase inhibitory region as well as SH2 domain. Genes Cells 1999; 4: 339-51.

[153] Qing Y, Costa-Pereira AP, Watling D, Stark GR. Role of tyrosine 441 of interferon-gamma receptor subunit 1 in SOCS-1-mediated attenuation of STAT1 activation. J Biol Chem 2005; 280: 1849-53.

[154] Yamamoto K, Yamaguchi M, Miyasaka N, Miura O. SOCS-3 inhibits IL-12-induced STAT4 activation by binding through its SH2 domain to the STAT4 docking site in the IL-12 receptor beta2 subunit. Biochem Biophys Res Commun 2003; 310: 1188-93.

[155] Bertholet S, Dickensheets HL, Sheikh F, *et al*. *Leishmania donovani*-induced expression of suppressor of cytokine signaling 3 in human macrophages: a novel mechanism for intracellular parasite suppression of activation. Infect Immun 2003; 71: 2095-01.

[156] Antoniazi S, Price HP, Kropf P, *et al*. Chemokine gene expression in toll-like receptor-competent and -deficient mice infected with *Leishmania major*. Infect Immun 2004; 72: 5168-74.

[157] Forget G, Matte C, Siminovitch KA, *et al.* Regulation of the *Leishmania*-induced innate inflammatory response by the protein tyrosine phosphatase SHP-1. Eur J Immunol 2005; 35: 1906-17.

[158] Teixeira MJ, Teixeira CR, Andrade BB, *et al.* Chemokines in host-parasite interactions in leishmaniasis. Trends Parasitol 2006; 22: 32-40.

[159] Rousseau D, Demartino S, Anjuere F, *et al.* Sustained parasite burden in the spleen of *Leishmania infantum*-infected BALB/c mice is accompanied by expression of MCP-1 transcripts and lack of protection against challenge. Eur Cytokine Netw 2001; 12: 340-07.

[160] Liew FY, Millott S, Parkinson C, *et al.* Macrophage killing of *Leishmania* parasite in vivo is mediated by nitric oxide from L-arginine. J Immunol 1990; 144: 4794-97.

[161] Murray HW. Cell-mediated immune response in experimental visceral leishmaniasis. II. Oxygen-dependent killing of intracellular *Leishmania donovani amastigotes*. J Immunol 1982; 129: 351-57.

[162] Marletta MA, Yoon PS, Iyengar R, *et al.* Macrophage oxidation of L-arginine to nitrite and nitrate - nitric-oxide is an intermediate. Biochemistry 1988; 27: 8706-11.

[163] Hibbs JB, Taintor RR, Vavrin Z, Rachlin EM. Nitric-oxide - a cyto-toxic activated macrophage effector molecule. Biochem Biophys Res Commun 1988; 157: 87-94.

[164] Green SJ, Meltzer MS, Hibbs JB, Jr., Nacy CA. Activated macrophages destroy intracellular *Leishmania major* amastigotes by an L-arginine-dependent killing mechanism. J Immunol 1990; 144: 278-83.

[165] Bogdan C, Rollinghoff M, Diefenbach A. Nitric Oxide and infection. Kluwer Academic/ Plenum Publishers, NY, USA 1999.

[166] Bourguignon SC, Alves CR, Giovanni-De-Simone S. Detrimental effect of nitric oxide on Trypanosoma cruzi and *Leishmania major* like cells. Acta trop 1997; 66: 109-18.

[167] Lemesre JL, Sereno D, Daulouede S, *et al. Leishmania* spp.: nitric oxide-mediated metabolic inhibition of promastigote and axenically grown amastigote forms. Exp Parasitol 1997; 86: 58-68.

[168] Cunningham AC. Parasitic adaptive mechanisms in infection by leishmania. Exp Mol Pathol 2002; 72: 132-41.

[169] Stenger S, Thuring H, Rollinghoff M, Bogdan C. Tissue expression of inducible nitric oxide synthase is closely associated with resistance to *Leishmania major*. J Exp Med 1994; 180: 783-93.

[170] Murray HW, Nathan CF. Macrophage microbicidal mechanisms in vivo: reactive nitrogen versus oxygen intermediates in the killing of intracellular visceral *Leishmania donovani*. J Exp Med 1999; 189: 741-6.

[171] Buchmuller-Rouiller Y, Mauel J. Impairment of the oxidative metabolism of mouse peritoneal macrophages by intracellular *Leishmania* spp. Infect Immun 1987; 55: 587-93.

[172] Olivier M, Baimbridge KG, Reiner NE. Stimulus-response coupling in monocytes infected with *Leishmania*. Attenuation of calcium transients is related to defective agonist-induced accumulation of inositol phosphates. J Immunol 1992 ; 148: 1188-96.

[173] Sorensen AL, Hey AS, Kharazmi A. *Leishmania major* surface protease Gp63 interferes with the function of human monocytes and neutrophils in vitro. APMIS 1994; 102: 265-71.

[174] Lodge R, Diallo TO, Descoteaux A. *Leishmania donovani* lipophosphoglycan blocks NADPH oxidase assembly at the phagosome membrane. Cell Microbiol 2006; 8: 1922-31.

[175] Lodge R, Descoteaux A. Phagocytosis of *Leishmania donovani* amastigotes is Rac1 dependent and occurs in the absence of NADPH oxidase activation. Eur J Immunol 2006; 36: 2735-44.

[176] Fontayne A, Dang PM, Gougerot-Pocidalo MA, El-Benna J. Phosphorylation of p47phox sites by PKC alpha, beta II, delta, and zeta: effect on binding to p22phox and on NADPH oxidase activation. Biochemistry 2002; 41: 7743-50.

[177] De Titto EH, Catterall JR, Remington JS. Activity of recombinant tumor necrosis factor on *Toxoplasma gondii* and *Trypanosoma cruzi*. J Immunol 1986; 137: 1342-5.

[178] Czuprynski CJ, Brown JF, Young KM, *et al.* Effects of murine recombinant interleukin 1 alpha on the host response to bacterial infection. J Immunol 1988; 140: 962-8.

[179] Bermudez LE, Young LS. Tumor necrosis factor, alone or in combination with IL-2, but not IFN-gamma, is associated with macrophage killing of Mycobacterium avium complex. J Immunol 1988; 140: 3006-13.

[180] Ozaki Y, Ohashi T, Minami A, Nakamura S. Enhanced resistance of mice to bacterial infection induced by recombinant human interleukin-1a. Infect Immun 1987; 55: 1436-40.

[181] Del Vecchio M, Bajetta E, Canova S, *et al.* Interleukin-12: biological properties and clinical application. Clin Cancer Res 2007; 13: 4677-85.

[182] Reiner NE, Ng W, Wilson CB, *et al.* Modulation of in vitro monocyte cytokine responses to *Leishmania donovani*. Interferon-gamma prevents parasite-induced inhibition of interleukin 1 production and primes monocytes to respond to *Leishmania* by producing both tumor necrosis factor-alpha and interleukin 1. J Clin Invest 1990; 85: 1914-24.

[183] Frankenburg S, Leibovici V, Mansbach N, *et al.* Effect of glycolipids of *Leishmania* parasites on human monocyte activity. Inhibition by lipophosphoglycan. J Immunol 1990; 145: 4284-9.

[184] Hatzigeorgiou DE, Geng J, Zhu B, *et al.* Lipophosphoglycan from *Leishmania* suppresses agonist-induced interleukin 1 beta gene expression in human monocytes via a unique promoter sequence. Proc Natl Acad Sci U S A 1996; 93: 14708-13.

[185] Matte C, Olivier M. *Leishmania*-induced cellular recruitment during the early inflammatory response: Modulation of proinflammatory mediators. J Infec Dis 2002; 185: 673-81.

[186] Carrera L, Gazzinelli RT, Badolato R, *et al*. *Leishmania* promastigotes selectively inhibit interleukin 12 induction in bone marrow-derived macrophages from susceptible and resistant mice. J Exp Med 1996; 183: 515-26.

[187] Weinheber N, Wolfram M, Harbecke D, Aebischer T. Phagocytosis of *Leishmania mexicana* amastigotes by macrophages leads to a sustained suppression of IL-12 production. Eur J Immunol 1998; 28: 2467-77.

[188] Marth T, Kelsall BL. Regulation of interleukin-12 by complement receptor 3 signaling. The J Exp Med 1997; 185: 1987-95.

[189] Sutterwala FS, Noel GJ, Clynes R, Mosser DM. Selective suppression of interleukin-12 induction after macrophage receptor ligation. J Exp Med 1997; 185: 1977-85.

[190] Abu-Dayyeh I, Shio MT, Sato S, *et al*. *Leishmania*-Induced IRAK-1 Inactivation Is Mediated by SHP-1 Interacting with an Evolutionarily Conserved KTIM Motif. PLoS Negl Trop Dis 2008; 2: e305.

[191] Murray RK, Granner DK, Mayes PA, Rodwell VW. Harper's Biochemistry. 25th ed. Norwalk: Appelton & Lange 1999.

[192] Belley A, Chadee K. Eicosanoid production by parasites: from pathogenesis to immunomodulation? Parasitol Today 1995; 11: 327-34.

[193] Farrell JP, Kirkpatrick CE. Experimental cutaneous leishmaniasis. II. A possible role for prostaglandins in exacerbation of disease in *Leishmania major*-infected BALB/c mice. J Immunol 1987; 138: 902-7.

[194] Reiner NE, Malemud CJ. Arachidonic acid metabolism in murine Leishmaniasis (*Donovani*): *ex-vivo* evidence for increased cyclooxygenase and 5-lipoxygenase activity in spleen cells. Cell Immunol 1984; 88: 501-10.

[195] Reiner NE, Malemud CJ. Arachidonic acid metabolism by murine peritoneal macrophages infected with *Leishmania donovani*: in vitro evidence for parasite-induced alterations in cyclooxygenase and lipoxygenase pathways. J Immunol 1985; 134: 556-63.

[196] Matte C, Maion G, Mourad W, Olivier M. *Leishmania donovani*-induced macrophages cyclooxygenase-2 and prostaglandin E-2 synthesis. Parasite Immunol 2001; 23: 177-84.

[197] Anstead GM, Chandrasekar B, Zhao W, *et al*. Malnutrition alters the innate immune response and increases early visceralization following *Leishmania donovani* infection. Infect Immun 2001; 69: 4709-18.

[198] Teicher BA. Transforming growth factor-beta and the immune response to malignant disease. Clin Cancer Res 2007; 13: 6247-51.

[199] Bogdan C, Rollinghoff M. The immune response to *Leishmania*: mechanisms of parasite control and evasion. Int J Parasitol 1998; 28: 121-34.

[200] Scharton-Kersten T, Afonso LC, Wysocka M, *et al*. IL-12 is required for natural killer cell activation and subsequent T helper 1 cell development in experimental leishmaniasis. J Immunol 1995;154 : 5320-30.

[201] Gantt KR, Schultz-Cherry S, Rodriguez N, *et al*. Activation of TGF-beta by *Leishmania chagasi*: importance for parasite survival in macrophages. J Immunol. 2003; 170: 2613-20.

[202] Somanna A, Mundodi V, Gedamu L. Functional analysis of cathepsin B-like cysteine proteases from *Leishmania donovani* complex. Evidence for the activation of latent transforming growth factor beta. J Bio Chem 2002; 277: 25305-12.

[203] Moore KW, de Waal Malefyt R, Coffman RL, O'Garra A. Interleukin-10 and the interleukin-10 receptor. Annu Rev Immunol 2001; 19: 683-765.

[204] Sutterwala FS, Noel GJ, Salgame P, Mosser DM. Reversal of proinflammatory responses by ligating the macrophage Fcgamma receptor type I. J Exp Med 1998; 188: 217-22.

[205] Groux H, Cottrez F, Rouleau M, *et al*. A transgenic model to analyze the immunoregulatory role of IL-10 secreted by antigen-presenting cells. J Immunol 1999; 162: 1723-29.

[206] Kane MM, Mosser DM. The role of IL-10 in promoting disease progression in leishmaniasis. J Immunol 2001; 166: 1141-47.

[207] De Almeida MC, Cardoso SA, Barral-Netto M. *Leishmania* (*Leishmania*) *chagasi* infection alters the expression of cell adhesion and costimulatory molecules on human monocyte and macrophage. Int J Parasitol 2003; 33: 153-62.

[208] Reiner NE, Ng W, McMaster WR. Parasite-accessory cell interactions in murine leishmaniasis. II. *Leishmania donovani* suppresses macrophage expression of class I and class II major histocompatibility complex gene products. J Immunol 1987; 138: 1926-32.

[209] Reiner NE, Ng W, Ma T, McMaster WR. Kinetics of gamma interferon binding and induction of major histocompatibility complex class II mRNA in *Leishmania*-infected macrophages. Proc Natl Acad Sci U S A 1988; 85: 4330-34.

[210] Fruth U, Solioz N, Louis JA. *Leishmania major* interferes with antigen presentation by infected macrophages. J Immunol 1993; 150: 1857-64.

[211] Prina E, Jouanne C, de Souza Lao S, *et al*. Antigen presentation capacity of murine macrophages infected with *Leishmania amazonensis* amastigotes. J Immunol 1993; 151: 2050-61.

[212] Kaye PM, Rogers NJ, Curry AJ, Scott JC. Deficient expression of co-stimulatory molecules on *Leishmania*-infected macrophages. Eur J Immunol 1994; 24: 2850-54.

[213] Saha B, Das G, Vohra H, *et al*. Macrophage-T cell interaction in experimental visceral leishmaniasis: failure to express costimulatory molecules on *Leishmania*-infected macrophages and its implication in the suppression of cell-mediated immunity. Eur J Immunol 1995; 25: 2492-98.

[214] Kamanaka M, Yu P, Yasui T, *et al*. Protective role of CD40 in *Leishmania major* infection at two distinct phases of cell-mediated immunity. Immunity 1996; 4: 275-81.

[215] Campbell KA, Ovendale PJ, Kennedy MK, *et al*. CD40 ligand is required for protective cell-mediated immunity to *Leishmania major*. Immunity 1996; 4: 283-9.

[216] Soong L, Xu JC, Grewal IS, *et al*. Disruption of CD40-CD40 ligand interactions results in an enhanced susceptibility to *Leishmania amazonensis* infection. Immunity 1996;4: 263-73.

[217] Heinzel FP, Rerko RM, Hujer AM. Underproduction of interleukin-12 in susceptible mice during progressive leishmaniasis is due to decreased CD40 activity. Cell Immunol 1998; 184: 129-42.

[218] Campos MA, Almeida IC, Takeuchi O, *et al*. Activation of Toll-like receptor-2 by glycosylphosphatidylinositol anchors from a protozoan parasite. J Immunol 2001; 167: 416-23.

[219] Ropert C, Gazzinelli RT. Regulatory role of Toll-like receptor 2 during infection with *Trypanosoma cruzi*. J Endotoxin Res 2004; 10: 425-30.

[220] Oliveira AC, Peixoto JR, de Arruda LB, *et al*. Expression of functional TLR4 confers proinflammatory responsiveness to *Trypanosoma cruzi* glycoinositolphospholipids and higher resistance to infection with *T. cruzi*. J Immunol 2004; 173: 5688-96.

[221] Ropert C, Almeida IC, Closel M, *et al*. Requirement of mitogen-activated protein kinases and I kappa B phosphorylation for induction of proinflammatory cytokines synthesis by macrophages indicates functional similarity of receptors triggered by glycosylphosphatidylinositol anchors from parasitic protozoa and bacterial lipopolysaccharide. J Immunol 2001; 166: 3423-31.

[222] Ropert C, Closel M, Chaves AC, Gazzinelli RT. Inhibition of a p38/stress-activated protein kinase-2-dependent phosphatase restores function of IL-1 receptor-associate kinase-1 and reverses Toll-like receptor 2- and 4-dependent tolerance of macrophages. J Immunol 2003; 171: 1456-65.

[223] de Veer MJ, Curtis JM, Baldwin TM, *et al*. MyD88 is essential for clearance of *Leishmania major*: possible role for lipophosphoglycan and Toll-like receptor 2 signaling. Eur J Immunol 2003; 33: 2822-31.

[224] Becker I, Salaiza N, Aguirre M, *et al*. *Leishmania* lipophosphoglycan (LPG) activates NK cells through toll-like receptor-2. Mol Biochem Parasitol 2003; 130: 65-74.

[225] Flandin JF, Chano F, Descoteaux A. RNA interference reveals a role for TLR2 and TLR3 in the recognition of *Leishmania donovani* promastigotes by interferon-gamma-primed macrophages. Eur J Immunol 2006; 36: 411-20.

[226] Krishnegowda G, Hajjar AM, Zhu J, *et al*. Induction of proinflammatory responses in macrophages by the glycosylphosphatidylinositols of *Plasmodium falciparum*: cell signaling receptors, glycosylphosphatidylinositol (GPI) structural requirement, and regulation of GPI activity. J Biol Chem 2005; 280: 8606-16.

[227] Naik RS, Branch OH, Woods AS, *et al*. Glycosylphosphatidylinositol anchors of *Plasmodium falciparum*: molecular characterization and naturally elicited antibody response that may provide immunity to malaria pathogenesis. J Exp Med 2000; 192: 1563-76.

[228] Debierre-Grockiego F, Campos MA, Azzouz N, *et al*. Activation of TLR2 and TLR4 by glycosylphosphatidylinositols derived from *Toxoplasma gondii*. J Immunol 2007; 179: 1129-37.

[229] Ouaissi A, Guilvard E, Delneste Y, *et al*. The *Trypanosoma cruzi* Tc52-released protein induces human dendritic cell maturation, signals via Toll-like receptor 2, and confers protection against lethal infection. J Immunol 2002; 168: 6366-74.

[230] Harris TH, Cooney NM, Mansfield JM, Paulnock DM. Signal transduction, gene transcription, and cytokine production triggered in macrophages by exposure to trypanosome DNA. Infect Immun 2006; 74: 4530-07.

[231] Shoda LK, Kegerreis KA, Suarez CE, *et al*. DNA from protozoan parasites *Babesia bovis*, *Trypanosoma cruzi*, and *T. brucei* is mitogenic for B lymphocytes and stimulates macrophage expression of interleukin-12, tumor necrosis factor alpha, and nitric oxide. Infect Immun 2001; 69: 2162-71.

[232] Brown WC, Corral RS. Stimulation of B lymphocytes, macrophages, and dendritic cells by protozoan DNA. Microbes Infect 2002; 4: 969-74.

[233] Bafica A, Santiago HC, Goldszmid R, *et al*. Cutting edge: TLR9 and TLR2 signaling together account for MyD88-dependent control of parasitemia in *Trypanosoma cruzi* infection. J Immunol 2006; 177: 3515-19.

[234] Drennan MB, Stijlemans B, Van den Abbeele J, *et al*. The induction of a type 1 immune response following a *Trypanosoma brucei* infection is MyD88 dependent. J Immunol 2005; 175: 2501-09.

[235] Jaramillo M, Gowda DC, Radzioch D, Olivier M. Hemozoin increases IFN-gamma-Inducible macrophage nitric oxide generation through extracellular signal-regulated kinase- and NF-kappa B-dependent pathways. J Immunol 2003; 171: 4243-53.

[236] Jaramillo M, Plante I, Ouellet N, *et al*. Hemozoin-inducible proinflammatory events in vivo: Potential role in malaria infection. J Immunol 2004; 172: 3101-10.

[237] Coban C, Ishii KJ, Kawai T, *et al*. Toll-like receptor 9 mediates innate immune activation by the malaria pigment hemozoin. J Exp Med 2005; 201: 19-25.

[238] Parroche P, Lauw FN, Goutagny N, *et al*. Malaria hemozoin is immunologically inert but radically enhances innate responses by presenting malaria DNA to Toll-like receptor 9. Proc Natl Acad Sci U SA 2007; 104: 1919-24.

[239] Yarovinsky F, Zhang D, Andersen JF, *et al.* TLR11 activation of dendritic cells by a protozoan profilin-like protein. Science 2005; 308: 1626-29.

[240] Aosai F, Chen M, Kang HK, *et al. Toxoplasma gondii*-derived heat shock protein HSP70 functions as a B cell mitogen. Cell Stress Chaperones 2002; 7: 357-64.

[241] Del Rio L, Butcher BA, Bennouna S, *et al. Toxoplasma gondii* triggers myeloid differentiation factor 88-dependent IL-12 and chemokine ligand 2 (monocyte chemoattractant protein 1) responses using distinct parasite molecules and host receptors. J Immunol 2004; 172: 6954-60.

[242] Gazzinelli RT, Denkers EY. Protozoan encounters with Toll-like receptor signalling pathways: implications for host parasitism. Nature Rev 2006; 6: 895-06.

[243] Campos MA, Closel M, Valente EP, *et al.* Impaired production of proinflammatory cytokines and host resistance to acute infection with *Trypanosoma cruzi* in mice lacking functional myeloid differentiation factor 88. J Immunol 2004; 172: 1711-18.

[244] Muraille E, De Trez C, Brait M, *et al.* Genetically resistant mice lacking MyD88-adapter protein display a high susceptibility to *Leishmania major* infection associated with a polarized Th2 response. J Immunol 2003; 170: 4237-41.

[245] Scanga CA, Aliberti J, Jankovic D, *et al.* Cutting edge: MyD88 is required for resistance to *Toxoplasma gondii* infection and regulates parasite-induced IL-12 production by dendritic cells. J Immunol 2002; 168: 5997-01.

[246] Adachi K, Tsutsui H, Kashiwamura S, *et al. Plasmodium berghei* infection in mice induces liver injury by an IL-12- and toll-like receptor/myeloid differentiation factor 88-dependent mechanism. J Immunol 2001; 167: 5928-34.

[247] Kropf P, Freudenberg MA, Modolell M, *et al.* Toll-like receptor 4 contributes to efficient control of infection with the protozoan parasite *Leishmania major.* Infect Immun 2004; 72: 1920-08.

[248] Kropf P, Freudenberg N, Kalis C, *et al.* Infection of C57BL/10ScCr and C57BL/10ScNCr mice with *Leishmania major* reveals a role for Toll-like receptor 4 in the control of parasite replication. J Leukoc Biol 2004; 76: 48-57.

[249] Grazia Cappiello M, Sutterwala FS, Trinchieri G, *et al.* Suppression of Il-12 transcription in macrophages following Fc gamma receptor ligation. J Immunol 2001; 166: 4498-06.

[250] Urban BC, Willcox N, Roberts DJ. A role for CD36 in the regulation of dendritic cell function. Proc Natl Acad Sci U S A 2001; 98: 8750-05.

[251] Ocana-Morgner C, Mota MM, Rodriguez A. Malaria blood stage suppression of liver stage immunity by dendritic cells. J Exp Med 2003; 197: 143-51.

[252] Perry JA, Olver CS, Burnett RC, Avery AC. Cutting edge: the acquisition of TLR tolerance during malaria infection impacts T cell activation. J Immunol 2005; 174: 5921-25.

[253] Urban BC, Ferguson DJ, Pain A, *et al. Plasmodium falciparum*-infected erythrocytes modulate the maturation of dendritic cells. Nature 1999; 400: 73-77.

[254] Butcher BA, Denkers EY. Mechanism of entry determines the ability of *Toxoplasma gondii* to inhibit macrophage proinflammatory cytokine production. Infect Immun 2002; 70: 5216-24.

[255] Denkers EY, Kim L, Butcher BA. In the belly of the beast: subversion of macrophage proinflammatory signalling cascades during *Toxoplasma gondii* infection. Cell Microbiol 2003; 5: 75-83.

[256] McKee AS, Dzierszinski F, Boes M, *et al.* Functional inactivation of immature dendritic cells by the intracellular parasite *Toxoplasma gondii.* J Immunol 2004 ; 173: 2632-40.

[257] Bennouna S, Sukhumavasi W, Denkers EY. *Toxoplasma gondii* inhibits toll-like receptor 4 ligand-induced mobilization of intracellular tumor necrosis factor alpha to the surface of mouse peritoneal neutrophils. Infect Immun 2006; 74: 4274-81.

[258] Williams L, Bradley L, Smith A, Foxwell B. Signal transducer and activator of transcription 3 is the dominant mediator of the anti-inflammatory effects of IL-10 in human macrophages. J Immunol 2004; 172: 567-76.

[259] Butcher BA, Kim L, Panopoulos AD, *et al.* IL-10-independent STAT3 activation by *Toxoplasma gondii* mediates suppression of IL-12 and TNF-alpha in host macrophages. J Immunol 2005; 174: 3148-52.

[260] Kim L, Butcher BA, Denkers EY. *Toxoplasma gondii* interferes with lipopolysaccharide-induced mitogen-activated protein kinase activation by mechanisms distinct from endotoxin tolerance. J Immunol 2004; 172: 3003-10.

[261] Butcher BA, Kim L, Johnson PF, Denkers EY. *Toxoplasma gondii* tachyzoites inhibit proinflammatory cytokine induction in infected macrophages by preventing nuclear translocation of the transcription factor NF-kappa B. J Immunol 2001; 167: 2193-01.

[262] Shapira S, Speirs K, Gerstein A, *et al.* Suppression of NF-kappaB activation by infection with *Toxoplasma gondii.* J Infec Dis 2002; 185: S66-72.

[263] Shapira S, Harb OS, Margarit J, *et al.* Initiation and termination of NF-kappaB signaling by the intracellular protozoan parasite *Toxoplasma gondii.* J Cell Sci 2005; 118: 3501-08.

[264] Richards RL, Rao M, Wassef NM, *et al.* Liposomes containing lipid A serve as an adjuvant for induction of antibody and cytotoxic T-cell responses against RTS,S malaria antigen. Infect Immun 1998; 66: 2859-65.

[265] Skeiky YA, Coler RN, Brannon M, *et al.* Protective efficacy of a tandemly linked, multi-subunit recombinant leishmanial vaccine (Leish-111f) formulated in MPL adjuvant. Vaccine 2002; 20: 3292-03.

[266] Zhang WW, Matlashewski G. Immunization with a Toll-like receptor 7 and/or 8 agonist vaccine adjuvant increases protective immunity against *Leishmania major* in BALB/c mice. Infect Immun 2008; 76: 3777-83.

[267] Araujo AF, de Alencar BC, Vasconcelos JR, *et al.* CD8+-T-cell-dependent control of *Trypanosoma cruzi* infection in a highly susceptible mouse strain after immunization with recombinant proteins based on amastigote surface protein 2. Infect Immun 2005; 73: 6017-25.

[268] Stacey KJ, Blackwell JM. Immunostimulatory DNA as an adjuvant in vaccination against *Leishmania major*. Infect Immun 1999; 67: 3719-26.

[269] Coban C, Ishii KJ, Stowers AW, *et al.* Effect of CpG oligodeoxynucleotides on the immunogenicity of Pfs25, a *Plasmodium falciparum* transmission-blocking vaccine antigen. Infect Immun 2004; 72: 584-88.

[270] Cunha MG, Rodrigues MM, Soares IS. Comparison of the immunogenic properties of recombinant proteins representing the *Plasmodium vivax* vaccine candidate MSP1(19) expressed in distinct bacterial vectors. Vaccine 2001; 20: 385-96.

[271] Kumar S, Jones TR, Oakley MS, *et al.* CpG oligodeoxynucleotide and Montanide ISA 51 adjuvant combination enhanced the protective efficacy of a subunit malaria vaccine. Infect Immun 2004; 72: 949-57.

[272] McSorley SJ, Ehst BD, Yu Y, Gewirtz AT. Bacterial flagellin is an effective adjuvant for CD4+ T cells in *vivo*. J Immunol 2002; 169: 3914-19.

[273] Arevalo I, Ward B, Miller R, *et al.* Successful treatment of drug-resistant cutaneous leishmaniasis in humans by use of imiquimod, an immunomodulator. Clin Infect Dis 2001; 33:1847-51.

[274] Buates S, Matlashewski G. Treatment of experimental leishmaniasis with the immunomodulators imiquimod and S-28463: efficacy and mode of action. J Infect Dis 1999; 179: 1485-94.

[275] Flynn B, Wang V, Sacks DL, *et al.* Prevention and treatment of cutaneous leishmaniasis in primates by using synthetic type D/A oligodeoxynucleotides expressing CpG motifs. Infect Immun 2005; 73: 4948-54.

CHAPTER 11

Immune Responses to *Leishmania guyanensis* Infection in Humans and Animal Models

Catherine Ronet[1, 2], Annette Ives[2], Eliane Bourreau[3], Nicolas Fasel[2], Pascal Launois*[,1,2,4] and Slavica Masina[2]

[1]*WHO-IRTC, Chemin des Boveresses 155,1066 Epalinges, Switzerland;* [2]*Department of Biochemistry, University of Lausanne, Chemin des Boveresses 155,1066 Epalinges, Switzerland;* [3]*Immunologie des Leishmanioses, Institut Pasteur de la Guyane, 97306 Cayenne, French Guyana and* [4]*Special Programme for Research and Training in Tropical Diseases (TDR), Avenue Apia,20, 1211 Geneva 27, Switzerland*

Abstract: Cutaneous Leishmaniasis caused by *Leishmania guyanensis* parasites is endemic in the North-East South America. There is, however, little information available concerning *L. guyanensis* infectivity and the immune response associated with different stages of the disease. In the following chapter we discuss the results obtained in human research with regard to the involvement of different types of immune cells and their roles during the development of infection with *L. guyanensis* parasites. We also provide a résumé on the status of animal models of *L. guyanensis* infection and emphasize how essential these models are so as to increase our knowledge of immunopathogenesis in the host and thus provide an indispensable tool to test new therapeutic strategies.

INTRODUCTION

Human cutaneous leishmaniasis is caused by many different species of *Leishmania* having different geographical distribution and spectra of disease. In the Old world, *Leishmania major*, *Leishmania tropica* and *Leishmania aethiopica* cause cutaneous leishmaniasis. In the New World, cutaneous leishmaniasis is due to species from either the *Leishmania mexicana* complex (*Leishmania mexicana* and *Leishmania amazonensis*) or to the *Leishmania Viannia* subgenus (*Leishmania guyanensis*, *Leishmania braziliensis*, *Leishmania peruviana* and *Leishmania panamensis*). After an initial infection, *Leishmania* parasites induce transitory cutaneous lesions in the host and develop an immune response that renders it, in the majority of cases, immune to re-infection.

Mechanisms of the immune response have been analyzed in detail in experimental murine models of dermal leishmaniasis after infection with specific strains of *Leishmania*. During these studies, the most widely used strain was *Leishmania major* (*L. major*). Following infection with *L. major*, mice from most inbred strains (C3H/He, CBA, C57BL/6, 129Sv/Ev) develop cutaneous lesions that heal spontaneously. These mice do not develop lesions after a second inoculation of *L. major* and are characterized as having a resistant phenotype. Mice from a few strains (BALB/c, DBA/2) develop severe and uncontrollable lesions and do not become immune to re-infection, and are representative of the susceptible phenotype. T lymphocytes, in particular CD4[+] T cells, have been identified as key players in determining resistance or susceptibility to *L. major*, since infection triggers predominantly a CD4[+] response [1]. Naive CD4[+] T cells can differentiate into a variety of effector subsets after encounter with antigens, including classical T helper type 1 cells (Th1), Th2 cells, and regulatory T cells (Treg cells). Th1 and Th2 subsets are distinguished by the mutually exclusive patterns of cytokines produced following their reactivation. Th1 cells are characterized by the production of interleukin (IL)-2, interferon-γ (IFN-γ) and lymphotoxin (LT) whereas Th2 cells produce IL-4, IL-5 and IL-13. During the immune response, tight regulations of effector T cell responses are controlled by Treg cells. Using the murine model of infection with *L. major*, a correlation was found between resistance to infection and development of a CD4[+] Th1 response, and susceptibility to infection is associated with the development of a CD4[+] Th2 response on the other hand [1].

HUMAN IMMUNE RESPONSE TO *L. GUYANENSIS* INFECTION

It is generally considered that patients with cutaneous leishmaniasis present a heterogeneous cellular immune response with a predominant CD4[+] Th1 type immune response upon healing of the lesion either due to treatment, or spontaneous

*Corresponding Author: Pascal Launois, WHO-IRTC, Chemin des Boveresses 155,1066 Epalinges, Switzerland, Tel:(+41) 22 791 26 59; Fax: :(+41) 22 791 48 54 ; Email : launoisp@who.int

Emilio Jirillo (Ed)
All rights reserved - © 2010 Bentham Science Publishers Ltd.

regression. The subsets of T cells (CD4$^+$ or CD8$^+$), and their function within lesions is still, however, under debate. *Leishmania* specific CD4$^+$ T cells and CD8$^+$ T cells have been demonstrated both in skin lesions and in PBMCs (peripheral blood mononucelar cells) during the acute phase of infection due to New and Old World dermotropic *Leishmania* such as *L. braziliensis* [2], *L. major* [3] and *L. aethiopica* [4]. Implication of CD8 responses could be important due to the emergence of patients with a decreased or a total absence of CD4$^+$ T cells, during co-infection of Leishmania and HIV [5]. Analysis of cytokine expression has been performed during human infection with different *Leishmania* species either in PBMCs or at the site of infection. The presence of IFN-γ is most often associated with cure of the infection and the presence of IL-4 and IL-13 are associated with non-healing lesions analogous to results obtained in the murine model of infection with *L. major*. However, the levels of IFN-γ do not always correlate with resistance, as similar levels of this cytokine were observed following leishmanization in subjects, regardless of lesion development [6]. Moreover, the preferential participation of Th1 or Th2 responses during human infection with *Leishmania* is not completely understood. It should be noted that in most human studies, the stage of disease is not specified, and this could be an important information as it is known that an immune response evolves during infection.

The immunopathogenesis of clinical leishmaniasis due to New World *Leishmania* species and the immunological mechanisms of resistance to these parasites are undefined. Thus, the role of the cytokine network in human infection with these *Leishmania* species requires better definition. With this aim, we have analyzed the role of cytokines during different phases of infection with *L. guyanensis*, a *Leishmania* species endemic in the North-East South America. We have determined cytokine production in PBMCs and at the site of infection in different human populations, namely subjects who have never been exposed to *Leishmania,* subjects exposed recently to *Leishmania* and patients developing the disease. All results presented in the following sections are summarized in Table **1** (for PBMC results) and in Fig. **1** (for cells present in the cutaneous lesions).

Cytokine Production by PBMCs from Unexposed Subjects

Absence of prior exposure to *Leishmania* in healthy subjects was assessed based on (a) the absence of scars due to leishmaniasis upon clinical examination, (b) no history of any stay in an endemic country, and (c) no reactivity against soluble *L. guyanensis* antigens (SLA). That is, healthy subjects do not develop IFN-γ reactivity and specific Abs against soluble *Leishmania* antigens.

When PBMCs from these unexposed healthy subjects were stimulated with live *L. guyanensis*, CD4$^+$ and CD8$^+$ T cell expansion was detected as following stimulation with *L. major* [7], *L. aethiopica* [8], *L. guyanensis* [9] and *L. amazonensis* [10]. Following stimulation with live *L. guyanensis,* PBMCs produced IFN-γ and TGF-β but not IL-4 and IL-13 [9, 11]. Cells that produce IFN-γ in response to live *L. guyanensis* are generated from naïve CD8$^+$ T cells and require the presence of whole *L. guyanensis* parasites (live or UV irradiated) and SLA stimulation is not sufficient to induce IFN-γ production [9]. Interestingly, these IFN-γ producing CD8$^+$ T cells recognize a specific antigen, the *Leishmania* homologue of receptors of Activated C Kinase (LACK) [9] and express preferentially the Vβ14 T cell repertoire (TCR) gene family [12]. In addition, these LACK-specific IFN-γ producing CD8$^+$ T cells express CLA (Cutaneous Lymphocyte-associated Antigen) and CCR4, two molecules involved in migration of T cells into cutaneous sites, suggesting that these LACK-specific T cells are able to migrate into the skin where infection with *Leishmania* can occur [12].

Very low or undetectable levels of IL-10 were produced by PBMCs stimulated with live *L. guyanensis*. However, a strong IL-10 response was detected in purified memory CD45RA$^-$CD4$^+$ T cells in response to LACK, suggesting that suppressive cytokine(s), other than IL-10 are produced by PBMCs in response to live *L. guyanensis* which could in turn inhibit the IL-10 production by memory CD4$^+$ T cells [9, 13]. The role of TGF-β, a well known immuno-suppressive cytokine, on IL-10 production was analyzed in PBMCs from naïve subjects stimulated with live *L. guyanensis*. Neutralization of TGF-β *in vitro* induced IL-10 production in both CD4$^+$ and CD8$^+$ T cells [13]. Interestingly, both IL-10 producing CD4$^+$ and CD8$^+$ T cells are LACK-specific [9, 14].

Altogether, IFN-γ producing CD8$^+$ T cells together with IL-10 producing CD4$^+$ T cells and CD8$^+$ T cells (when TGF-β is neutralized) are detected in PBMCs from subjects who have never been exposed to *Leishmania*. Although IFN-γ is a key molecule for anti-*Leshmania* effector function [15], IL-10 is able to down-regulate IFN-γ production and/or function and consequently promote disease progression. The precise role of these distinct IFN-γ and IL-10 sub-populations during the establishment of an appropriate immune response to contain *L. guyanensis* infection is not well understood.

Cytokine Production by PBMCs from Exposed Healthy Subjects

Thus, to analyze the role of IFN-γ producing T cell subpopulations detected in PBMCs from unexposed subjects, we monitored the immune response against *L. guyanensis* in a population of subjects exposed to this parasite. Healthy subjects were followed during 7 months before and after their stay in the rain forest in French Guyana (South America), a natural environment endemic for *L. guyanensis*. Among these subjects, some became responsive to *Leishmania* following their stay in the rain forest. Indeed, and in contrast to unexposed subjects, PBMCs of these subjects produced IFN-γ in response to SLA. We were unable, however, to detect IL-4 or IL-13 cytokine production in supernatants of SLA-stimulated PBMCs from subjects who became IFN-γ responders, thus we considered the unique IFN-γ increase in response to SLA stimulation as a signature of exposure to *Leishmania* [16].

Table 1: Type and characterisitics of human PBMCs secreting cytokines before or after infection with *Leishmania guyanensis*.
Stimuli required to induce cytokine production are indictated: *L. guyanensis*, soluble leishmania antigen (SLA) or LACK antigen.
+ = positive reaction; - = negative reaction.

	Naïve	Infected	
		Early (< 1 month)	Late (>1 month and < 6 months)
IFN-γ	**Naïve CD8⁺ T cells** *L. guyanensis* + SLA - LACK + (Vβ14⁺, CLA⁺, CCR4⁺)	**CD4⁺/ CD8⁺ T cells** *L. guyanensis* + SLA + LACK + (CLA⁺)	**CD4⁺/ CD8⁺ T cells** *L. guyanensis* + SLA + (CLA+)
IL-4	*L. guyanensis* -	*L. guyanensis* +/ - SLA-	*L. guyanensis* - SLA-
IL-13	*L. guyanensis* -	*L. guyanensis* +/ - SLA-	*L. guyanensis* - SLA-
TGF-β	**Total PBMC** *L. guyanensis* +	*L. guyanensis* -	*L. guyanensis* -
IL-10	**CD4⁺ memory T cells** LACK + **CD4⁺and CD8⁺ memory T cells** when TGF-β neutralised	**CD4⁺/ CD8⁺ T cells** LACK +	**CD4⁺/ CD8⁺ T cells** SLA + LACK +

Furthermore, an increase in IFN-γ production by PBMCs following LACK stimulation was also detected in subjects who were exposed to *L. guyanensis* [17]. However, contrary to the results obtained in subjects never exposed to *Leishmania*, both CD4⁺ and CD8⁺ T cells were responsible for IFN-γ production in response to LACK stimulation in exposed individuals [17]. Moreover, LACK-reactive IFN-γ production by CD4⁺ T cells was detected in these subjects prior to SLA-reactive IFN-γ production by CD4⁺ T cells, suggesting that the former readout assay could be used as an early predictive immunological marker of exposure to *Leishmania* in subjects who were exposed to *Leishmania* parasites but did not present with clinical disease [17]. Additionally, both SLA and LACK-specific CD4⁺ T cells express CLA, suggesting that these cells are able to migrate to the skin at the site of *Leishmania* infection [9, 17]. In contrast to IFN-γ, levels of IL-10 produced by LACK specific CD4⁺ T cells in subjects exposed to *Leishmania* remained identical to those observed in subjects unexposed to *Leishmania* [18].

Cytokine Production by PBMCs from Localized Cutaneous Leishmaniasis Patients

Unlike subjects who have never been exposed to *Leishmania*, PBMCs from localized cutaneous leishmaniasis (LCL) patients are able to produce IFN-γ and IL-10 but not TGF-β in response to *L. guyanensis* [13, 16]. IFN-γ was produced at high levels following *L. guyanensis* stimulation in all patients, IFN-γ was produced in response to LACK stimulation only during the early phase of infection (less than 30 days) [17]. IFN-γ producing cells in response to LACK were both CD4⁺ and CD8⁺ T cells and only that of the CD4⁺ type in response to SLA [18].

It is not clear why T cells producing IFN-γ in response to LACK are no longer detected in blood 30 days after initial lesion development. One explanation for the loss of detection of T cells producing IFN-γ in the circulation could be due to cellular recruitment to the site of *Leishmania* infection. Indeed, at the site of infection, Th2 responses predominate during the early phase of infection in LCL patients and precede the development of a Th1 response [18]. Thus, the Th1 response detected in the skin during the late phase of infection could be due to the migration of IFN-γ producing T cells to the site of infection. In support of this, results obtained in our laboratory have shown that IFN-γ producing CD8[+] T cells in response to LACK in unexposed subjects express the Vβ14 TCR gene, together with CLA and CCR4 molecules allowing them to migrate to the skin. Furthermore, Vβ14 TCR gene expression is increased in most lesions from LCL patients [12], particularly during the late phase of infection. This is in accordance with the hypothesis of migration and accumulation of LACK-specific IFN-γ producing cells to the inflamed skin.

The levels of IFN-γ produced by LACK-specific PBMCs and the phenotype of LACK-reactive CD4[+] T cells producing IFN-γ, that is CD45RA[-], CD62L[-] and CLA[+], are identical in subjects who have never been exposed to *Leishmania* [17] and in *Leishmania*-positive patients [9, 17]. Thus, the role of LACK-specific CD4[+] T cells producing IFN-γ is debatable in terms of protection to infection. The production of immunosuppressive factors inhibits the protective role of IFN-γ and could explain the development of disease in subjects infected with *Leishmania*. Considering that TGF-β and IL-4 are not detected in supernatants of PBMCs from LCL patients stimulated with *L. guyanensis*, two cytokines, namely IL-10 and IL-13 have been further evaluated for their immunosuppressive functions during human infection with *L. guyanensis*.

IL-10 production in response to SLA stimulated PBMCs was lower than in LACK-stimulated PBMCs, nevertheless, IL-10 was still detectable and produced by both CD4[+] and CD8[+] T cells in LCL patients [14]. The homing capacities of IL-10 producing T cells are not known, yet, the extremely low levels of IL-10 mRNA expression in LCL lesions suggests that these cells did not migrate to the skin. In addition, IL-10 producing CD4[+] T cells in PBMCs express particular TCR gene families (Vβ3, Vβ5.1, Vβ16 and Vβ20). The fact that the expression of these Vβ TCR genes are rarely detected in lesions of LCL patients reinforces our hypothesis that these cells do not migrate to the skin [12]. Finally, the expression of CD62L on IL-10 producing T cells confirms that these cells are able to migrate to the LN (lymph node), and in some circumstances, the migration of IL-10 producing T cells can be directed towards inflamed site of infection. Indeed, high intra-lesional IL-10 mRNA expression is detected in lesions of patients prior to any treatment and in those who respond poorly to treatment, when compared to those who respond well to treatment [11, 19]. Factors responsible for the preferential recruitment of IL-10 secreting T cells in the skin from patients that are non-responders to treatment have yet to be characterized.

Low levels of the Th2 cytokines IL-4 and IL-13 are expressed in lesions. Nevertheless IL-13 is the main cytokine expressed within the lesion at the early phase of infection [20]. Considering that IL-13 could induce IL-12 unresponsiveness in specific T cells by inducing down-regulation of the IL-12Rβ2 chain [20], IL-13 may thus contribute to the development of the Th2 cells detected in lesions during the early phase of infection (less than 1 month of infection). Additionally, IL-13 is also produced by CD4[+] T cells in response to SLA but not with LACK stimulation in PBMCs from LCL patients [16]. Altogether these observations suggest that IL-13 may be responsible for the maintenance of infection with *L. guyanensis*.

Regulatory T cells (Tregs)

In the past few years, the notion of there being subpopulations of T cells specialized in the suppression of immune responses has been revisited. Considerable attention has been given to a minor subpopulation of CD4[+] T cells constitutively expressing CD25, the α-chain of the IL-2 receptor. Two main subsets of Treg cells have been described namely, natural Treg cells (nTregs), which develop in the thymus and regulate self-reactivity in the periphery, and inducible Treg cells (iTregs) which can develop from conventional CD4[+] T cells after exposure to antigen and specific signals. Treg cells are capable of suppressing the proliferation of effector T cells in mice and humans [21]. CD4[+]CD25[+] T cells express markers that can be up-regulated on activated T cells, these markers include CTLA-4, glucorticoid-induced TNF receptor (GITR), CD103, CD45B[low], CD62L, OX-40, LAG-3, neuropilin-1 and CCR4, therefore the phenotypic definition of these cells is not specific [22]. However, the transcription factor Foxp3 was recently shown to be a specific marker for CD4[+] CD25[+] T cells [23-25]. Tregs have also been shown to regulate immunity against pathogens [26] and more particularly in murine models of infection with *L. major*.

To date, limited information is available on the role of Treg cells during human infection with *Leishmania*. Treg cells with immunosuppressive functions have been detected in lesions of LCL patients due to *L. braziliensis* [27] and in PBMCs from acute and cured patients infected with *L. braziliensis* [28].

<u>Tregs in Subjects Never Exposed to *Leishmania*</u>

We demonstrated that CD4[+]CD25[+] T cells produced TGF-β but not IL-10 in response to live *L. guyanensis*. In PBMCs of subjects who have never been exposed to *Leishmania*, CD4[+]CD25[+] T cells producing TGF-β are clearly Treg cells since they express CD25, CD45RO and HLA-DR markers at their surface [13] and Foxp3 at the RNA and protein levels [29]. They also have immunosuppressive properties since they are able to inhibit IL-2 and IL-10 production by CD4$^+$CD25$^-$ T cells in an *in vitro* co-culture assay [13].

The role played by TGF-β in the suppression mediated by Treg cells was determined *in vitro* using neutralizing mAbs. The neutralization of TGF-β abrogated the suppressive activity of these CD4$^+$CD25$^+$ T cells, since restoration of IL-10 but not IFN-γ production was possible *in vitro* in CD4$^+$CD25$^-$ T cells. In addition, subjects who have never been exposed to *Leishmania*, neutralization of TGF-β induced IL-10 production in memory CD8$^+$ T cells. Furthermore, TGF-β produced by Treg cells maintains CCR4 and CLA expression on these IFN-γ producing CD8$^+$ T cells.

In conclusion, subjects who have never been exposed to *Leis*hmania, PBMC derived CD4$^+$CD25$^+$ Treg cells produce TGF-β, and its neutralization induces IL-10 production by CD4$^+$ and CD8$^+$ T cells.

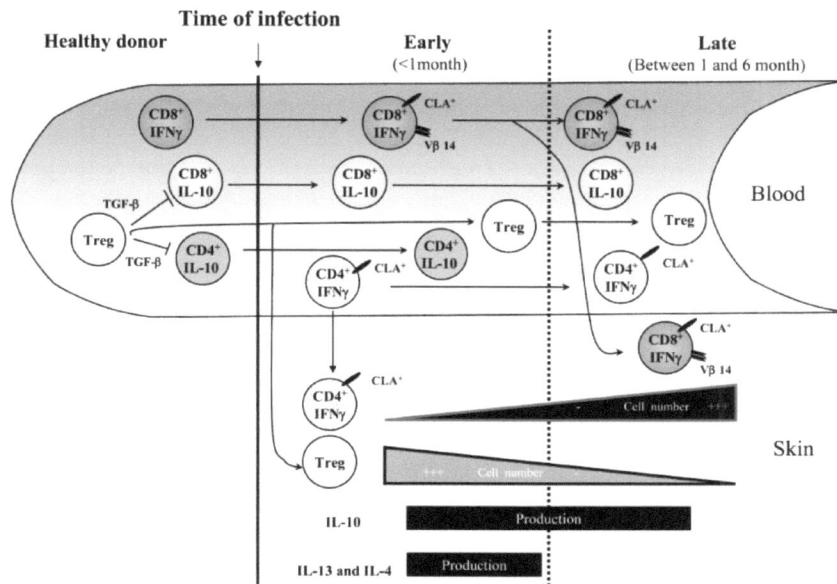

Figure 1: Summary of the cells present in the blood or in the skin before or after *Leishmania guyanenesis* infection.

Tregs in LCL Patients

Although non-exposed subjects were shown to produce TGF-β after stimulation with L*eishmania* parasites, we were unable to detect TGF-β production by CD4$^+$CD25$^+$ T cells in PBMCs of LCL patients, and the percentage of CD4$^+$ T cells expressing Foxp3 was lower in LCL patients as compared to controls [29]. CD4$^+$CD25$^+$T cells detected in PBMCs from unexposed subjects express CLA and CCR4, suggesting that they are able to migrate to the skin where *Leishmania* is located. To confirm that Treg cells migrate to the site of infection, we determined the levels of Treg cells within the lesion by analyzing the Foxp3 mRNA expression. We confirmed, as previously described during infection with *L. braziliensis* [27] that Treg cells accumulate during the early phase of infection (lesion duration of less than 1 month) in lesions of LCL patients due to *L. guyanenesis* [29]. Treg cells were shown to have suppressive functions *in vitro*, since they inhibited IFN-γ production by CD4$^+$CD25$^-$ T cells from the same patient in response to *L. guyanensis* stimulation. IL-10 production by intra-lesional Treg cells was quite low and is partially responsible for the suppressive activity observed previously. Intra-lesional Treg cells are unable to produce TGF-β after stimulation by *L. guyanensis* suggesting that other mechanisms are involved that could account for Treg suppressive activities. One possibility could be that 2,3-indoleamine dioxygenase (IDO), a molecule with demonstrated suppressive activities [30], is involved. Treg cells have been demonstrated to induce IDO expression in APCs and to maintain its expression by IL-10. Interestingly IDO mRNA expression is detected in lesions from LCL patients with the highest level during the early phase of infection (less than 30 days) as was observed with Foxp3 mRNA expression [29]. One hypothesis could be that IDO is one of the immunosuppressive molecules induced by intra-lesional Treg cells. The immunosuppressive role of IDO could be explained by different mechanisms, namely the deprivation of tryptophan compromising the function of effector T cells, the production of tryptophan metabolites, such as 3-

OH-kyrunenine and 3-OH-anthralinic acid, which demonstrate some anti-proliferative activity, and the induction of apoptosis of Th1 cells but not Th2 cells [30].

Although the presence of intra-lesional Treg cells in early lesions (less than 1 month) due to *L. guyanensis* could be predictive of a favorable clinical evolution after treatment, their persistence in lesions (between 1 and 6 months) might be an indicator of poor response to therapy [19]. High levels of Treg cells with suppressive functions were detected within lesions from patients with chronic Cutaneous Leishmaniasis (CCL) due to *L. guyanensis* [29]. These observations suggest that the chronicity of lesions due to *L. guyanensis* infection is associated with local immunosuppression due to the presence of Treg cells, suggesting in turn that Treg cells could have a role in the down-regulation of local *Leishmania*-specific immune responses. If this hypothesis is confirmed, the chronicity of the disease might be the consequence of the excessive down-regulation of a successful effector response. In support of this, the level of IDO mRNA expression is elevated in CCL lesions [29]. Since this high level of IDO mRNA expression is associated with high levels of Foxp3 mRNA, it reinforces our previous hypothesis that IDO might be one of the immunosuppressive molecules induced by Treg cells during human leishmaniasis.

Taken together, the results obtained allow a better understanding of immunological mechanisms involved following *L. guyanensis* infection. This research on patients must be pursued in order to identify the implication of new cells types or molecular mechanisms involved in *Leishmania* infection. Unfortunately, albeit understandably this type of research is restricted due to sample material for testing, and ethical constraints. For these reasons, the development of animal models is justified and seems to be appropriate to improve our knowledge in the field and to test new therapeutics.

EXPERIMENTAL MODELS OF *LEISHMANIA GUYANENSIS* INFECTION

Rodents and primates are susceptible to infection with most *Leishmania* species. Studies indicate that the development of leishmaniasis is dependent on the combination of the host genetic background, parasite virulence and the parasite-induced host immune response. Parasites from the *Leishmania Viannia* sub-genus, namely, *L. braziliensis*, *L. guyanensis* and *L. panamensis* give rise, in humans, to cutaneous leishmaniasis (CL). In up to 10% of CL cases a secondary manifestation of disease known as mucocutaneous leishmaniasis (MCL) develops in the naso-pharyngeal area of the face. Due to the unavailability of adequate experimental animal models of infection for the parasites belonging to the *L. Viannia* sub-genus, research describing the identification of the mechanisms responsible for resistance, or susceptibility, is scarce.

In this chapter, progress in the development of experimental models following infection with *L (V). guyanensis* parasites will be discussed. Due to the limited number of studies performed with *L (V). guyanensis* parasites, reference will also be given to what can be learnt from experimental models based on the closely related *L (V). braziliensis* and *L (V). panamensis* parasites.

Mouse Models of *Leishmania Viannia* Infection

It is without doubt that mice are a convenient and economical laboratory model for the investigation of disease development, the host response to parasites, and for research into the action of potential anti-leishmanial drugs and vaccines.

With the aim of covering the broad spectrum of human disease, murine models of leishmaniasis have been developed. In genetically defined strains of mice, *Leishmania* species produce distinguishable and characteristic patterns of disease. The most studied murine model is that of CL caused by *L. major,* whereby BALB/c mice are susceptible and C57BL/6 mice are resistant to infection. It has been proven that the resistance phenotype is attributed to the elimination of the parasite by nitric oxide (NO) produced by macrophages that have been activated by IFN-γ from CD4$^+$T cells when a Th1 immune response is generated. Susceptibility, on the other hand, is determined by the absence of NO and the production of IL-4, IL-13, and/or IL-10 in the context of CD4$^+$T cell type 2 (Th2) response [31, 32]. However, the paradigms of protection and pathogenesis established in the *L. major* mouse model does not explain resistance or susceptibility to all species of *Leishmania.*

Leishmania *guyanensis* Infection in Mice

Work performed by Sousa-Franco and colleagues [33] was the first and only published report, to our knowledge, describing *in vivo* mouse infection experiments with *L. guyanensis* parasites. In this study the authors used the M4147 strain of *L. guyanensis* derived from a human case of CL to infect footpads of BALB/c mice. Following the 20 weeks of observation, infected mice did not develop progressive lesions. There was a well preserved inflammatory cell population and tissue architecture in the footpads, and limiting dilution analysis showed a very low number of parasites at the site of infection. The parasites used were apparently infectious as they were able to infect hamsters. The authors then went on to describe that *L. guyanensis* parasites were efficiently eliminated by reactive oxygen intermediates (ROI) formed from NADPH oxidase that was elicited following the *in vitro* infection of bone marrow derived macrophages. The authors further determined that the amastigotes within the macrophage died in an apoptotic manner induced by the exposure to ROI. Taken together, the work by Sousa-Franco *et al.*, postulates that an innate immune mechanism is responsible for the rapid control of *L. guyanensis* parasite burden, during the acute phase prior to the establishment of an adaptive immune response *in vivo*.

L. panamensis Infection in Mice

The resistance observed in the above mentioned study on BALB/c leishmaniasis is striking for a mouse strain that is highly susceptible to most species of *Leishmania*. Interestingly, the closely related *L. panamensis* parasites behave like most *Leishmania* species in BALB/c mice, and induces footpad swelling that evolves to form a tumor-like lesion that does not heal, nor necrose. [34, 35]. In the study by Guervara- Mendoza *et al.* [36] an early induction of IFN-γ with minimal amounts of detectable IL-4 was detected at 24 hours post-infection in the draining LN of mice infected with *L. panamensis* parasites. Interestingly, at 7 days post-infection there was a significant reduction in IFN-γ and an up-regulation of IL-4. Unfortunately, recent and more thorough studies examining the immune response in mice following infection with *L. panamensis* have not been documented and thus we do not have a complete understanding of the processes involved in the progression of infection and immune status of the host.

It is known that one of the major problems in establishing a susceptible phenotype with *Leishmania* promastigotes is retaining infectivity of the parasite culture. The growth kinetics and point of maximum infectivity differ among species. *Leishmania* of the *Viannia* subgenus, unlike *L. major*, do not show strict growth-phase dependent infectivity and conversion of these parasites to metacyclics under standard culture conditions is inefficient [37], thus requiring that a large inoculum of parasites be used to achieve infection. Differences in infectivity are an important consideration when experimentally analyzing pathogenicity and/or virulence, since some expressions of disease are linked to the dose and route of the infective inoculum. In light of this, what we can ascertain from the studies performed with *L. panamensis* is that footpad swelling in susceptible mice was observed from 20 days post infection with an exponential increase in lesion size after day 40. There was no ulceration, necrosis, or dissemination of the lesions at any point for up to 6 months post infection. The dose of inoculum was high at 10^8 parasites per footpad [34], compared with the 5×10^6 parasites used in the study by Sousa-Franco, [39] with *L. guyanensis*. Interestingly, draining lymph node proliferation with *Leishmania* antigen peaked in a bi-phasic manner at day 20 and about 4 months post-infection. It was between 1 to 4 months post-infection (during the refractory phase of lymphocyte proliferation) that the footpad lesions peaked correlating in turn with a peak in antibody response. Thus suggesting, as for *L. major* [38, 39], that a cellular immune response, and not a humoral one, plays a role in resistance to infection with *L. panamensis*. Hopefully, the *L. panamensis* model in mice will be reinvestigated in the future, as the production of a significant lesion size over a long period is ideal to study the mechanisms that control disease outcome and for experimental chemotherapeutic studies to detect drug action.

L. braziliensis Infection in Mice

Cutaneous footpad infections with *L. braziliensis* require a high dose (1×10^7) of parasites to give a transient small lesion in BALB/c mice that heals within 6 weeks [40, 41]. Thus as an alternative, an ear dermis model was developed [42] based on the model described for *L. major* [43]. The advantage of this model is that it mimics a more natural course of infection using an inoculation with a low number of parasites (10^5) into ear dermis following brief *in vitro* passage. Infection in the ear dermis with *L. braziliensis* [42] also lead to transient small lesions until about the 4th or 5th week following infection. Despite complete clinical resolution of infection, parasite persistence was observed in the draining lymph nodes [42, 44]. The control of *L. braziliensis* was due to the IL-12 dependent generation of IFN-γ by CD4+ and CD8+ T cells [40, 42, 44, 45]. Self healing skin lesions were also accompanied by the expression of a broad spectrum of chemokines that are known to attract neutrophils, monocytes/macrophages, NK cells and CD4+ and CD8+ T cells [42, 46]. The rapid killing of *L. braziliensis* in infected macrophages by IFN-γ was likely to be possible due to the lack of IL-4 production in these mice when compared to *L. major* infected mice [40]. It was further demonstrated that IL-12 and Stat4 were necessary to prevent visceralization of the parasite and that an increased expression of iNOS (inducible nitric oxide synthase), when compared with susceptible *L. major* infected mice, could explain the rapid healing of skin lesions following *L. braziliensis* infection [44].

It is known that the origin of the parasite strain may also influence progression of disease [47], together with the composition of the inoculum. For example, a study by Samuelson *et al.* [48], described an *L. braziliensis* model where they co-injected sandfly saliva together with parasites from human CL in footpads of BALB/c mice. These mice produced progressive lesions, which showed no evidence of resolution 120 days post infection. The difficulty, however, to acquire sufficient amounts of sandfly salivary gland lysate may explain why future studies have not been reported using this model with *L. braziliensis.*

Despite the drawback of not having long established lesions following experimental infection with *L. braziliensis* parasites the footpad model was used in cross protection studies whereby mice that were previously infected with *L. braziliensis* were completed protected when challenged with *L. major.* This suggests that there are cross reactive antigenic epitopes between the two species which elicit a protective Th1 response against future infection [41]. Furthermore, the ear dermis model, though requiring expertise and training for the intra-dermal ear injections was more recently used [49], with the aim to test recombinant protein vaccine candidates against *L. braziliensis* and as a model using *L. major* parasites to optimize topical treatments of drug therapy against localized cutaneous leishmaniasis [50].

Hamster

Unlike mice, hamsters are a susceptible host to parasites of the *L. Viannia* sub-genus. Studies to characterise the immune response and the mechanisms responsible for resistance or susceptibility to this species are however limited as the hamster has an immune system that is poorly characterized compared to mice and for which few immunological reagents are available.

L. Viannia infection in the golden hamster gives rise to primary cutaneous lesions at the site of infection and, depending on the infecting species, secondary lesions at sites distal to that of the inoculum [51, 52]. Studies aiming to improve the hamster model and gain insight into the cellular immune response of the host following infection with parasites from the *L. Viannia* complex was explored by Osorio *et al* [53] and Gamboa *et al* [54]. In the former study the Authors took advantage of the recent development of primers and probes for hamster cytokines and examined the cellular immune response in this model at the transcript level by semi-quantitative real time PCR. It was evidenced that the more severe snout lesions were associated with an impaired antigen-specific spleen cell proliferative response, together with an increased expression of IFN-γ, IL-12p40, IL-10 and TGF-β in lesions, in the absence of a significant increase in IL-4. Studies at the protein level were, however, lacking to support this data especially when considering that TGF-β is post-transcriptionally regulated. Nevertheless, there appears to be a co-expression of type 1 and type 2 cytokines in the hamster, and that production of immunosuppressive molecules (such as IL-10) could be controlling the inflammatory effect of IFN-γ, as has been seen in human lesions of CL and MCL [55-57]. Currently, reagents for neutralization experiments, such as anti-hamster-IL-10, are unavailable to further study the *in vivo* role of this cytokine.

Factors such as trauma enhance multiplication at the inoculation site, or trigger renewed replication at secondary sites, and apparently potentiate the development of metastatic lesions [51, 52]. The metastatic capability of *L. (V.) panamensis* and *L. (V.) guyanensis* and *L. (V.) braziliensis* in golden hamsters was investigated by Martinez and colleagues [58] and Weigle and Saravia [59]. The secondary metastatic lesions are most evident in *L. (V.) guyanensis* infection and least in *L. (V.) braziliensis.* In human infection, the opposite is true with *L. (V.) braziliensis* producing the most frequent and severe form of metastatic lesions. The golden hamster model has supported human studies in that the development of disseminated or metastatic lesions was accompanied by lymphatic involvement, and that parasites are able to disseminate via the lymphatic system and or the blood [58, 60].

The retention of the metastatic phenotype described above in hamsters, following cloning and upon sequential passage *in vivo* in the hamster, was first demonstrated by Martinez *et al.* [61]. In this investigation the authors described that a single metastatic strain, namely *L. guyanenseis* M5313, was constituted by populations of parasites that differed in their ability to disseminate throughout the lymphoid tissues and to produce cutaneous metastasis. Cloned populations of parasites isolated from metastatic lesions and reinoculated into hamsters showed the metastatic and non-metastatic trait to be reproducible. Infections were in the snout following no more than 2 *in vitro* passages from a cutaneous metastatic lesion and repeated for 5 *in vivo* generations. The reproducible expression of the metastatic phenotype was lost following long-term *in vitro* culture. Dissemination to draining and distant lymph nodes occurred for most clones. 13 of 20 clones produced cutaneous metastatic lesions with multiple lesions being common. This work indicated that there are intrinsic differences in parasites that are able to only disseminate and those that disseminate and induce metastatic lesion development. The immune status of the hamsters was not, however, examined.

Using the golden hamster model with parasites from the *L. Viannia* complex has enabled the identification of highly metastatic strains and developed a model system to analyze cutaneous and metastatic pathogenesis. With advances in genetics of the hamster new molecular and immunological tools will allow for more thorough investigations of the underlying mechanisms leading to clinical disease caused by parasites of this sub-genus.

Non-Human Primates

Non-human primates appear to have a significant advantage over conventional laboratory animals in terms of modeling human leishmaniasis for purposes of drug evaluation as they tend to better reproduce human metabolism, disease and the immune response to infection. When it comes to infection with parasites from the *L. Viannia* sub-genus, non-human primates have demonstrated to be susceptible to disease; however, only a few experiments of this nature have been performed.

A study by Lainson and Shaw [62] used parasites which at the time of investigation were given the nomenclature of *L. braziliensis guyanensis, L. braziliensis braziliensis, L. mexicana mexicana and L. mexicana amazonensis* in cross protection studies in the *Cebus apella apella* species of monkey. Interestingly, *L. b. guyanensis* protected against challenge with *L. b. braziliensis* and *L .m. amazonensis* but not *vice versa*, thus showing the important role that *L. guyanensis* may play in vaccine trails. Another observation made, which exemplified the difference between the above strains, was that almost all monkeys infected with *L. guyanensis* on the ear showed metastatic spread to other regions of the ear in the form of separate nodules. There was no such spread with monkeys infected with *L. braziliensis*. Thus, the monkey similar to the hamster, may be a potential model for *L. guyanensis*-dependent metastatic cutaneous lesion development.

Subsequent studies using *L. guyanensis* parasites as the infecting agent in Simian species have not, to our knowledge, been documented. The most thoroughly performed studies have been with *L. braziliensis* parasites as the infecting agent in rhesus monkeys [63-65]. The aim of the former paper was to establish an experimental model for MCL and to help to understand the nature of parasite metastatic events and immunopathology. The latter two papers used this model in cross protection studies and to analyze the efficacy of a low dose compared to a standard dose of pentavalent antimony in *L. (V.) braziliensis* infected rhesus monkeys. The rhesus monkey model is a suitable model for CL as all monkeys infected with parasites isolated from either CL or MCL lesions developed chronic ulcerative CL that persisted between 6 months to 3 years [64]. One of the five monkeys infected with the CL isolate developed skin metastasis in non-mucosal sites and long standing mucosal disease in the face. This monkey also showed increased antibody titers, IFN-γ responses and DTH reactions when compared with the other monkeys that developed only CL, supporting the notion of a modulatory role for antibody as found in human infection with MCL [66].

The Authors were unable to reproduce MCL using parasites isolated from the MCL monkey upon reinfection unlike the reproducible metastatic phenotype developed in hamsters [61].

Thus it appears that the rhesus monkey may be a suitable model for cutaneous leishmaniasis caused by parasites from the *L. Viannia* complex. The scarcity of studies using primate models are likely due to the high cost for maintenance, the need for expert handling and the fact that monkeys are not readily available in large numbers for purposes of scientific investigation in all countries. Furthermore, a limited number of animals can be used per experimental group and all these factors taken together limits the ability to perform repeated experiments and to therefore achieve statistically relevant data.

In summary, it is clear that a suitable experimental model for infection with *L. guyanensis* parasites and for other members of the *L. Viannia* sub-genus is lacking. There are advantages and disadvantages to using the different models described above; importantly however, the development of an experimental model for infection by leishmaniasis of the subgenus *Viannia* would provide a biological system for the study of latent infection and the pathogenesis of metastatic and recurrent disease. Such information is essential for the development of research into testing new drugs to treat human cutaneous and mucocutaneous leishmaniasis.

Conflict of Interest

The Authors have no financial conflict of interest.

Funding

CR and PL were supported by Grant 310030-120325 from the Swiss National Foundationand , PL and EB by Institut Pasteur, and the French Ministry of Research (Programme de Recherche Fondamentale, Microbiologie Maladies

Infectieuses et Parasitaires du Ministère de l'Enseignement Supérieur et de la Technologie), AI and NF by Grant 31003A-116665 from the Swiss National Foundation and the Pierre-Mercier Foundation to SM

ACKNOWLEDGEMENTS

We thank the group of Prof Couppie at the Institut Guyanais de Dermatologie Tropicale, Centre Hospitalier Andrée Rosemon, Cayenne, French Guyana, who provide us with patient samples.

REFERENCES

[1]   Gumy A, Louis JA, Launois P, *et al.* The murine model of infection with *Leishmania major* and its importance for the deciphering of mechanisms underlying differences in Th cell differentiation in mice from different genetic backgrounds. Int J Parasitol 2004; 34: 433-44.

[2]   Da-Cruz AM, Conceicao-Silva F, Bertho AL, *et al. Leishmania*-reactive CD4+ and CD8+ T cells associated with cure of human cutaneous leishmaniasis. Infect Immun 1994; 62: 2614-8.

[3]   Gaafar A, Veress B, Permin H, *et al.* Characterization of the local and systemic immune responses in patients with cutaneous leishmaniasis due to *Leishmania major*. Clin Immunol 1999; 91: 314-20.

[4]   Maasho K, Sanchez F, Schurr E, *et al.* Indications of the protective role of natural killer cells in human cutaneous leishmaniasis in an area of endemicity. Infect Immun 1998; 66: 2698-704.

[5]   Cruz I, Nieto J, Moreno J, *et al. Leishmania*/HIV co-infections in the second decade. Indian J Med Res 2006; 123: 357-88.

[6]   Nylen S, Khamesipour A, Mohammadi A, *et al.* Surrogate markers of immunity to *Leishmania major* in leishmanin skin test negative individuals from an endemic area re-visited. Vaccine 2006; 24: 6944-54.

[7]   Rogers KA, Titus RG. Characterization of the early cellular immune response to *Leishmania major* using peripheral blood mononuclear cells from *Leishmania*-naive humans. Am J Trop Med Hyg 2004; 71: 568-76.

[8]   Maasho K, Satti I, Nylen S, *et al.* A Leishmania homologue of receptors for activated C-kinase (LACK) induces both interferon-gamma and interleukin-10 in natural killer cells of healthy blood donors. J Infect Dis 2000; 182: 570-8.

[9]   Bourreau E, Collet M, Prevot G, *et al.* IFN-gamma-producing CD45RA+CD8+ and IL-10-producing CD45RA-CD4+ T cells generated in response to LACK in naive subjects never exposed to Leishmania. Eur J Immunol 2002; 32: 510-20.

[10]   Russo DM, Chakrabarti P, Higgins AY. Leishmania: naive human T cells sensitized with promastigote antigen and IL-12 develop into potent Th1 and CD8(+) cytotoxic effectors. Exp Parasitol 1999; 93: 161-70.

[11]   Bourreau E, Prevot G, Gardon J, *et al.* High intralesional interleukin-10 messenger RNA expression in localized cutaneous leishmaniasis is associated with unresponsiveness to treatment. J Infect Dis 2001;184: 1628-30.

[12]   Kariminia A, Bourreau E, Ronet C, *et al.* Selective expression of the V beta 14 T cell receptor on *Leishmania guyanensis*--specific CD8+ T cells during human infection. J Infect Dis 2007; 195: 739-47.

[13]   Kariminia A, Bourreau E, Pascalis H, *et al.* Transforming growth factor beta 1 production by CD4+ CD25+ regulatory T cells in peripheral blood mononuclear cells from healthy subjects stimulated with *Leishmania guyanensis*. Infect Immun 2005; 73: 5908-14.

[14]   Bourreau E, Ronet C, Couppie P, *et al.* IL-10 producing CD8+ T cells in human infection with *Leishmania guyanensis*. Microbes Infect 2007; 9:1034-41.

[15]   Liew FY, Li Y, Moss D, *et al.* Resistance to *Leishmania major* infection correlates with the induction of nitric oxide synthase in murine macrophages. Eur J Immunol 1991; 21: 3009-14.

[16]   Bourreau E, Prevot G, Gardon J, *et al.* LACK-specific CD4(+) T cells that induce gamma interferon production in patients with localized cutaneous leishmaniasis during an early stage of infection. Infect Immun 2002; 70: 3122-9.

[17]   Bourreau E, Pascalis H, Prevot G, *et al.* Increased production of interferon-gamma by Leishmania homologue of the mammalian receptor for activated C kinase-reactive CD4+ T cells among human blood mononuclear cells: an early marker of exposure to Leishmania? Scand J Immunol 2003; 58: 201-10.

[18]   Pascalis H, Lavergne A, Bourreau E, *et al.* Th1 cell development induced by cysteine proteinases A and B in localized cutaneous leishmaniasis due to *Leishmania guyanensis*. Infect Immun 2003; 71: 2924-6.

[19]   Bourreau E, Ronet C, Darsissac E, *et al.* In leishmaniasis due to *Leishmania guyanensis* infection, distinct intralesional interleukin-10 and Foxp3 mRNA expression are associated with unresponsiveness to treatment. J Infect Dis 2009; 199: 576-9.

[20]   Bourreau E, Prevot G, Pradinaud R, Launois P. Interleukin (IL)-13 is the predominant Th2 cytokine in localized cutaneous leishmaniasis lesions and renders specific CD4+ T cells unresponsive to IL-12. J Infect Dis 2001; 183: 953-9.

[21]   Shevach EM. CD4+ CD25+ suppressor T cells: more questions than answers. Nat Rev Immunol 2002; 2: 389-400.

[22]   McHugh RS, Whitters MJ, Piccirillo CA, *et al.* CD4(+) CD25(+) immunoregulatory T cells: gene expression analysis reveals a functional role for glucocorticoid-induced TNF receptor. Immunity 2002; 16: 311-23.

[23]   Fontenot JD, Gavin MA, Rudensky AY. Foxp3 programs the development and function of CD4+CD25+ regulatory T cells. Nat Immunol 2003; 4: 330-6.

[24]   Hori S, Nomura T, Sakaguchi S. Control of regulatory T cell development by the transcription factor Foxp3. Science 2003; 299: 1057-61.

[25]   Khattri R, Cox T, Yasayko SA, Ramsdell F. An essential role for Scurfin in CD4+CD25+ T regulatory cells. Nat Immunol 2003; 4: 337-42.

[26]   Belkaid Y. Regulatory T cells and infection: a dangerous necessity. Nat Rev Immunol 2007; 7: 875-88.

[27]   Campanelli AP, Roselino AM, Cavassani KA, *et al*. CD4+CD25+ T cells in skin lesions of patients with cutaneous leishmaniasis exhibit phenotypic and functional characteristics of natural regulatory T cells. J Infect Dis 2006; 193: 1313-22.

[28]   Salhi A, Rodrigues V, Jr., *et al*. Immunological and genetic evidence for a crucial role of IL-10 in cutaneous lesions in humans infected with *Leishmania braziliensis*. J Immunol 2008; 180: 6139-48.

[29]   Bourreau E, Ronet C, Darcissac E, *et al*. Intralesional regulatory T-cell suppressive function during human acute and chronic cutaneous leishmaniasis due to *Leishmania guyanensis*. Infect Immun 2009; 77: 1465-74.

[30]   Mellor AL, Munn DH. IDO expression by dendritic cells: tolerance and tryptophan catabolism. Nat Rev Immunol 2004; 4: 762-74.

[31]   Alexander J, McFarlane E. Can type-1 responses against intracellular pathogens be T helper 2 cytokine dependent? Microbes Infect 2008; 10: 953-9.

[32]   Sacks D, Noben-Trauth N. The immunology of susceptibility and resistance to *Leishmania major* in mice. Nat Rev Immunol 2002; 2: 845-58.

[33]   Sousa-Franco J, Araujo-Mendes E, Silva-Jardim I, *et al*. Infection-induced respiratory burst in BALB/c macrophages kills *Leishmania guyanensis* amastigotes through apoptosis: possible involvement in resistance to cutaneous leishmaniasis. Microbes Infect 2006; 8: 390-400.

[34]   Goto H, Rojas JI, Sporrong L, *et al*. *Leishmania (viannia) panamensis*-induced cutaneous leishmaniasis in susceptible and resistant mouse strains. Rev Inst Med Trop Sao Paulo 1995;37(6):475-81.

[35]   Rojas JI, Tani E, Orn A, *et al*. *Leishmania (Viannia) panamensis*-induced cutaneous leishmaniasis in Balb/c mice: pathology. Int J Exp Pathol 1993; 74: 481-91.

[36]   Guevara-Mendoza O, Une C, Franceschi Carreira P, Orn A. Experimental infection of Balb/c mice with *Leishmania panamensis* and *Leishmania mexicana*: induction of early IFN-gamma but not IL-4 is associated with the development of cutaneous lesions. Scand J Immunol 1997; 46: 35-40.

[37]   Pinto-da-Silva LH, Camurate M, Costa KA, *et al*. *Leishmania (Viannia) braziliensis* metacyclic promastigotes purified using *Bauhinia purpurea* lectin are complement resistant and highly infective for macrophages in vitro and hamsters in vivo. Int J Parasitol 2002; 32: 1371-7.

[38]   Liese J, Schleicher U, Bogdan C. The innate immune response against Leishmania parasites. Immunobiology 2008; 213: 377-87.

[39]   von Stebut E. Cutaneous Leishmania infection: progress in pathogenesis research and experimental therapy. Exp Dermatol 2007; 16: 340-6.

[40]   DeKrey GK, Lima HC, Titus RG,. Analysis of the immune responses of mice to infection with *Leishmania braziliensis*. Infect Immun 1998; 66: 827-9.

[41]   Lima HC, DeKrey GK, Titus RG. Resolution of an infection with *Leishmania braziliensis* confers complete protection to a subsequent challenge with *Leishmania major* in BALB/c mice. Mem Inst Oswaldo Cruz 1999; 94: 71-6.

[42]   de Moura TR, Novais FO, Oliveira F, *et al*. Toward a novel experimental model of infection to study American cutaneous leishmaniasis caused by *Leishmania braziliensis*. Infect Immun 2005; 73: 5827-34.

[43]   Belkaid Y, Kamhawi S, Modi G, *et al*. Development of a natural model of cutaneous leishmaniasis: powerful effects of vector saliva and saliva preexposure on the long-term outcome of *Leishmania major* infection in the mouse ear dermis. J Exp Med 1998; 188: 1941-53.

[44]   Rocha FJ, Schleicher U, Mattner J. Cytokines, signaling pathways, and effector molecules required for the control of *Leishmania (Viannia) braziliensis* in mice. Infect Immun 2007; 75 : 3823-32.

[45]   de Souza-Neto SM, Carneiro CM, Vieira LQ, Afonso LC. *Leishmania braziliensis*: partial control of experimental infection by interleukin-12 p40 deficient mice. Mem Inst Oswaldo Cruz 2004; 99: 289-94.

[46]   Teixeira MJ, Fernandes JD, Teixeira CR, *et al*. Distinct *Leishmania braziliensis* isolates induce different paces of chemokine expression patterns. Infect Immun 2005; 73: 1191-5.

[47]   Oliveira CC, Lacerda HG, Martins DR, *et al*. Changing epidemiology of American cutaneous leishmaniasis (ACL) in Brazil: a disease of the urban-rural interface. Acta Trop 2004; 90: 155-62.

[48]   Samuelson J, Lerner E, Tesh R, *et al*. A mouse model of *Leishmania braziliensis braziliensis* infection produced by coinjection with sand fly saliva. J Exp Med 1991; 173: 49-54.

[49]   Salay G, Dorta ML, Santos NM, *et al*. Testing of four Leishmania vaccine candidates in a mouse model of infection with *Leishmania (Viannia) braziliensis*, the main causative agent of cutaneous leishmaniasis in the New World. Clin Vaccine Immunol 2007; 14: 1173-81.

[50] Lecoeur H, Buffet P, Morizot G, *et al.* Optimization of Topical Therapy for *Leishmania major* Localized Cutaneous Leishmaniasis Using a Reliable C57BL/6 Model. PLoS Negl Trop Dis 2007; 1:e34.

[51] Travi B, Rey-Ladino J, Saravia NG. Behavior of *Leishmania braziliensis* s.l. in golden hamsters: evolution of the infection under different experimental conditions. J Parasitol 1988; 74 : 1059-62.

[52] Travi BL, Osorio Y, Saravia NG. The inflammatory response promotes cutaneous metastasis in hamsters infected with *Leishmania* (*Viannia*) *panamensis*. J Parasitol 1996; 82: 454-7.

[53] Osorio Y, Melby PC, Pirmez C, *et al.* The site of cutaneous infection influences the immunological response and clinical outcome of hamsters infected with *Leishmania panamensis*. Parasite Immunol 2003; 25:1 39-48.

[54] Gamboa D, Torres K, De Doncker S, *et al.* Evaluation of an in vitro and in vivo model for experimental infection with *Leishmania* (*Viannia*) *braziliensis* and *L.* (*V.*) *peruviana*. Parasitology 2008; 135: 319-26.

[55] Faria DR, Gollob KJ, Barbosa J, *et al.* Decreased in situ expression of interleukin-10 receptor is correlated with the exacerbated inflammatory and cytotoxic responses observed in mucosal leishmaniasis. Infect Immun 2005; 73: 7853-9.

[56] Gaze ST, Dutra WO, Lessa M, *et al.* Mucosal leishmaniasis patients display an activated inflammatory T-cell phenotype associated with a nonbalanced monocyte population. Scand J Immunol 2006; 63: 70-8.

[57] Gomes-Silva A, de Cassia Bittar R, Dos Santos Nogueira R, *et al.* Can interferon-gamma and interleukin-10 balance be associated with severity of human *Leishmania* (*Viannia*) *braziliensis* infection? Clin Exp Immunol 2007; 149: 440-4.

[58] Martinez JE, Travi BL, Valencia AZ, Saravia NG. Metastatic capability of *Leishmania* (*Viannia*) panamensis and *Leishmania* (*Viannia*) *guyanensis* in golden hamsters. J Parasitol 1991; 77: 762-8.

[59] Weigle K, Saravia NG. Natural history, clinical evolution, and the host-parasite interaction in New World cutaneous Leishmaniasis. Clin Dermatol 1996;14 : 433-50.

[60] Almeida MC, Cuba-Cuba CA, Moraes MA, Miles MA. Dissemination of *Leishmania* (*Viannia*) *braziliensis*. J Comp Pathol 1996; 115: 311-6.

[61] Martinez JE, Valderrama L, Gama V, Leiby DA, Saravia NG. Clonal diversity in the expression and stability of the metastatic capability of *Leishmania guyanensis* in the golden hamster. J Parasitol 2000; 86: 792-9.

[62] Lainson R, Shaw JJ. Leishmaniasis in Brazil: XII. Observations on cross-immunity in monkeys and man infected with *Leishmania mexicana mexicana*, *L. m. amazonensis*, *L. braziliensis braziliensis*, *L. b. guyanensis* and *L. b. panamensis*. J Trop Med Hyg 1977; 80: 29-35.

[63] Porrozzi R, Teva A, Amaral VF, Santos da Costa MV, Grimaldi G, Jr. Cross-immunity experiments between different species or strains of Leishmania in rhesus macaques (*Macaca mulatta*). Am J Trop Med Hyg 2004; 71: 297-305.

[64] Teva A, Porrozzi R, Cupolillo E, *et al. Leishmania* (*Viannia*) *braziliensis*-induced chronic granulomatous cutaneous lesions affecting the nasal mucosa in the rhesus monkey (*Macaca mulatta*) model. Parasitology 2003; 127(Pt 5): 437-47.

[65] Teva A, Porrozzi R, Oliveira-Neto MP, Grimaldi GJ. Responses of *Leishmania* (*Viannia*) *braziliensis* cutaneous infection to N-methylglucamine antimoniate in the rhesus monkey (*Macaca mulatta*) model. J Parasitol 2005; 91: 976-8.

[66] Saravia NG, Valderrama L, Labrada M, *et al.* The relationship of *Leishmania braziliensis* subspecies and immune response to disease expression in New World leishmaniasis. J Infect Dis 1989; 159: 725-35.

INDEX

Emilio Jirillo (Ed)
All rights reserved - © 2010 Bentham Science Publishers Ltd.

www.ingramcontent.com/pod-product-compliance
Lightning Source LLC
Chambersburg PA
CBHW041702210326
41598CB00007B/505

* 9 7 8 1 6 0 8 0 5 6 7 8 1 *